AF688444

Autoimmune Disorders and Secondary Plant Metabolites

(Part 1)

Edited by

M.S. Ashawat
Department of Pharmaceutics
Laureate Institute of Pharmacy
Kangra, Himachal Pradesh, India

Aditi Kaushik
Department of Pharmaceutical Chemistry
Laureate Institute of Pharmacy
Kangra, Himachal Pradesh, India

Akash Jain
Department of Pharmacology
M.M. College of Pharmacy, M.M. (Deemed to be University)
Mullana, Ambala, Haryana, India

Jasmine Chaudhary
Department of Pharmaceutical Chemistry
M.M. College of Pharmacy, M.M. (Deemed to be University)
Mullana, Ambala, Haryana, India

&

Manish Kaushik
Department of Pharmacology
SBS College of Pharmacy
Kangra, Himachal Pradesh, India

Autoimmune Disorders and Secondary Plant Metabolites *(Part 1)*

Editors: M.S. Ashawat, Aditi Kaushik, Akash Jain, Jasmine Chaudhary and Manish Kaushik

ISBN (Online): 979-8-89881-234-8

ISBN (Print): 979-8-89881-235-5

ISBN (Paperback): 979-8-89881-236-2

© 2025, Bentham Books imprint.

Published by Bentham Science Publishers Pte. Ltd. Singapore, in collaboration with
Eureka Conferences, USA. All Rights Reserved.

First published in 2025.

BENTHAM SCIENCE PUBLISHERS LTD.

End User License Agreement (for non-institutional, personal use)

This is an agreement between you and Bentham Science Publishers Ltd. Please read this License Agreement carefully before using the ebook/echapter/ejournal (**"Work"**). Your use of the Work constitutes your agreement to the terms and conditions set forth in this License Agreement. If you do not agree to these terms and conditions then you should not use the Work.

Bentham Science Publishers agrees to grant you a non-exclusive, non-transferable limited license to use the Work subject to and in accordance with the following terms and conditions. This License Agreement is for non-library, personal use only. For a library / institutional / multi user license in respect of the Work, please contact: permission@benthamscience.org.

Usage Rules:

1. All rights reserved: The Work is the subject of copyright and Bentham Science Publishers either owns the Work (and the copyright in it) or is licensed to distribute the Work. You shall not copy, reproduce, modify, remove, delete, augment, add to, publish, transmit, sell, resell, create derivative works from, or in any way exploit the Work or make the Work available for others to do any of the same, in any form or by any means, in whole or in part, in each case without the prior written permission of Bentham Science Publishers, unless stated otherwise in this License Agreement.
2. You may download a copy of the Work on one occasion to one personal computer (including tablet, laptop, desktop, or other such devices). You may make one back-up copy of the Work to avoid losing it.
3. The unauthorised use or distribution of copyrighted or other proprietary content is illegal and could subject you to liability for substantial money damages. You will be liable for any damage resulting from your misuse of the Work or any violation of this License Agreement, including any infringement by you of copyrights or proprietary rights.

Disclaimer:

Bentham Science Publishers does not guarantee that the information in the Work is error-free, or warrant that it will meet your requirements or that access to the Work will be uninterrupted or error-free. The Work is provided "as is" without warranty of any kind, either express or implied or statutory, including, without limitation, implied warranties of merchantability and fitness for a particular purpose. The entire risk as to the results and performance of the Work is assumed by you. No responsibility is assumed by Bentham Science Publishers, its staff, editors and/or authors for any injury and/or damage to persons or property as a matter of products liability, negligence or otherwise, or from any use or operation of any methods, products instruction, advertisements or ideas contained in the Work.

Limitation of Liability:

In no event will Bentham Science Publishers, its staff, editors and/or authors, be liable for any damages, including, without limitation, special, incidental and/or consequential damages and/or damages for lost data and/or profits arising out of (whether directly or indirectly) the use or inability to use the Work. The entire liability of Bentham Science Publishers shall be limited to the amount actually paid by you for the Work.

General:

1. Any dispute or claim arising out of or in connection with this License Agreement or the Work (including non-contractual disputes or claims) will be governed by and construed in accordance with the laws of Singapore. Each party agrees that the courts of the state of Singapore shall have exclusive jurisdiction to settle any dispute or claim arising out of or in connection with this License Agreement or the Work (including non-contractual disputes or claims).
2. Your rights under this License Agreement will automatically terminate without notice and without the

need for a court order if at any point you breach any terms of this License Agreement. In no event will any delay or failure by Bentham Science Publishers in enforcing your compliance with this License Agreement constitute a waiver of any of its rights.

3. You acknowledge that you have read this License Agreement, and agree to be bound by its terms and conditions. To the extent that any other terms and conditions presented on any website of Bentham Science Publishers conflict with, or are inconsistent with, the terms and conditions set out in this License Agreement, you acknowledge that the terms and conditions set out in this License Agreement shall prevail.

Bentham Science Publishers Pte. Ltd.
No. 9 Raffles Place
Office No. 26-01
Singapore 048619
Singapore
Email: subscriptions@benthamscience.net

BENTHAM SCIENCE

CONTENTS

FOREWORD

The contents of the book "Autoimmune disorders and Secondary Plant Metabolites" have been read in detail by me and it contains highly useful information on the important functions of the secondary plant metabolites in the management of various autoimmune disorders. The editors of this book are the experts who have been working in the field of Pharmaceuticals for years and are known in the subjects of their specializations. Their focused and multidisciplinary approach aims to introduce the basic insights of the book and emphasizes the comprehensive use of the secondary plant metabolites.

All the chapters have been authored by a group of dedicated academicians and scientists who actively engaged in the field of the design and development of novel pharmaceuticals in the management of different autoimmune disorders. As a medical expert for more than 20 years, I foresee that this book will be of great value not only to postgraduates, teachers and research scholars in the field of Pharmaceuticals, but also to the industrial and scientific communities. This work contains substantial data for emphasizing herbal therapeutics as one the newer approach for the design and development of novel pharmacophore and their derivatives in the management of various autoimmune disorders.

In this post-COVID era, phytotherapy would be effectively utilized for the treatment of various diseases more effectively. The overall detail of the subject by the various authors in the different chapters of this book would go a long way in throwing new light on the area of autoimmune disorders.

I sincerely hope this venture is a great success, as it reflects the devotion, dedication and hard work of the team of editors. I am confident that this book will be very useful and gain enough attention from research scholars and academicians working in the field of medical and pharmaceuticals.

May the spirit of discovering better future remedies and optimizing phytopharmaceuticals provide superior medication to the benefit of humanity.

Nor Farid Bin Mohd Noor
Faculty of Medicine
Universiti Sultan Zainal Abidin (UniSZA)
Medical Campus, Jalan Sultan Mahmud
Kuala Terengganu 20400, Terengganu
Malaysia

PREFACE

The human immune system is a multi-faceted network of functionally diverse cells expressing a broad array of receptors that collectively function to respond to infection, eliminate precancerous cells, and maintain metabolic health. The breakdown of this delicately poised immune response is typically life-limiting; however, even subtle changes in its ability to distinguish an invading pathogen from the host can give rise to a spectrum of autoimmune diseases. Indeed, autoimmune diseases affect approximately 5%–8% of the world population and cause tremendous suffering to patients while also representing a major global socioeconomic issue. Although detailed molecular, immunological, genetic, and clinical studies have provided an increasingly sophisticated understanding of the mechanisms that underpin some autoimmune diseases, the drivers of human autoimmune diseases, including environmental triggers and the ensuing pathogenesis, remain poorly understood. In general, current immune-modulatory drugs used in the treatment of autoimmune diseases are broadly acting, non-disease specific, and, consequently, associated with side effects such as infection and malignant disease. Furthermore, it is clear that the majority of patients are not responding optimally to these therapies. Thus, there is a pressing need for the development of new drugs or repositioning of drugs based on a molecular and clinical understanding of the specific autoimmune diseases in individual patients in combination with high-throughput analysis of integrated datasets. Such personalized medicines may go hand in hand with the inclusion of new diagnostics, leading to a better disease understanding and more patient-centric clinical trials that also consider ethnic diversity and patient-reported outcome measures. Prevention should also be part of future early intervention. This book's perspective will highlight the different types of current therapies and showcase how future basic studies, new technologies, and clinical trials could dynamically and reciprocally inform each other, leading to a better understanding of disease mechanisms and, hence, more refined treatments.

Treatment of autoimmune diseases has drastically changed over the last 20 years with development and routine clinical use of synthetic or biologic drugs that block various pathways and components of the immune system, such as cytokines, cell adhesion molecules, and co-stimulatory molecules, or delete entire immune cell populations.

The novelty intensifies in this book's content, reflecting growing interest in exploring herbal alternatives as complementary or alternative therapies for autoimmune diseases. While these herbal options show promise, it is essential to consult with a healthcare professional before incorporating them into your treatment plan. Individual responses may vary, and personalized approaches are crucial for managing autoimmune disorders effectively. Always prioritize safety and work closely with your healthcare provider to find the best combination of therapies for your specific condition. The different plant's secondary metabolites play a significant role in modern therapy, including the treatment of autoimmune disorders. Insides of book where the attempt is made to focus on the Plants secondary metabolites, have gained prominence due to their relative safety and multifunctionality. Phytoconstituents offer better pharmacokinetic profiles and reduced adverse effects compared to synthetic drugs. Hundreds of phytoconstitutents have shown promising results in biochemical and cell line studies. Certain phytoconstitutents have been studied for their potential in managing autoimmune disorders. In summary, plant secondary metabolites offer a diverse array of therapeutic possibilities, making them valuable allies in the quest for better health. Thus, the research in the field of autoimmune disorders and secondary metabolites increased the hope of the scientific community. This book is focused on the role of various secondary plant metabolites in the management of different autoimmune disorders. The contents are divided into two sections wherein the first section focuses on the basics of autoimmunity as well as the interrelationship between autoimmune disorders, medicinal plants and drug discovery. The second section of this book strikes, therefore, a great balance at the described role of the secondary plant metabolites in different autoimmune disorders.

M.S. Ashawat
Department of Pharmaceutics
Laureate Institute of Pharmacy
Kangra, Himachal Pradesh, India

Aditi Kaushik
Department of Pharmaceutical Chemistry
Laureate Institute of Pharmacy
Kangra, Himachal Pradesh, India

Akash Jain
Department of Pharmacology
M.M. College of Pharmacy, M.M. (Deemed to be University)
Mullana, Ambala, Haryana, India

Jasmine Chaudhary
Department of Pharmaceutical Chemistry
M.M. College of Pharmacy, M.M. (Deemed to be University)
Mullana, Ambala, Haryana, India

&

Manish Kaushik
Department of Pharmacology
SBS College of Pharmacy
Kangra, Himachal Pradesh, India

List of Contributors

Ashwani K. Dhingra	Department of Pharmaceutical Chemistry, Global Research Institute of Pharmacy, Radaur, Yamuna Nagar 135133, Haryana, India
Ashna Gupta	Department of Pharmaceutics, Guru Gobind Singh College of Pharmacy, Yamunanagar, India
Asbar Banu Bazeer	Department of Medical Biotechnology, Aarupadai Veedu Medical College & Hospital, Vinayaka Mission's Research Foundation (Deemed to be University), Kirumampakkam, Puducherry 607403, India
Bipindra Pandey	Department of Pharmacy, Madan Bhandari Academy of Health Sciences, Hetauda, Nepal
Balaji Govindaswamy	Department of Biotechnology, Bhupat and Jyoti Mehta School of Biosciences, Indian Institute of Technology Madras, Chennai 600042, Tamil Nadu, India
Chandrasekar Ponnusamy	Department of Biotechnology, Rathinam College of Arts and Science, Coimbatore 641021, Tamil Nadu, India
Divya Dhawal Bhandari	Department of Pharmaceutical Chemistry, University Institute of Pharmaceutical Sciences, Panjab University, Chandigarh, Punjab, India
Ekambaram Gayathiri	Department of Plant Biology and Plant Biotechnology, Guru Nanak College (Autonomous), Chennai 600042, India
Jasmeen Kaur	Department of Pharmaceutics, Global Research Institute of Pharmacy, Radaur, Yamuna Nagar 135133, Haryana, India
Kulvinder Kaur	Department of Pharmacy, Global Research Institute of Pharmacy, Radaur, Yamuna Nagar 135133, Haryana, India
Kirtik Ramadoss	Department of Medical Biotechnology, Aarupadai Veedu Medical College & Hospital, Vinayaka Mission's Research Foundation (Deemed to be University), Kirumampakkam, Puducherry 607403, India
Megha Ashawat	Department of Pharmaceutics, Bansthali Vidyapith University, Newai Jaipur, India
Mahalakshmi Suresha Biradar	Department of Pharmaceutical Chemistry, Al-Ameen College of Pharmacy, Bengaluru, India
Manisha Bhatia	Department of Pharmacognosy, MM College of Pharmacy, Maharishi Markandeshwar (Deemed to be University), Mullana, Ambala, India
Murugappan Kumarappan	Department of Biotechnology, School of Biotechnology and Genetic Engineering, Bharathidasan University, Tiruchirappalli 620024, Tamil Nadu, India
Pratima Rao	Department of Applied Sciences, Laureate Institute of Pharmacy, Kangra, India
Prerna Sarup	Department of Pharmacognosy, University Institute of Pharmaceutical Sciences, Panjab University, Chandigarh, Punjab, India
Parul Gupta	Department of Pharmaceutics, Guru Gobind Singh College of Pharmacy, Yamunanagar, India

Palanisamy Prakash	Department of Botany, Periyar University, Periyar Palkalai Nagar, Salem 636011, Tamil Nadu, India
Poorna Chandrika Sabapathy	Directorate of Medical Research, Research and Innovation Lab, Aarupadai Veedu Medical College & Hospital, Vinayaka Mission, India
Prithiviraj Nagarajan	Department of Medical Biotechnology, Aarupadai Veedu Medical College & Hospital, Vinayaka Mission's Research Foundation (Deemed to be University), Kirumampakkam, Puducherry 607403, India
Ravindra Khadka	School of Health and Allied Sciences, Pokhara University, Kaski, Pokhara, Nepal
Rashmi Bhamra	Department of Pharmacy, Global Research Institute of Pharmacy, Radaur, Yamuna Nagar 135133, Haryana, India
Rupa Devi	Department of Pharmaceutics, Global Research Institute of Pharmacy, Radaur, Yamuna Nagar 135133, Haryana, India
Rohit Kamboj	Department of Pharmaceutics, Guru Gobind Singh College of Pharmacy, Yamunanagar, India
Ramachandran Kaliaperumal	Department of Biochemistry, Sri Manakula Vinayagar Medical College and Hospital, Madagadipet, Kalitheerthalkuppam, Puducherry 605107, India
Shankar Thapa	Department of Pharmacy, Madan Bhandari Academy of Health Sciences, Hetauda, Nepal
Sarath Perumal	Department of Biotechnology, School of Bio-science and Technology, Vellore Institute of Technology, Vellore 632014, Tamil Nadu, India
Sweta Kamboj	Department of Pharmaceutics, Guru Gobind Singh College of Pharmacy, Yamunanagar, India
Shikha Kamboj	Department of Pharmaceutics, Guru Gobind Singh College of Pharmacy, Yamunanagar, India
Suganya Kannan	Central Research Laboratory for Biomedical Research and Molecular Biology, Vinayaka Mission's Medical College and Hospital, Vinayaka Mission's Research Foundation, Karaikal, Puducherry 609609, India
Sharangouda J. Patil	Department of Zoology, NMKRV College for Women, Bengaluru 560011, Karnataka, India
Vishakha Saini	Department of Pharmaceutics, Global Research Institute of Pharmacy, Radaur, Yamuna Nagar 135133, Haryana, India
Varinder Kaur	Department of Pharmacy, Global Research Institute of Pharmacy, Radaur, Yamuna Nagar 135133, Haryana, India

CHAPTER 1

Introduction to Immunology and Autoimmune Disorders

Megha Ashawat[1] and **Pratima Rao**[2,*]

[1] *Department of Pharmaceutics, Bansthali Vidyapith University, Newai Jaipur 304021, Rajasthan, India*

[2] *Department of Applied Sciences, Laureate Institute of Pharmacy, Kangra 176031, Himachal Pradesh, India*

Abstract: From the very moment our heart starts to beat, and we take our first breath, there is an army of cells and tissues that make up organs and a system that stands in our defense called the **'Immune system.'** The immune system responds to foreign molecules like viruses, bacteria, or any other organic molecule that is not familiar to the body and the extrinsic particles that, however, can cause us damage whilst not attacking its cells with specific identifiers. This remarkable and intricate network is called the immune system, and as complex as it is, it is fascinating. To study this system, we have a very delicate and integral part of the medical field called **'Immunology.'** Several physiological processes are intertwined with the elaborate defensive system, like clotting, wound healing, maintenance of body temperature, and much more. This chapter will walk you through the fundamentals of immunology, like diverse types of immunities, and what can happen if the body attacks its own cells, such as accidental betrayal. The accident is medically called **the 'Autoimmune disorder,'** which occurs as a result of neglected self-tolerance, leading to attacking the body's own tissues and network systems. Factors like genetics, environment, and lifestyle are generally taken into consideration to diagnose and further treat an autoimmune disorder. Though this is not an event that is often experienced in the body, it might occur sometimes, which leads us to study it and prevent it. Additionally, we will be talking about why and how this accidental betrayal usually happens.

Keywords: Antibodies, Autoimmune disorder, Bacteria, Body defense, Cells, Clotting process, Defense system, Diagnostics, Environment factors, Foreign molecules, Genetics, Immune response, Immune system, Immunology, Lifestyle factors, Pathogens, Physiological processes, Self-tolerance, Tissue network, Wound healing.

* **Corresponding author Pratima Rao:** Laureate Institute of Pharmacy, Kathog, Kangra, Himachal Pradesh, India; E-mail: pratimalgs@gmail.com

M.S. Ashawat, Aditi Kaushik, Akash Jain, Jasmine Chaudhary & Manish Kaushik (Eds.)
All rights reserved-© 2025 Bentham Science Publishers

WONDERFUL WORLD OF IMMUNITY

Ever wondered what it looks like on the inside of our body? Let us open that door today. Imagine a highly trained bodyguard, never resting and protecting you 24/7 from when you are surrounded by germs and harmful foreign substances. That is what our immune system is...

The word immunity comes from the Greek word *"Immunis,"* which, if laid down into basic terms, means protection. Immunity is one's bodily ability to protect oneself from diseases by becoming resistant to them. It is an in-built system for our body, just like the respiratory or cardiovascular system [1 - 5]. The system is extensively evolving to shield human bodies from harmful microorganisms and those invading foreign substances that can potentially cause harm to the delicate system. The cells and molecules in the immune system work together as a network and relay between two major activities called recognition and response. The ability of the immune system to recognize and differentiate between self and non-self makes it so prolifically specific. After recognizing whether the substance is self or non-self, the next major activity is response. Once the system recognizes the foreign substance as harmful, it sends an army of cells and molecules to produce an appropriate response without affecting the body's own cells [6, 7]. But, like every other thing in the world, this system can also go wrong sometimes, which can diverge into two cases, namely, immunodeficiency and hypersensitivity. Immunodeficiency can result in extreme weakness of the system, which is generally caused by Human Immunodeficiency Virus (HIV), which therefore turns the body into a fragile system that can be fatal even after a common cold. On the other hand, if the system gets hyperactive, it turns into an allergy that is deadly if not treated in time [8] [9].

HISTORY OF IMMUNIZATION

Immunization dates back centuries, when, in the late fifth century BC, a plague struck Athens. The Europeans mentioned the concept for the first time. Thucydides, in his writings, observed that- "only those who have recovered from the illness can nurse the sick as the disease cannot attack the same person twice, at least not fatally". This was an astute and significant observation that made people recognize the concept of immunization [10].

Similarly, the Chinese used to powder the skin lesions of people recovering from smallpox and then make children inhale that to make them immune to the disease. As the technique began to expand its way to Asia, Europe, and Africa, progress was only made in the late seventeenth century. Cotton Mather, with his friend Dr. Zabdiel Boylston, in 1721 decided to inoculate his patients with smallpox pustules. People adopted the technique enthusiastically to immunize their children when the Prince of Wales, U.K., in 1722 had their children immunized with smallpox residues [11].

In 1798, came Edward Jenner famously known as the Father of Vaccination, created the world's first successful vaccine. He analyzed and adopted techniques from previous studies and observed that housekeepers in the era who contracted cowpox once were particularly safe from the smallpox infection too. In the year 1786, Jenner inoculated an eight-year-old boy with cowpox lesions, allowing the system to develop immunity. Later, he infected the same boy with infectious smallpox pus, but the disease did not produce any notable effect on the boy. This experiment finally concluded the theory given by Thucydides in 430 B.C. The technique was called 'vaccination'. The term was derived from a Latin word, '*Vacca*', meaning 'cow', highlighting the significance of cowpox in the discovery process [12].

Although this discovery represented a monumental breakthrough in the field of immunology, the scientists were not able to comprehend how the system brings about protection. In 1879, Louis Pasteur conducted another similar experiment to study the pathogenesis of bacteria *(Pasteurella multocida)* that causes cholera. In the meantime, he contributed to an astute observation as to how vaccines work. It all started when he went on a vacation and told his assistant to inject the chicken in an experiment with the bacterial culture. Somehow, the process got delayed, resulting in an aged bacterial culture to inject. To their astonishment, they found that the inoculated chicken had not died. The immune chickens survived the second dose of bacterial culture, too. This remarkable insight clicked as the phenomenon of vaccination once again. It was then concluded that chickens injected with dead and aged culture bacteria were protected against the disease. The discovery marked the successful invention of the vaccine against rabies and *Bacillus anthracis* [13].

Although the nineteenth century laid the foundation for prolific advancements, the twentieth century witnessed some tremendous developments, including Karl Landsteiner's strong advancements in the field of immunology, as depicted in Table **1**. He discovered the four primary blood groups and received a Nobel Prize for them. In 1943, along with Merrill Chase, he discovered 'delayed hypersensitivity'.

INTRODUCTION

Immunity refers to resistance or exemption from disease. By recognition and response, the system identifies and eliminates harmful substances from the body. The immune system mechanisms are divided into two categories called Innate and Acquired immunity.

Table 1. Scientific discoveries related to immunology.

Year	Winner(s)	Birth Country	Prize Awarded For
1901	Emil von Behring	Germany	Discovery of serum therapy (antibodies)
1903	NielsRyberg Finsen	Denmark	Treatment of lupus vulgaris with concentrated light radiation (early phototherapy)
1908	Paul Ehrlich (Germany) &Elie Metchnikoff (Russian Empire/France)	Germany & Russia/France	Phagocytosis and humoral immunity development
1919	Jules Bordet	Belgium	Discovery of the complement system (immune response)
1929	Christiaan Eijkman	Netherlands	Discovery of vitamin B1 (thiamine)
1930	Karl Landsteiner	Austria	Discovery of human blood groups
1934	George Hoyt Whipple (USA), George Richards Minot (USA) & William Parry Murphy (USA)	USA	Treatment of pernicious anemia with liver therapy
1945	Howard Florey (Australia/UK), Ernst Boris Chain (Germany/UK) & Alexander Fleming (UK)	Australia/UK, Germany/UK & UK	Discovery of penicillin (revolutionized treatment of bacterial infections)
1946	Wendell Stanley	USA	Crystallization of a virus (demonstrating viral nature)
1957	Daniel Bovet	Switzerland	Discovery of synthetic compounds that inhibit the action of certain toxins
1960	Sir Frank Macfarlane Burnet (Australia) & Peter Medawar (UK)	Australia & UK	Acquired immune tolerance
1963	John Eccles (Australia), Alan Hodgkin (UK) & Andrew Huxley (UK)	Australia & UK	Discoveries concerning the synaptic mechanisms in the transmission of nerve impulses
1970	Julius Axelrod (USA) and Ulf von Euler (Sweden)	USA & Sweden	Discovery of the transmitters in nerve synapses and the synthesis and storage mechanisms in nerve endings
1972	Gerald Edelman (USA) & Rodney Porter (UK)	USA & UK	Structure of antibodies and chemistry of immunoglobulins
1980	Baruj Benacerraf (Venezuela), Jean Dausset (France) & George Snell (USA)	Venezuela, France & USA	Discovery of major histocompatibility complex (MHC)
1983	Georges Jean LeFranc	France	Pioneering work in the field of immunogenetics
1984	Niels Jerne (Denmark), Georges Köhler (western Germany) & César Milstein (Argentina/UK)	Denmark, western Germany &Argentina/UK	Development of monoclonal antibodies

(Table 1) cont.....

Year	Winner(s)	Birth Country	Prize Awarded For
1996	Peter Doherty (Australia) & Rolf Zinkernagel (Switzerland)	Australia & Switzerland	How the immune system recognizes virus-infected cells
1997	Stanley Prusiner (USA)	USA	Discovery of prions (infectious proteins causing brain diseases)
2018	TasukuHonjo (Japan) & James Allison (USA)	Japan & USA	Discovery of cancer therapy by inhibiting immune checkpoints

Innate Immunity

The human body is exposed to millions of pathogens every day *via* ingestion, inhalation, and damaged skin barriers. Innate immunity is the first line of defense, which includes the exterior barriers to the entry of foreign substances. This immunity has been present in the individual since birth as a gift to resist infections. As this is already there when we are born, it is also called *native, natural, or nonspecific immunity.* Innate immune responses are not pathogen-specific; instead of reacting to a particular invader, they eliminate every foreign substance they recognize while on patrol. Responses in the innate system do not get better with multiple infections or develop over time. This dynamic network of cells and organs is much faster (minutes to hours) and includes several components as [14 - 16]

- Anatomical defenses
- Cellular defenses
- Biochemical defenses
- Genetic defenses

i. **Anatomical defenses:** These generally involve the extrinsic membranes, salivary and teary action, and cilia in the respiratory passages. These form a charming network that prevents the entry of microorganisms into the body.

a. **Skin:** The skin, being the largest organ and the covering of the entire body, protects the body from any invading pathogens that may enter. The vast surface prevents the microorganisms from penetrating, growing, or infecting the insides. The uppermost layer of the skin, called the epidermis is subdivided into four distinct layers, with stratum corneum as the outermost horny layer acting as a protective shield. The layer contains epithelial cells rich in proteolytic enzymes and microbicidal compounds. These specialized layers work together as a network to prevent the proliferation of the invading pathogen. An example of this can be stated as to when the skin is exposed to wounds or burns, it is advised to cover it up and treat it accordingly, because if the tissues are in contact with the environment, the probability of infections getting in increases, as represented in Fig. (**1**) [17].

b. **Cilia:** These are small hair-like projections that have persistent movement. These tiny shreds are present in epithelial tissues like the respiratory tract, which trap the invading pathogens in the mucus and sweep them off by coughing or sneezing. The response being non-specific eliminates any particles that irritate the throat or nose cilia [18].
c. **Salivary and teary action:** Flushing of the lacrimal gland in the eye is called a tear, which frees the eyes of any big particles that particularly rupture the layers of the eye. Saliva contains lysozymes, which have antimicrobial activity that breaks down any microorganisms entering *via* the mouth. Hence, when a person suffers from dry mouth (a condition in which saliva production edges to a negligible quantity), invasion of microorganisms increases and as a result, the oral cavity stinks with bad breath [18].
d. **Mucus membrane:** The mucosal membrane, consisting of epithelial cells, forms a layer like a cling wrap and protects the body from any damage or invasion from microbes and other pathogens. Present in the digestive tract, oral cavity, respiratory tract, and other tracts, this membrane is thick enough to prevent pathogens from entering the outermost layer [18].
e. **Coughing and sneezing actions:** These actions help in flushing the foreign particles out of the body, which may cause irritation and can be a potential harm to the body.

ii. **Biochemical defenses:** The chemical substances or toxins released from the body of the host contribute to the biochemical barriers of the immune system. These include body secretions like secretions from the digestive tract, skin, mammary glands, nasal passage, *etc.*
   a. **Skin secretion:** Our sweat essentially has a high amount of salt in it, which enables the skin to possess antibacterial activity. The sebaceous and sweat gland secretions also contain some fatty acids with lactic acid that tend to have antiseptic and fungicidal properties to some extent. The alkaline gaps of our body, namely the soles of the feet, which are deficit in sweat secretion, are more prone to be attacked by fungus and therefore should be vigilantly taken care of [19].
   b. **Mammary gland secretion:** Human milk is produced by female mammary glands used to feed infants at the time of birth because it contains essential amino acids, IgA antibody, protecting the child from early intestinal infections caused by *E.coli*. Lactoferritin and neuraminic acid are also predominantly found in the mother's milk, which are antibacterials in nature. Hence, human milk serves as the primary

antibody manufacturer for the infant [20].

c. **Lysozyme:** Lysozyme is a mucolytic enzyme found in every secretion of the body, like tears, saliva, nasal secretions, and tissue fluids (except for cerebrospinal fluid). This enzyme is secreted by the lysosome when the phagocytic cell finally ingests the invading pathogen and helps digest it because of its low molecular weight basic protein that can easily break sugars off Gram-positive bacteria. This was first observed by Fleming in 1922.

d. **Properdin:** Proteins are a part of normal healthy serum and contribute to resisting infections. Unlike lysozyme, this group of proteins attacks the gram-negative bacteria [21].

e. **Acute phase proteins:** These proteins are present in the plasma and are seen to be elevated in case of infection. One of these can be explained by the example of a CRP (C-Reactive Protein) that essentially binds to the C-protein of the pneumococci and acts as an opsonin, facilitating phagocytosis [22].

iii. Cellular defenses: When the host body cannot defend itself by anatomical and biochemical barriers, then the cells create an intricate process and protect us from the invading microorganism. Macrophages and phagocytic cells are large cells in the human body that act as highly trained muscular guards and eat up any invader that comes their way. There are special substances called ***opsonins*** that attach to cells or pathogens to increase the susceptibility to phagocytosis.

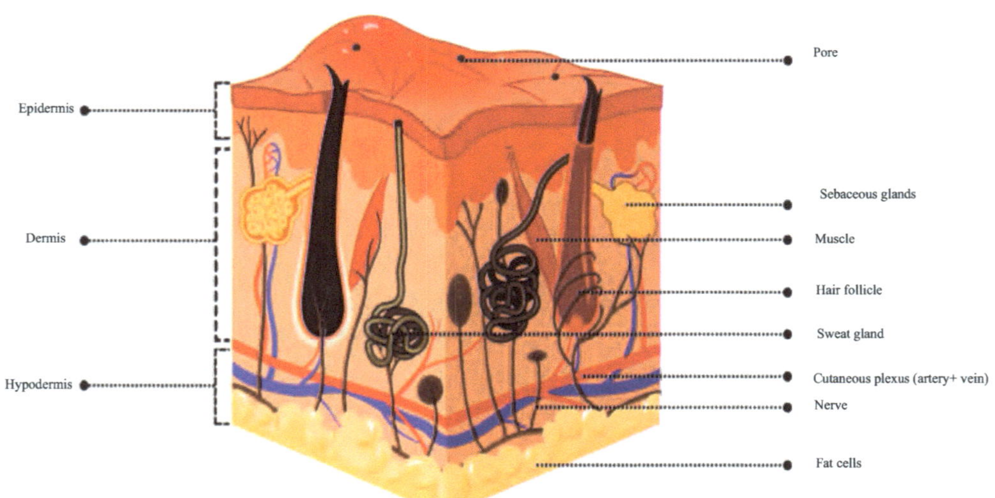

Fig. (1). Diagram of skin and underlying glands.

- **Macrophages or phagocytes:** In 1838, the groundbreaking discovery was made of phagocytic cells, namely microphages and macrophages. Macrophages belong to the 'mononuclear phagocytic system,' also known as the 'reticulo-endothelial system.' The cells originate from the bone marrow, which then differentiate into monocytes and finally into macrophages. The mechanism of phagocytosis occurs in different steps explained below in Fig. (**2**) [22].
  1. **Chemotaxis:** The step involves the movement of phagocytic cells to the action site.
  2. **Attachment:** Binding is initiated through special molecules called opsonins, which coat the antigen and facilitate the formation of a surrounding layer.
  3. **Ingestion:** As soon as the attachment is done, the phagocytes start with cell eating (ingestion/phagocytosis). Pseudopodia (false feet) start to show up and coil around the antigen. The false feet then surround the entire invader and take it into their 'arms', and hence the particle is entirely packed into the vacuole created, which is called the phagosome. The newly made phagosome then fuses with the lysosome inside the cell, forming a secondary lysosome called the 'phagolysosome.'
  4. **Intracellular killing:** Now that the antigen is inside the phagocytic cell, the lysosome releases antimicrobial substances, including lysozyme and hydrogen peroxide.
  5. **Digestion:** For the ultimate step, the killed particle is digested well by the hydrolytic enzymes produced by the lysosome and then excreted out of the cell.

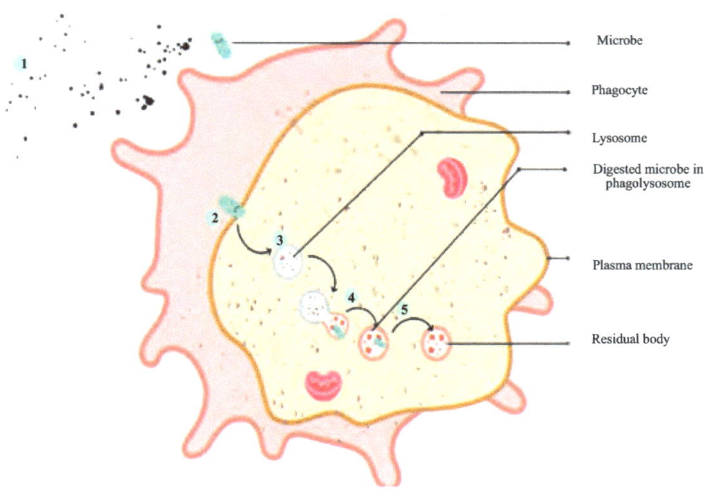

Fig. (2). Phagocytosis phases.

Several Types of Cells with a Defensive Nature are Elaborated Below

a. **Natural killer cells:** These are nonspecific antigen killer cells that can eliminate several types of virally infected cells or tumors. The viral cells come with glycoproteins that are recognized by the killer cells, and before they can proliferate inside the host cell, they are eliminated. When the natural killer cells are triggered, they bring with them some chemicals and release them between the two cells. The most important of all chemicals is perforin, also called cytolysis, which brings about the lysis of virus-infected cells [23].
b. **Neutrophils:** They make up the largest population in the WBC pool, around 60-70%. These tiny cells are short-lived, but their contribution is not. They have large weaponry of antibiotic proteins stored in granules, namely *azurophilic* (primary) and *specific* (secondary). These cytotoxic releases help in the step where the ingested invader must be digested and excreted out of the cell [24, 25].
c. **Eosinophils:** These cells generally have a bilobed nucleus and cytoplasmic granules, which are stained by acidic dyes. The proportion they take up is about 2-5% in healthy, non-infected people. Eosinophils are not primarily deployed for phagocytosis, but it comes under their scope of action in certain conditions. When large pathogens occur, the cells degranulate to fuse with the plasma membrane, which leads to the release of granular contents into the extracellular environment. This process is not a usual event as it is only triggered when the pathogen cannot be phagocytosed [26, 27].
d. **Basophils:** These are a type of white blood cell, consisting of about 0.4% of white cells. Basophil cells are an essential part of the network, especially in terms of hypersensitivity and inflammation. The granulocytes contain heparin, histamine, serotonin, platelet-activating factor and other amines. Basophils participate in the body's hypersensitivity reactions. They help build an immune response to the irritant by releasing certain mediators and attracting other cells of the arsenal to the site of action [28].
e. **Antigen Presenting Cells (APCs):** APCs are a class of leucocytes found mainly in skin, lymph nodes and the thymus. The APCs present the antigen before the T lymphocytes and activate the immune response. Antigen-presenting cells play a crucial role in adaptive immunity: they internalize foreign particles through phagocytosis or endocytosis, degrade them into peptide fragments, and then load those peptides onto either MHC-I or MHC-II molecules, depending on the requirements of the immune response [29].
f. **Platelets:** The non-nucleated cells derived from the bone marrow megakaryocytes are colorless, small cells that play an intensively significant role in the blood clotting process. Apart from this, platelet is also involved in inflammation. They contain granules that particularly release histamine and serotonin and contribute to the immediate hypersensitive reactions [30].

iv. Genetic defenses: Natural or innate immunity also depends on the genetic conditions, differing at several levels like races, species, and individuals.

a. **Species immunity:** Some diseases and pathogens only attack a certain species, like measles targets only humans and will never go toward non-primates. Rats are insusceptible to diphtheria, while guinea pigs and humans are more prone to the same. By these examples, we can establish the fact that certain species develop their natural immunity to some diseases and pathogens.
b. **Racial immunity:** Different races can also show levels of immunity while belonging to the same species. A study observed that in the USA, black people are more susceptible to tuberculosis as compared to white people.
c. **Individual immunity:** Even individuals belonging to the same race can have diverse levels of immunity. Studies showed that the homozygous twins are identical in susceptibility and immunity.

Inflammation: When the tissue damage is caused by any intruding pathogen or abrasions, a complex and intrinsic series of events occurs, called inflammation or inflammatory response. This is a non-specific and defensive set of events. The four fundamental symptoms of inflammation are *rubor* (redness), *dolor* (pain), *calor* (increased temperature) and *tumor* (swelling). After the inflammatory actions have taken place, two things happen: either the invader is swept out of the body, or an immune response is triggered if the severity of the antigen is estimated. Now, as we have already established the fact that inflammation is non-specific, then the action against a small scratch would be similar to burns or viral infection, too, keeping the extent of activity the same throughout. The four cardinal symptoms, as listed above, are caused by some triggers or substances discussed below:

a. **Histamine:** This is one of the key mediators of inflammation. Histamine is released by injured cells, which initiates inflammation by vasodilation and enhances permeability. When macrophages are at the target site, they call histamine for help, which causes pain and itching in the area.
b. **Leukotrienes(LTs):** These are produced by mast cells and basophils. They are derived from a polyunsaturated fatty acid called Arachidonic acid. They participate in the constriction of bronchioles, helping in asthma and other allergens. It makes the target site attractive for white blood cells to initiate a response by attaching the phagocytes to pathogens.
c. **Kinins:** Bradykinin is a popular example of this kind. Kinins are polypeptides formed in blood from the inactive precursors known as kininogens. These tend to cause vasodilation, leading to enhanced permeability.
d. **Prostaglandins (PGs):** These are kinins and the derivatives of arachidonic

acid. These are the lipids released by injured cells and elevate the effect of histamine and kinins, including pain reception and sensitivity to stimuli. PGs also cause the migration of macrophages through the walls of the capillaries [30].

ACQUIRED IMMUNITY

This is the resistance to infections or diseases which is developed over time and is acquired or gained from the surroundings. When antigens attack a host body for the first time, they are analyzed and recorded by the cells of the immune system, which facilitates the triggering of an immune response for the next time that specific antigen encounters the receptors, and the response only gets better with each successive encounter. The successive response is called the 'secondary response', which is explicitly better than the previous one as the humoral and cell-mediated mechanisms are more developed than before. This is the basic principle of adaptive or acquired immunity. Acquired immunity is broadly divided into classes as shown in Fig. (**3**) [31].

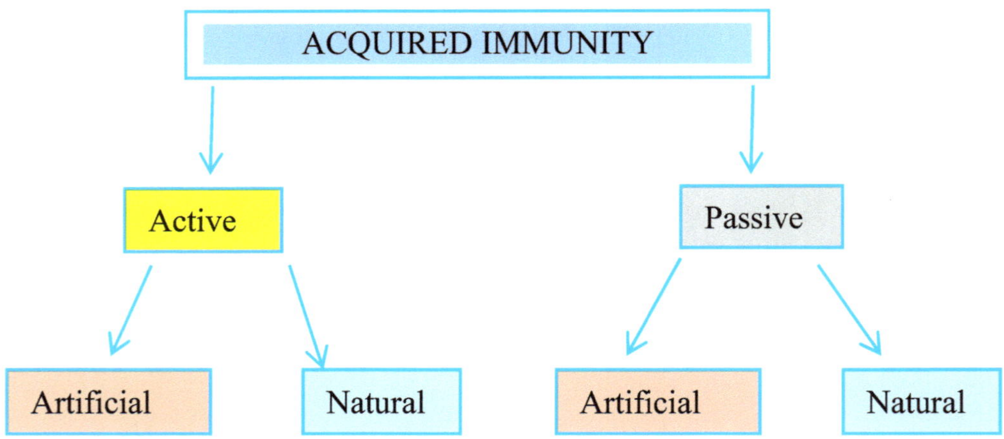

Fig. (3). Flowchart depicting classification of acquired immunity.

1. **Active immunity:** It is referred to as the resistance developed by the host when it encounters a pathogen attack. Active immunity is triggered when an antigen either invades the body *via* an infection or is injected for immunization purposes *via* a vaccine. Immunity can be developed by two basic mechanisms, namely, humoral and cell-mediated immunity [32].

   a. **Humoral immunity:** Humor is the body's fluid that contains enzymes and cells to help fight infection. Antibodies are then released into the bodily fluids, including lymph or plasma. The antibodies thus produced are antigen-specific; hence, this type is also called 'specific immunity.' The killed or dumped invaders then must go through phagocytosis to neutralize the toxic effects. It comes into play after a certain period after the attack as the immunological machinery gears itself to produce the specific antibodies. This phase of no action is also called the Lag phase or the latent period. The primary response is therefore divided into four major phases, namely [33, 34].

- **Lag phase:** This phase is immediate after the entry of the pathogen. In this phase, no antibodies are produced and is also referred to as 'latent' or 'induction' period.
- **Log phase:** The level of antibodies elevates gradually in this step. The primary response is all about IgM antibodies mainly whose half-life is approximately ~5days.
- **Plateau phase:** antibody level is steady in the third phase without any significant increase or decrease.
- **Decline phase:** This phase marks the decrease in the levels of antibodies throughout. The equilibrium is disrupted and the rate of catabolism of antibodies is much greater than their production.

Antibody

An antibody is an immunoglobulin that is produced in the serum and fluids of the body. Majorly, three kinds of globulins exist in the body, namely alpha, gamma and beta. The antibodies fall into the gamma category. They protect the body from infection in numerous ways, like preventing the adhesion of pathogens onto the membranes in the host body. They also neutralize the toxins produced by viruses or antigens. In the 1890s, scientists Von Behring and Kitasato proved that antibodies do exist in physical form. This was inferred by analyzing the serum obtained from diphtheria-infected rabbits. The results showed that the serum obtained could prevent diseases in mice caused by the same pathogens. The substance found to provide protection was later named 'antitoxin' by another pair of scientists, namely Tizzoni and Cattani, in 1891. After this discovery, curiosity took a deep dive, and it was figured out that this protection can also be provided against cells like erythrocytes, so a more inclusive term was needed, and hence the protective substance was called 'antibody.' Each of these consists of four polypeptide chains (heavy and light; two of each). Additionally, it has two carbohydrate chains on either side attached to the heavy chains in the stem region. There are two types of light chains, essentially named Kappa and Lambda, but each of the immunoglobulin has only one type, which is the basis of division into K-type and L-type antibodies, as shown in Table **2**. While K-type antibodies constitute 60% of the serum, the L-type antibodies are approximately 40% [32 - 35] (Fig. **4**).

Table 2. Different types of antibodies and their characteristics.

Antibody	Characteristics
IgG	About 80% of the antibodies are constituted of these. Found in the lymph, blood, and intestines. It is a monomeric structure. Protecting against viruses by enhancing phagocytosis and triggering the rest of the system for a better response.
IgA	About 10-13% in the blood. Majorly found in secretions like sweat, tears, saliva, and mother's milk. Can be both monomeric and dimeric structures. Protects against local attacks from invaders on the mucous membrane.
IgM	About 10% in the blood. It is the largest of all occurring as pentamers. It is the first antibody that is released when an antigen attacks the body. It causes agglutination followed by lysis of the microbe.
IgD	About 0.2% in the blood. Mainly found on the surface of B cells and activates them when needed. It is a monomeric structure.
IgE	Less than 0.1% in the blood. Present on the surface of basophils and mast cells. Occurs as a monomeric unit. Responsible for triggering allergic reactions.

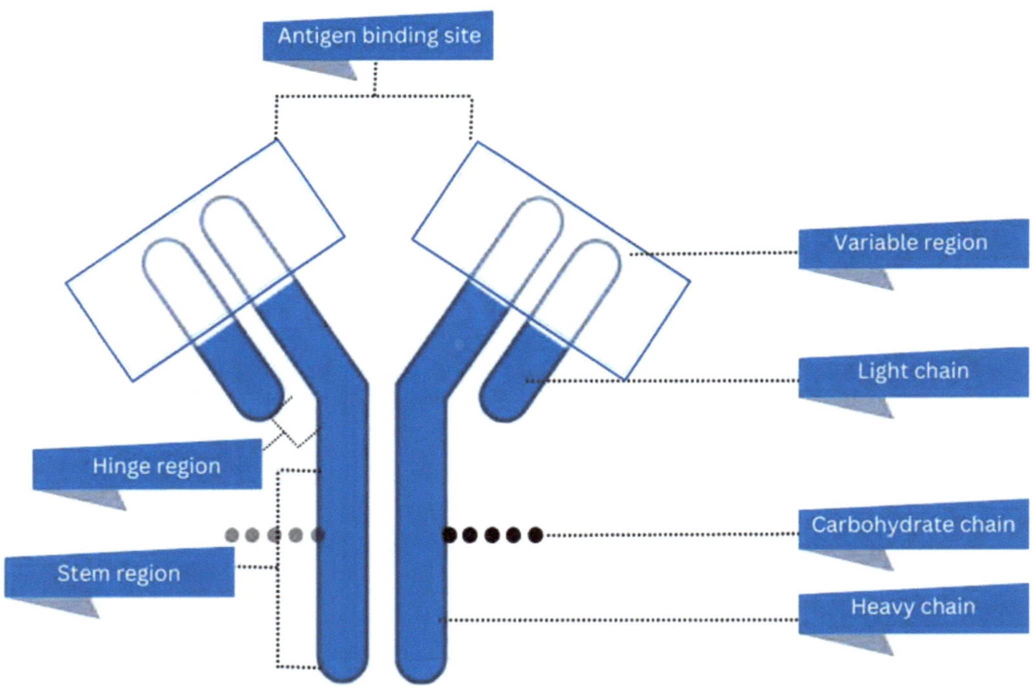

Fig. (4). Structure of a typical IgG antibody.

Antigen

An antigen is any substance that causes the immune system to respond when it is complete. The antigen gets its name from its function: *anti-* as in antibody and *gen*-generating. An incomplete antigen (called a hapten), however, cannot generate an immune response but can only bind with the antibodies unless it is adhered to a carrier [36]. In order to be a complete antigen, it has to have two main properties: immunogenicity and reactivity. **Immunogenicity** is the ability to trigger an immune response, which will eventually lead to the production of antibodies and differentiation of T cells. Reactivity, on the other hand, is when the antigen can react with the provokes antibodies [37]. Examples of antigens can be chemical components of the bacterial body, like flagella or capsules. Non-antigenic substances can be pollen and dust that only have a partial effect on the immune system. There are also substances that may be a complete antigen in some species of animals but a hapten in others, like the pneumococcal polysaccharide, which is an antigen in mice and humans but a hapten in rabbits. There are determinants for antigenic activity called the epitopes, the smallest fundamental unit that reacts with the antibody's active site, called the paratopes. These are usually more than one in number present on the surface of the antigen [38]. However, denaturation and unfolding studies have revealed that the antigen also contains latent or hidden epitopes. The number of functional epitopes present on the surface of the antigen is referred to as the valency. Antigens can usually weigh around 10,000 Daltons and compounds like cellulose, containing starch and are non-antigenic and hence are used for intrinsic valves and restore artificial activity in the body [39, 40] (Fig. **5**).

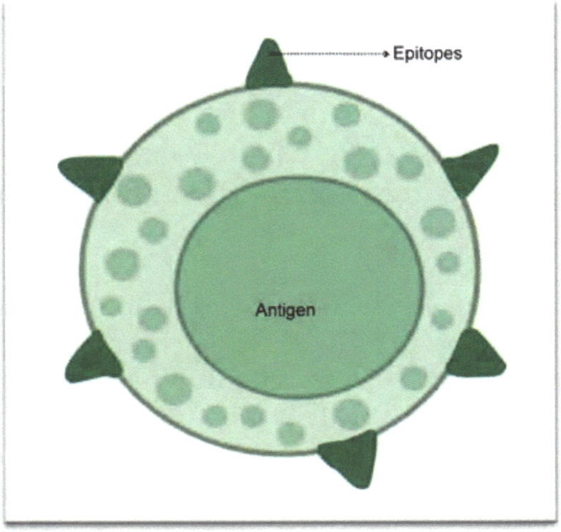

Fig. (5). Antigen structure.

Natural Active Immunity

Natural active immunity occurs when an individual encounters a pathogen and produces its antibodies in its defense. After the infection is cleared out of the body, the memory cells remain there and protect the body if the same pathogen ever attacks again. A classic example of the same is when a person recovers from chicken pox after a long period of immunity from the infection [41].

Artificial Active Immunity

This immunity is induced artificially when the person is exposed to pathogens deliberately, followed by the production of antibodies in the host body to create the scenario of an infection and eventually have a bunch of memory cells lined up for the next similar pathogenic invasion. An example of this is the MMR vaccine for a trio of deadly diseases, measles, mumps, and rubella [42].

a. **Cell-mediated immunity:** No antibodies are produced in this type of immunity; rather, sensitive lymphocytes participate in the process. They react with antigens that attack, and then phagocytosis occurs to eliminate them from the host's body. It all starts with the activation of T-cells when an invasion occurs. Then, it differentiates into several cells called the **'effector cells'** which then recognize and response by triggering a defense. The system needs two basic signals to get started on the attack. First is recognition of the antigen to analyze the situation and severity of invasion. The second signal is co-stimulation. Costimulation is basically a second signal given after the T cell adheres to the antigen. Some of the costimulatory substances are cytokines and interleukins [43].

T cells: These are the T-lymphocytes produced in the thymus. Then, these differentiate into memory cells, CD4 and CD8 cells. The lymph produces a large army of these antigen-specific T cells, which, when needed, mitigate the invasion by pathogens. Once activated, the T cells differentiate into an arsenal of effector cells [43, 44].

There are three main types of T cells that participate in the immune response.

i. Helper T cells: The CD4 T cells often exhibit CD4. When in the resting phase, they recognize the intruder initiating the attack with the help of fragments in association with MHC-II. The CD4 protein helps the T cells encounter the Antigen Presenting Cells (APCs), followed by costimulation and hence activating the T cells. After the second signal of costimulation, the active T cells start releasing several cytokines into the space. One of the major triggers of the T cell proliferation is the Interleukin-2 (IL-2) cytokine. This cytokine also plays an essential role in awakening the dormant T cells and the cytotoxic cells [45].

a. **Th1 Cells:** These activate the macrophagic cells to fight and eliminate the intracellular invaders, like bacteria. During the action of Th1 cells, cytokines such as Interferon-gamma (IFN-gamma) are released.
b. **Th2 Cells:** The Th2 cells are at the heart of the humoral immunity, which facilitates the B cell differentiation into an antibody-producing factory. In this, too, cytokines are released like IL-4. IL-5, which activates the eosinophils, *etc.* These cells play a vital role in allergic reactions.
c. **T Follicular helper (Tfh) cells:** These are produced in the lymphoid tissues of the human body. T follicular cells basically assist B cells to proliferate in specialized centers in the lymphoid organs called the germinal centers. These special cells help the B cells grow into better antibodies to combat the infection.

ii. Cytotoxic Cells: These kinds of cells generally exhibit the CD8 protein and hence the name. The cytotoxic cells destroy the host cells when they encounter an infection. They are also called the 'killer T cells', which execute the basic immune response of eliminating the enemy. After these cells are activated, certain cytotoxic granules are released, packed with perforin and granzymes. These substances make the target cell porous, leading to apoptosis. Additionally, to this activity, these cells also facilitate phagocytic action by releasing cytokines, which enhance inflammation [46].

iii. Regulatory cells: These are also known as 'Tregs' and maintain homeostasis within the immune system. These are basically the peacekeepers of the system, making sure the immune system cells do not attack their own cells. They do it by talking directly to other immune cells and signaling them to stop whenever necessary, or they also have the authority to take away what they need to survive, causing them to die [47].

iv. Memory T cells: Now, these are like the guards protecting our body's intrinsic system from intruders. These are long-lived cells differentiated from T cells. Keeping in mind what antigen caused what harm to us is what they do. If the same pathogen comes back, it is easy for the system to fight it back. These cells tend to provide a rapid response as they patrol in the bloodstream as well as the lymphoid tissues. They further differentiate into two types, namely, central memory T cells (T_{cm}) and effector memory T cells (T_{em}). Where T_{cm} provides long-term memory while camping in the lymphoid organs, the T_{em} provides immediate response and protection by reaching the site of action in no time [48] (Fig. **6**).

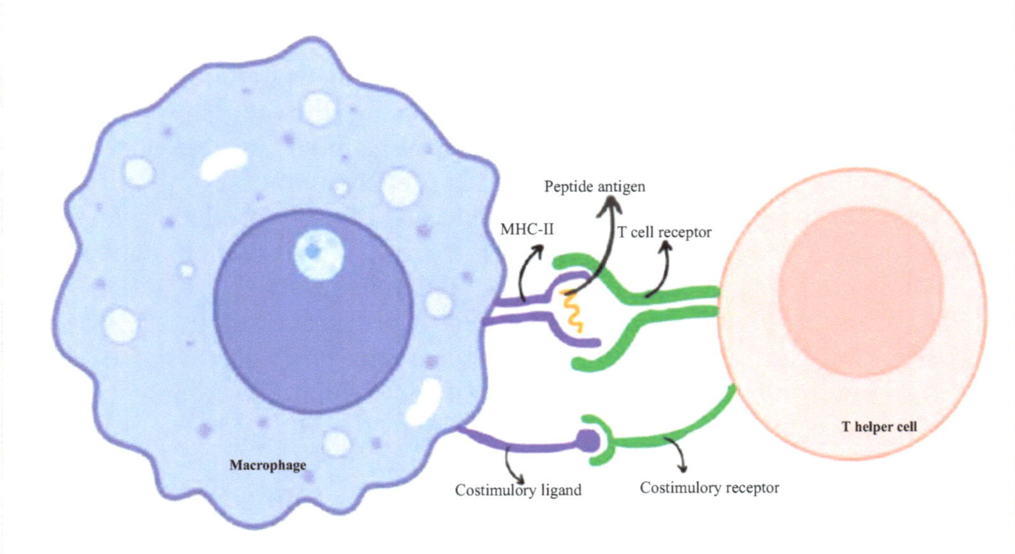

Fig. (6). Activation of Macrophage *via* T helper cell.

Passive Immunity

Passive immunity is outsourcing your defense system and ammunition. Instead of producing antibodies in-house, this immunity allows us to borrow the shield to fight off pathogens. It is deployed when there is an elevated risk of infection, and no time can be spared for the vaccine to work. Although it has a temporary action and there is no memory of the infection to fight it the second time as no memory cells are involved, but it has some advantages like first, it supports the system when the body has no time left to build its army of antibodies and secondly, it provides immediate protection against invaders as it has no latent period. We can have this immunity in two ways [49]:

a. **Natural Passive Immunity:** This type of immunity is passed to a child by his mother when antibodies pass through the mother's milk or even the placenta. This facilitates the baby to have the same immunity to the diseases the mother is immune to. For example, breast milk, colostrum, the first milk produced after childbirth, contains several antibodies, especially IgA antibodies, which protect the child from pathogens.
b. **Artificial Passive Immunity:** Artificial immunity, as the name suggests, involves the medical injection of antibodies from the outside. For example, an injection of gamma globulin contains the protection a baby needs by supplying all the essential gamma globulin antibodies. This immunity can be induced by two main methods:

i. **Immune globulin therapy**: When human plasma is used as a pool for concentrated antibodies to protect the host against a broad spectrum of diseases. It is generally used for people prone to infection or exposed to pathogens frequently.
ii. **Antiserum therapy**: The process of this technique is more complex than just harvesting antibodies and putting them into the host body. In this technique, antibodies are first harvested from other species that have been previously immunized to a particular antigen or disease. Although this is an effective method, it can cause severe allergic reactions.

BASIS OF AUTOIMMUNITY

Imagine a war raging between your friend and his brother. The situation is even worse because the attacking party is your friend's inner circle. If we come to think of it, this is an unfortunate reality for those millions of humans out there suffering from autoimmune disorders.

The term 'autoimmune' is self-explanatory in nature, meaning auto (self) and immune (immune system), when the individual's own system internally starts to attack its own cells, and the sense of differentiating identities is lost. As stated by Paul R. Ehrlich (1901), an immune reaction towards the "self" can produce antibodies that may be detrimental to the person. As per his renowned concept of "horror autotoxicus," the body needs a defense mechanism to safeguard itself from the threats posed by self-autoantibodies [50].

When the body identifies the cell components as non-self, it elicits an immune response. This results in the destruction of the body's own cells, often leading to fatal consequences. In 1904, Donath and Landsteiner observed autoimmune disease for the first time. This was discovered during the study of paroxysmal cold hemoglobinuria. The antibodies in this case bind to the RBCs while the temperature is low and cause subsequent hemolysis when the temperature is gradually increased. The intensity of this phenomenon matters a lot, as if the level of autoimmunity is low, then it may be significant to identify CD8+ cells in its initial stages of development [51]. Women are more likely to develop autoimmune diseases than men, and there are so many possible factors like hormonal changes, X-chromosome differences, sex hormones, genetic factors, environmental factors, *etc*. Other factors are also responsible for the same as poor diet, lack of exercise, increased stress, *etc* [52].

Hereditary factors for autoimmune diseases are heightened in genetic regulatory areas specific to T cells. Contemporary T cell datasets facilitate association studies linking Single-Nucleotide Polymorphisms (SNPs) to various molecular traits, such as chromatin accessibility, gene expression, transcriptional programs,

T Cell Antigen Receptor (TCR) amino acid utilization, and cell state levels. These investigations have revealed numerous Quantitative Trait Loci (QTLs) in T cells that overlap with genetic susceptibility to autoimmune disorders [53, 54]. Variations in genetic risk for autoimmune diseases are commonly found in T cell-specific regulatory areas of the genome, and they are disproportionately located near genes that have T cell-specific functions. These results indicate that T cells are crucial for the progression of autoimmune diseases [55, 56]

Factors Affecting Autoimmunity

1. **Genetic susceptibility:** Some people are genetically liable to autoimmune diseases. This vulnerability is associated with many genes and other hazard elements. Individuals with a genetic predisposition do not continually develop autoimmune diseases. Three important genes are notion to be involved in many autoimmune diseases concerning T cells, MHC-II, and immunoglobulins. People with a family history of the same are more likely to have this phenomenon. Moreover, HLA (Human Leukocyte Antigen) genes also contribute to the case, located on the cell surface; HLA genes help the immune system to distinguish between self and non-self. These are often related to specific diseases, such as HLA-B27 is associated with Ankylosing spondylitis (spondyloarthropathies), which is an inflammatory disease belonging to the class of rheumatoid arthritis mainly affecting the spine and bones of the axial skeleton [57].
2. **Environment**: Infections can be triggered by the pathogens present in the environment. The resting T cells come into play as autoreactive when self-antigens are released from injured tissues. Also, when the pathogen mimics the body components, the immune system can mistakenly take it as a non-self-part [58].
3. **Chemicals:** Toxins like silica dust have a deteriorating impact on the defense system as it causes severe lung inflammation leading to a systemic chronic autoimmune disorder characterized by inflammation and damaging one's own tissues in most of the area in the body like brain, blood vessels, joints *etc.* called the lupus erythematosus [59].
4. **Hormones:** There is a considerable amount of difference between male and female hormone intensities. Women are more susceptible to autoimmune disorders because of their 'overworking hormones' in two major life events: pregnancy and menopause. Estrogen is the key hormone regulating all the feminine events. A shift in this can cause a woman's body to react abruptly. Estrogen can elevate the immune response, causing the T and B cells to get activated and influence the Th2 action, leading to lupus disorder. However, lower levels of androgens and progesterone can also cause the immune system to get triggered, as these are basically mild immunosuppressives. Pregnancy

often shifts the hormonal balance, contradicting the immune system, leading to its confusion. On one hand, the Th1 system, known as proinflammatory, helps regulate the symptoms of rheumatoid arthritis; on the other hand, the Th2 system, known as anti-inflammatory, tends to worsen the condition in lupus [60].

Classification of Autoimmune Disorders

There are hundreds of autoimmune disorders in existence, out of which the most clinically diverse are explained below and represented in Fig. (7). This classification of these is based on the intensity of the symptoms and to what extent the body is affected.

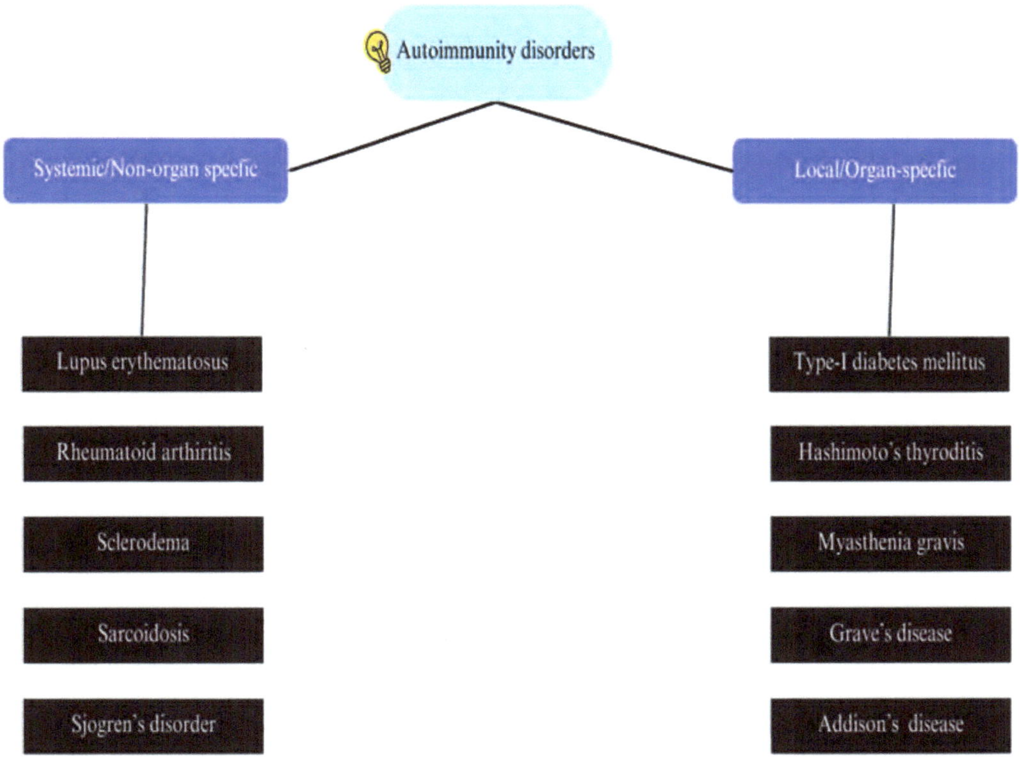

Fig. (7). Classification of Autoimmune Disorders.

1. Systemic disorders: systemic disorders are highly prevalent throughout the body and hence are non-organ specific. These can affect multiple organs of the body and are extensively spread across the system. Signs and symptoms of systemic disorders spread prolifically across the body. The conditions exhibit the production of autoantibodies, which are tested for when detecting the autoimmune disorder. Some of these are described below [60]:

a. Systemic Lupus Erythematosus (SLE): The disorder affects the kidneys, heart, and lungs by causing inflammation and damage to multiple tissues. It is observed primarily in African American women with a woman-to-man infection ratio of 10:1. Affected individuals produce antibodies against contrasting functions, shutting down the normal activities of the body. It tends to develop a type-III hypersensitivity reaction due to antigens adhering to the walls of blood vessels. Hydroxychloroquine, basically an anti-malarial drug, is effective in reducing flare-ups and aids in preventing organ damage [61].

b. Rheumatoid arthritis (RA): It is a common autoimmune disorder prevailing among women aged 40-60 years mainly affecting joint functioning. The cardinal signs include inflammation of joints, causing redness and swelling, stiffness, *etc.* In some rare cases, it can also affect other organs, such as the lungs or heart, making it non-organ-specific. Autoantibodies produced in RA react against the IgG antibody region and are called **rheumatoid factors.** An example of the rheumatoid factors is the IgM antibody. Non-steroidal drugs like ibuprofen have proven effectiveness for inflammation and pain, hence are given as first-line treatments [62].

c. Scleroderma: It affects the connective tissue all over the body, scleroderma elicits the release of collagen that leads to the petrification of the internal organs. One of the initial pieces of evidence includes Raynaud's syndrome, characterized by changes in the color of fingers due to vasoconstriction in response to cold or stress. The autoantibodies involved are Anti-Scl-70, also known as anti-topoisomerase antibodies, which are often associated with a substantial risk of lung infection. General measures include calcium channel blockers like the famous amlodipine or topical nitroglycerin applied on the affected areas to expand the blood flow locally and help with the changed color of the skin [63].

d. Sarcoidosis: A multisystem disease characterized by inflammation, and formation of clusters of granulomas across multiple organs, chest pain due to dry cough is also noticeable. Lungs are mostly affected in sarcoidosis, followed by the eyes, heart, skin, and other organs. One of the primary signs is swelling in lymph nodes, fatigue, and purple-colored lesions on the skin. Some of the autoantibodies involved are Antinuclear Antibodies (ANA), which work against the nucleus, and Angiotensin-Converting Enzyme (ACE), whose levels are tested for sarcoidosis diagnosis. The most common drug for first-line treatment is prednisone, which helps reduce redness and pain.

e. Sjogren's disorder: Like any other autoimmune disorder, Sjogren's disorder tends to attack its own endocrine system affecting mostly the salivary and lacrimal glands. Chronic in nature, the disorder presents symptoms of xerostomia and keratoconjunctivitis sicca. Glandular, along with extrinsic glandular activities, are primarily affected by this condition, which displays joint pain (arthralgia), muscle pain, and tender joints. The autoantibodies involved are Rheumatoid Factor (RF), which is tested as either positive or negative, indicating the presence of the disease, and anti-Ro/SSA, among others. First-line treatment in this case is interesting, artificial tears are used to restore the lubrication in the eyes, prescription drugs like cyclosporin ophthalmic emulsion also increase tear production and reduce inflammation. Just like artificial tears, over-the-counter saliva substitutes are also available to treat xerostomia [64].

2. Local disorders: These are characterized by the invasion confined to only one part of the body, leading to localized tissue damage. It results in more damage to a specific organ, sometimes completely shutting down its functionality and ultimately leading to organ failure. The antibodies hence produced may block or overexcite the activity of the target organ. Some of the common examples are discussed below:

a. Type-I diabetes mellitus: It is a chronic condition where the insulin producing beta-cells are destroyed by the own system, which leads to a significant decline in the insulin levels and hence called Insulin-Dependent Diabetes Mellitus (IDDM). As insulin is one of the vital hormones in the absorption of glucose to provide intracellular energy. The condition can be fatal as, without glucose as the energy source, our body starts to break fat for the same and that leads to production of ketones, acidic compounds by nature. IDDM can be caused by several factors, such as genetic factors, environmental factors, and most importantly, autoimmune dysfunction. This not only causes ketoacidosis but also has a deteriorating effect on the heart, increasing the chances of stroke. Fatigue, blurred vision, and increased thirst are some of the early signs and symptoms. First-line treatment of IDDM includes insulin therapy to replenish the levels. Insulin therapy can include both pumps and multiple daily injections [65].

b. Hashimoto's thyroiditis: Hashimoto's disease, also known as chronic lymphocytic thyroiditis, is a condition that invades the thyroid gland, leading to the gradual deterioration of the gland. Some of the cardinal signs include unexplained weight gain, a slower metabolism, and goiter, among others. An autoimmune response triggered can be diagnosed by testing for autoantibodies attacking the thyroid proteins. Several factors contribute to the occurrence, such as certain genes (HLA complex), excessive cytokine release signaling to inflammation and destruction of thyroid tissues. If left unmanaged for too long, the severity of complications can reach hypothyroidism, a life-threatening condition, and elevated thyroid levels, which are responsible for fatal cardiac issues. First-line treatments incorporate a synthetic form of thyroxine, levothyroxine, to replenish hormone levels. Lifestyle changes and constant medications help to restore normal conditions [66].

c. Myasthenia gravis: It is characterized by muscle weakness and chronic neuromuscular dysfunction. Myasthenia gravis is abbreviated as MG. The autoantibodies produced destroy the communication gateway of the neuromuscular junction. The severity varies from individual to individual. There are five levels of muscle weakness:

Class I: weakness limited to the eyes, showcasing drooping eyelids and heaviness.

Class II: weakness starts to propagate to other parts as well, leaving the daily activities unperturbed.

Class III: evident weakness takes over, but mildly. Makes it difficult to chew or swallow for the time being.

Class IV: severity increases and starts to obstruct daily activities of endurance, and muscle strength. Treatment is needed immediately.

Class V: muscle weakness has now reached your survival activities, like breathing making you visit the hospital for artificial ventilation.

Common symptoms include drooping eyelids, difficulty swallowing, *etc*. Muscle strength is often tested for diagnostic purposes. An electromyography can also be performed to test the electrical activity of the nerves. Although the causes are not fully known, genetic and environmental toxins can often lead to this autoimmune response. First-line treatment includes pyridostigmine (anticholinesterase agent) that improves the gateway between nerves and muscles, to calm the attacking autoimmune response, and prednisone is also administered [67].

d. Grave's disease: Graves' disease is a common disorder showcasing elevated thyroid levels. The disease targets the thyroid glands, making them overwork and produce hormones that essentially regulate heart rate and temperature. Despite diet and appetite, the individual experiencing weight loss due to hypermetabolism, tachycardia, and hand tremors is one of the key signs indicating Graves' disease. Elevated levels of cortisol, bacterial or viral infections, and the course of pregnancy are some of the factors that contribute to the occurrence of the disease. Primary autoantibodies include TSIs that act as thyroid-stimulating hormone signaling to overproduction of thyroid hormone. When the disease is due to pregnancy hormones then, propylthiouracil is used in the first trimester of the event to stabilize the hormonal levels, propranolol (beta blocker) is used to control the hand tremors [68].

e. Addison's disease: Addison's disease, also known as autoimmune adrenalitis, is characterized by declining levels of adrenal hormones as a result of an autoimmune attack. Unlike others, this is not a common disease to occur, but it can be fatal if left unaddressed for long. The condition primarily targets the bilateral adrenal cortex, resulting in low production of cortisol, aldosterone, and androgens. It is a chronic condition that gradually develops and creates life-threatening issues. Major signs and symptoms include low blood pressure, hypoglycemia, abdominal pain, darkening of skin, *etc*. As this is a hormone-related issue, to bring back the usual conditions, hormonal levels need to be stabilized. Therefore, hormone replacement therapy using hydrocortisone or dexamethasone is used to reinvigorate the hormonal level, which is the primary treatment followed by mineralocorticoids when and as needed [69].

BALANCE BETWEEN IMMUNITY AND STRESS

There is a delicate and intricate balance between the immune system and stress. Stress is laid down when a psychological trigger response is triggered by a situation we are unable to handle with ease. It exerts a great influence on the body's defense. Whether the immune system will improve or deteriorate will depend on the intensity and timeline of the stress. There is even a specialized branch assigned to study the relationship called **'psychoneuroimmunology' (PNI),** which deals with the strings between nervous, endocrine, and immune systems. When we are in an intense situation that triggers stress, the Hypothalamic-Pituitary-Adrenal (HPA) axis gets into motion, which further releases cortisol (often referred to as the 'stress hormone'). The stress hormone released from the adrenal gland comes into play, causing our immune system to shut down and back away momentarily. Prolonged elevated levels of cortisol lead the immune system to take a dip. To balance the dynamic network and stress, one should eat healthy, at regular intervals and stay away from intoxicants as much as possible, which is most likely to cause detrimental effects on the brain activity too. Sleep is also a vital factor in determining how strong your immune system is. Even if you sleep during the day, stealing some productive hours at night, affects the system in terms of efficacy, as it leads to insomnia and poor gut health, too. Keeping stress management in place with healthy eating habits and a regular sleep schedule helps a lot to improve the defense arsenal. Always remember that your body is a big space, and it needs to be cleaned frequently because it cannot afford to let the dust settle in [70].

CONCLUSION

The immune system, a complex network of cells and tissues, is essential for defending the body against pathogens like viruses and bacteria. It includes innate immunity, which is present from birth and acts as the first line of defense through different barriers. It is also known as specific immunity, as it responds rapidly without improving over time. The other immunity is the one that we acquire over time from the environment. Autoimmune disorders occur when the immune system mistakenly attacks the body's own cells, resulting in harmful consequences. This arises from a breakdown in self-tolerance, where the body identifies its own self as an invader. Women are more susceptible to autoimmune diseases due to factors like hormones, genetic predisposition, *etc*. Stress also plays an essential role in the immune function. It triggers the hypothalamic-pituitar--adrenal axis, releasing cortisol, which is a hormone that suppresses the immune activity. Chronic stress can weaken the immune system over time, making it more vulnerable. Hence, maintaining a balanced diet, regular sleep and stress management can help support the immune system.

Core Concepts

- *Acute phase protein:* Serum protein that elevates during the invasion of pathogens or inflammatory conditions.
- *Adaptive immunity*: This is a pathogen-specific response that develops over multiple infections from the same invader. The immunity that a human acquires over a period is called adaptive or acquired immunity.
- *Anaphylaxis*: It is an antigen-specific immune response and a multi-system allergic reaction that may or may not be fatal.
- *Antigen*: A substance that is particularly non-self and is recognized to elicit the immune response.
- *Antibodies*: These are proteins produced and released by B cells that bind to a specific antigen (such as a pathogen) and initiate its elimination.
- *B cells*: A kind of WBC that facilitates the production of antibodies. These are present in plasma and are a part of the humoral immune system.
- *Cell-mediated immunity*: T cells get triggered and rage the war against the pathogens to fight infections or even tumors.
- *Complement:* It is a group of serum proteins that centrally hold the inflammation and activation of phagocytes and the lytic attack on cell membranes.
- *Cytokines*: These are proteins that signal the release after the immune response has been triggered. The signaling molecules cause processes like inflammation and hematopoiesis to occur.
- *Dendritic cell*: A cell that analyses and reads the antigen and hands it over to T cells, which further initiates an immune response.

- *Innate Immunity:* The immunity that is present in the body by birth and protects the body from external particles that can cause potential harm to us. This system includes physical barriers and phagocytes.
- *Interferons (IFNs)*: Signaling molecules between cells of the network system.
- *Interleukin*: Molecules that signal between cells as well as protect them from viral infection.
- *Natural killer cells*: Lymphocyte cells which can identify and eliminate cells infested with virus and certain tumors.
- *Non-self:* These are the particles that invade our body and can cause harm to us. They are sometimes called foreign bodies. Non-self-particles, such as bacteria, viruses, and pollen grains, typically irritate the intrinsic membranes and trigger an immune response.
- *Humoral immunity:* This immunity is dependent on the antigen-antibody reaction, produced by B cell and is present in the body fluids.
- *Macrophage:* It is a large phagocytic cell discovered in 1838 that eats up extrinsic harmful particles.
- *Memory cell*: It is a type of lymphocyte that is retained in the body after the infection has been taken care of. This helps the system to register the infection and the pathogen that caused it so that it can fight it without generating everything from scratch the next time it attacks the body.
- *Major Histocompatibility Complex (MHC)*: It is a genetic region primarily responsible for rapid rejection of graft during tissue or organ transplants. It also acts as a signaling molecule between lymphocyte and cells which showcase antigen.
- *Self:* These are particles or molecules that are essentially a part of your body or originated from the body. Self-particles can be proteins or can be a part of the circulating system.
- *T cells:* A kind of WBC that is significant in adaptive/ acquired immunity and is a part of the mediated response.
- *Vaccination:* Immunization against diseases by bacterial or viral culture, which may or may not be viable.
- *Pathogen:* An invading organism that causes diseases like bacteria, viruses, or certain fungi.

REFERENCES

[1] Annual Review of Immunology. Immunology 1983; 1.

[2] Abbas AK, Lichtman AH, Pober JS. Cellular and Molecular Immunology. 3rd ed., Philadelphia, PA: W.B. Saunders Company 1997.

[3] Janeway CA, Travers P, Walport M, Capra JD. Immunobiology. London (UK): 4th ed Garland 1999.

[4] Paul WE, Ed. Fundamental Immunology. New York: Raven Press 1984.

[5] Kuby J Immunology. 3rd ed., Oxford: W.H. Freeman 1997.

[6] Nisinoff A. Introduction to Molecular Immunology. 2nd ed., 1985.

[7] Metchnikoff E. Immunity in the Infectious Diseases. New York: MacMillan 1905.

[8] Peakman M, Vergani D. Basic and Clinical Immunology. Edinburgh, UK: Churchill Livingstone 1997.

[9] Playfair JHL, Lydyard PM. Medical Immunology for Students. 2nd ed., Edinburgh, UK: Churchill Livingstone 2000.

[10] Roitt IM. Essential Immunology. 9th ed., Oxford, UK: Blackwell Scientific 1997.

[11] Davis BD, Dulbecco R, Eisen MN, Ginsberg MS. Microbiology. 4th ed. Philadelphia (PA): J.B. Lippincott Co.; 1990. Prusiner SB, Collinge J, Powell J, Anderton B, editors. Prion Diseases of Humans and Animals. New York: Ellis Morwood 1992.

[12] Medzhitov R, Janeway C Jr. Innate Immunity. N Engl J Med 2000; 343(5): 338-44. [http://dx.doi.org/10.1056/NEJM200008033430506] [PMID: 10922424]

[13] Paul W, Ed. Fundamental Immunology. 4th ed., Philadelphia, PA: Lippincott-Raven 1999.

[14] Kimbrell DA, Beutler B. The evolution and genetics of innate immunity. Nat Rev Genet 2001; 2(4): 256-67. [http://dx.doi.org/10.1038/35066006] [PMID: 11283698]

[15] Lawson PR, Reid KBM. The roles of surfactant proteins A and D in innate immunity. Immunol Rev 2000; 173(1): 66-78. [http://dx.doi.org/10.1034/j.1600-065X.2000.917308.x] [PMID: 10719668]

[16] Peiser L, Mukhopadhyay S, Gordon S. Scavenger receptors in innate immunity. Curr Opin Immunol 2002; 14(1): 123-8. [http://dx.doi.org/10.1016/S0952-7915(01)00307-7] [PMID: 11790542]

[17] Edelson RL, Fink JM. The immunologic function of skin. Sci Am 1985; 252(6): 46-53. [http://dx.doi.org/10.1038/scientificamerican0685-46] [PMID: 3923622]

[18] Weiss L. Cells and Tissues of the Immune System: Structure, Functions, Interactions Foundations of Immunology Series. Englewood Cliffs, NJ: Prentice-Hall 1972; pp. 88-9.

[19] Wekerle H, Ketelsen U-P, Ernst M. Thymic nurse cells. Lymphoepithelial cell complexes in murine thymuses: morphological and serological characterization. J Exp Med 1980; 151(4): 925-44. [http://dx.doi.org/10.1084/jem.151.4.925] [PMID: 6966312]

[20] Newman J. How breast milk protects newborns. Sci Am 1995; 273(6): 76-9. [http://dx.doi.org/10.1038/scientificamerican1295-76] [PMID: 8525349]

[21] Frazer JK, Capra JD. Immunoglobulins: structure and function. In: Paul WE, Ed. Fundamental Immunology. 4th ed., Philadelphia, PA: Lippincott-Raven 1999.

[22] Kraehenbuhl J, Neutra M. Transepithelial transport and mucosal defence II: secretion of IgA. Trends Cell Biol 1992; 2(6): 170-4. [http://dx.doi.org/10.1016/0962-8924(92)90036-M] [PMID: 14731986]

[23] Silverton EW, Navia MA, Davies DR. Three-dimensional structure of an intact human immunoglobulin. Proc Natl Acad Sci USA 1977; 74(11): 5140-4. [http://dx.doi.org/10.1073/pnas.74.11.5140] [PMID: 270751]

[24] Valentine RC, Green NM. Electron microscopy of an antibody-hapten complex. J Mol Biol 1967; 27(3): 615-7. [http://dx.doi.org/10.1016/0022-2836(67)90063-0] [PMID: 4167449]

[25] Amit AG, Mariuzza RA, Phillips SEV, Poljak RJ. Three-dimensional structure of an antigen-antibody complex at 2.8 A resolution. Science 1986; 233(4765): 747-53. [http://dx.doi.org/10.1126/science.2426778] [PMID: 2426778]

[26] Fearon DT, Carter RH. The CD19/CR2/TAPA-1 complex of B lymphocytes: linking natural to acquired immunity. Annu Rev Immunol 1995; 13(1): 127-49. [http://dx.doi.org/10.1146/annurev.iy.13.040195.001015] [PMID: 7542009]

[27] Mariuzza RA, Phillips SEV, Poljak RJ. The structural basis of antigen-antibody recognition. Annu Rev Biophys Biophys Chem 1987; 16(1): 139-59. [http://dx.doi.org/10.1146/annurev.bb.16.060187.001035] [PMID: 2439094]

[28] Audhya T, Kroon D, Heavner G, Viamontes G, Goldstein G. Tripeptide structure of bursin, a selective B-cell-differentiating hormone of the bursa of fabricius. Science 1986; 231(4741): 997-9. [http://dx.doi.org/10.1126/science.3484838] [PMID: 3484838]

[29] Barclay AN. The organization of B and T lymphocytes in lymph nodes. Immunol Today 1982; 3(12): 330-1. [http://dx.doi.org/10.1016/0167-5699(82)90017-2] [PMID: 25290675]

[30] Duijvestijn A, Hamann A. Mechanisms and regulation of lymphocyte migration. Immunol Today 1989; 10(1): 23-8. [http://dx.doi.org/10.1016/0167-5699(89)90061-3] [PMID: 2665769]

[31] Iwasaki A, Medzhitov R. Regulation of adaptive immunity by the innate immune system. Science 2010; 327(5963): 291-5. [http://dx.doi.org/10.1126/science.1183021] [PMID: 20075244]

[32] Burton DR. Antibody: the flexible adaptor molecule. Trends Biochem Sci 1990; 15(2): 64-9. [http://dx.doi.org/10.1016/0968-0004(90)90178-E] [PMID: 2186517]

[33] Blattner FR, Tucker PW. The molecular biology of immunoglobulin D. Nature 1984; 307(5950): 417-22. [http://dx.doi.org/10.1038/307417a0] [PMID: 6420708]

[34] Lane P. Development of B-cell memory and effector function. Curr Opin Immunol 1996; 8(3): 331-5. [http://dx.doi.org/10.1016/S0952-7915(96)80121-X] [PMID: 8793988]

[35] Davies DR, Metzger H. Structural basis of antibody function. Annu Rev Immunol 1983; 1(1): 87-115. [http://dx.doi.org/10.1146/annurev.iy.01.040183.000511] [PMID: 6399980]

[36] Berzofsky JA, Berkower JJ. Immunogenicity and antigen structure. In: Paul WE, Ed. Fundamental Immunology. 4th ed., Philadelphia, PA: Lippincott-Raven 1999.

[37] Grey HM, Sette A, Buus S. How T cells see antigen. Sci Am 1989; 261(5): 56-64. [http://dx.doi.org/10.1038/scientificamerican1189-56] [PMID: 2530628]

[38] Brodsky FM, Guagliardi LE. The cell biology of antigen processing and presentation. Annu Rev Immunol 1991; 9(1): 707-44. [http://dx.doi.org/10.1146/annurev.iy.09.040191.003423] [PMID: 1910692]

[39] Cantrell D. T cell antigen receptor signal transduction pathways. Annu Rev Immunol 1996; 14(1): 259-74. [http://dx.doi.org/10.1146/annurev.immunol.14.1.259] [PMID: 8717515]

[40] Clark EA, Ledbetter JA. How B and T cells talk to each other. Nature 1994; 367(6462): 425-8. [http://dx.doi.org/10.1038/367425a0] [PMID: 8107800]

[41] Landsteiner K. The Specificity of Serological Reactions. Cambridge, MA: Harvard University Press 1945.

[42] Laver WG, Air GM, Webster RG, Smith-Gill SJ. Epitopes on protein antigens: Misconceptions and realities. Cell 1990; 61(4): 553-6. [http://dx.doi.org/10.1016/0092-8674(90)90464-P] [PMID: 1693095]

[43] Romagnani S. Lymphokine production by human T cells in disease states. Annu Rev Immunol 1994; 12(1): 227-57.

[http://dx.doi.org/10.1146/annurev.iy.12.040194.001303] [PMID: 8011282]

[44] Mosmann TR, Coffman RL. TH1 and TH2 cells: different patterns of lymphokine secretion lead to different functional properties. Annu Rev Immunol 1989; 7(1): 145-73. [http://dx.doi.org/10.1146/annurev.iy.07.040189.001045] [PMID: 2523712]

[45] Barnett LA, Fujinami RS. Molecular mimicry: a mechanism for autoimmune injury. FASEB J 1992; 6(3): 840-4. [http://dx.doi.org/10.1096/fasebj.6.3.1740233] [PMID: 1740233]

[46] Sinha AA, Lopez MT, McDevitt HO. Autoimmune diseases: the failure of self tolerance. Science 1990; 248(4961): 1380-8. [http://dx.doi.org/10.1126/science.1972595] [PMID: 1972595]

[47] Steinman L. Autoimmune Disease. Sci Am 1993; 269(3): 106-14. [http://dx.doi.org/10.1038/scientificamerican0993-106] [PMID: 8211084]

[48] Vyse TJ, Kotzin BL. Genetic susceptibility to systemic lupus erythematosus. Annu Rev Immunol 1998; 16(1): 261-92. [http://dx.doi.org/10.1146/annurev.immunol.16.1.261] [PMID: 9597131]

[49] Feldmann M, Brennan FM, Maini RN. Role of cytokines in rheumatoid arthritis. Annu Rev Immunol 1996; 14(1): 397-440. [http://dx.doi.org/10.1146/annurev.immunol.14.1.397] [PMID: 8717520]

[50] Tienari PJ, Sajantila A, Peltonen L, Tienari PJ, Wikström J, Palo J. Genetic susceptibility to multiple sclerosis linked to myelin basic protein gene. Lancet 1992; 340(8826): 987-91. [http://dx.doi.org/10.1016/0140-6736(92)93007-A] [PMID: 1383661]

[51] Wilder RL. Neuroendocrine-immune system interactions and autoimmunity. Annu Rev Immunol 1995; 13(1): 307-38. [http://dx.doi.org/10.1146/annurev.iy.13.040195.001515] [PMID: 7612226]

[52] Liblau RS, Singer SM, McDevitt HO. Th1 and Th2 CD4+ T cells in the pathogenesis of organ-specific autoimmune diseases. Immunol Today 1995; 16(1): 34-8. [http://dx.doi.org/10.1016/0167-5699(95)80068-9] [PMID: 7880387]

[53] Epstein FH, Harris ED Jr. Rheumatoid Arthritis. N Engl J Med 1990; 322(18): 1277-89. [http://dx.doi.org/10.1056/NEJM199005033221805] [PMID: 2271017]

[54] Charreire J. Immune mechanisms in autoimmune thyroiditis. Adv Immunol 1989; 46: 263-334. [http://dx.doi.org/10.1016/S0065-2776(08)60656-2] [PMID: 2675564]

[55] Lockshin MD. Why women?. J Am Med Womens Assoc 1998; 53(1): 4-8. [PMID: 9458617]

[56] Eisenbarth GS. Type I diabetes: clinical implications of autoimmunity. Hosp Pract 1987; 22(9): 167-184, 174, 177 passim. [http://dx.doi.org/10.1080/21548331.1987.11703312] [PMID: 3114287]

[57] Ronald Kahn C. Autoimmunity and the aetiology of insulin-dependent diabetes mellitus. Nature 1982; 299(5878): 15-6. [http://dx.doi.org/10.1038/299015a0] [PMID: 7050728]

[58] Stuart JM, Cremer MA, Townes AS, Kang AH. Type II collagen-induced arthritis in rats. Passive transfer with serum and evidence that IgG anticollagen antibodies can cause arthritis. J Exp Med 1982; 155(1): 1-16. [http://dx.doi.org/10.1084/jem.155.1.1] [PMID: 7054355]

[59] Lopate G, Pestronk A. Autoimmune myasthenia gravis. Hosp Pract 1993; 28(1): 109-131, 115-117, 121-122 passim. [http://dx.doi.org/10.1080/21548331.1993.11442741] [PMID: 8380423]

[60] Steinman L, Mantegazza R. Prospects for specific immunotherapy in myasthenia gravis. FASEB J

1990; 4(10): 2726-31.
[http://dx.doi.org/10.1096/fasebj.4.10.2197152] [PMID: 2197152]

[61] Shoenfeld Y, Schwartz RS. Immunologic and genetic factors in autoimmune diseases. N Engl J Med 1984; 311(16): 1019-29.
[http://dx.doi.org/10.1056/NEJM198410183111605] [PMID: 6384779]

[62] Hang LM, Aguado MT, Dixon FJ, Theofilopoulos AN. Induction of severe autoimmune disease in normal mice by simultaneous action of multiple immunostimulators. J Exp Med 1985; 161(2): 423-8.
[http://dx.doi.org/10.1084/jem.161.2.423] [PMID: 3871835]

[63] Wu J, Zhou T, He J, Mountz JD. Autoimmune disease in mice due to integration of an endogenous retrovirus in an apoptosis gene. J Exp Med 1993; 178(2): 461-8.
[http://dx.doi.org/10.1084/jem.178.2.461] [PMID: 7688023]

[64] Lagattuta KA, Park HL, Rumker L, Ishigaki K, Nathan A, Raychaudhuri S. The genetic basis of autoimmunity seen through the lens of T cell functional traits. Nat Commun 2024; 15(1): 1204.
[http://dx.doi.org/10.1038/s41467-024-45170-w] [PMID: 38331990]

[65] Trynka G, Sandor C, Han B, *et al.* Chromatin marks identify critical cell types for fine mapping complex trait variants. Nat Genet 2013; 45(2): 124-30.
[http://dx.doi.org/10.1038/ng.2504] [PMID: 23263488]

[66] Amariuta T, Luo Y, Gazal S, *et al.* IMPACT: genomic annotation of cell-state-specific regulatory elements inferred from the epigenome of bound transcription factors. Am J Hum Genet 2019; 104(5): 879-95.
[http://dx.doi.org/10.1016/j.ajhg.2019.03.012] [PMID: 31006511]

[67] Samuels H, Malov M, Saha Detroja T, *et al.* Autoimmune disease classification based on PubMed text mining. J Clin Med 2022; 11(15): 4345.
[http://dx.doi.org/10.3390/jcm11154345] [PMID: 35893435]

[68] Marrie RA, Reider N, Cohen J, *et al.* A systematic review of the incidence and prevalence of autoimmune disease in multiple sclerosis. Mult Scler 2015; 21(3): 282-93.
[http://dx.doi.org/10.1177/1352458514564490] [PMID: 25533299]

[69] Miller FW. The increasing prevalence of autoimmunity and autoimmune diseases: an urgent call to action for improved understanding, diagnosis, treatment, and prevention. Curr Opin Immunol 2023; 80: 102266.
[http://dx.doi.org/10.1016/j.coi.2022.102266] [PMID: 36446151]

[70] Cao F, Liu YC, Ni QY, *et al.* Temporal trends in the prevalence of autoimmune diseases from 1990 to 2019. Autoimmun Rev 2023; 22(8): 103359.
[http://dx.doi.org/10.1016/j.autrev.2023.103359] [PMID: 37201621]

CHAPTER 2

Medicinal Plants and Drug Discovery

Bipindra Pandey[1], **Shankar Thapa**[1,*], **Mahalakshmi Suresha Biradar**[2] and **Ravindra Khadka**[3]

[1] *Department of Pharmacy, Madan Bhandari Academy of Health Sciences, Hetauda, Nepal*

[2] *Department of Pharmaceutical Chemistry, Al-Ameen College of Pharmacy, Bengaluru, India*

[3] *School of Health and Allied Sciences, Pokhara University, Kaski, Pokhara, Nepal*

Abstract: Plants have been used as a source of medicine for the treatment of different diseases for thousands of years. Bioprospecting of medicinal plants aims at the development of commercially valuable therapeutic goods, which could be used for the treatment of different diseases. The therapeutic values of medicinal plants are due to the presence of different bioactive secondary metabolites. The exploration of phytochemicals from the medicinal plants *via* ethnopharmacological, chemotaxonomical and random selection approach. The phytochemical-based drug discovery was performed by extraction, isolation, identification, bioassay, which further goes for target identification, target validation, lead identification, lead optimization, and clinical trials. The crucial step in drug discovery from the medicinal plant is lead identification and optimization due to their complex structural organization. This problem of drug discovery can be resolved by employing the concept of virtual screening and databases like COCONUT, TCMPG, IMPPAT 2.0, PMDB, PMhub, *etc*. Each of these steps has its specificities, limitations, and advances. In this regard, knowledge about combinatorial biosynthesis, chemical synthesis, and the technique of acquiring drugs from medicinal plants was gathered for this chapter. This chapter concludes by discussing a few significant facets of current case studies in relation to the discovery of novel bioactive compounds from medicinal plants and the creation of affordable, safe, and effective medications to combat the world's expanding list of illnesses.

Keywords: Advantages, Biological activity, Bioprospecting, Challenges, Disadvantages, Drug discovery process, Druggability characters, Ethnopharmacology approach, History, Human disease, Medicinal plant database, Medicinal plants, Modern methods, Natural product, Phytoconstituents, Plant selection approach, Random approach, Traditional medicine, Traditional methods, Zoopharmacognosy approach.

[*] **Corresponding author Shankar Thapa:** Department of Pharmacy, Madan Bhandari Academy of Health Sciences, Hetauda, Nepal; Tel: +977-9860352048; E-mail: tshankar551@gmail.com

M.S. Ashawat, Aditi Kaushik, Akash Jain, Jasmine Chaudhary & Manish Kaushik (Eds.)
All rights reserved-© 2025 Bentham Science Publishers

INTRODUCTION

Natural products are chemical compounds or substances produced by living organisms, found in nature. Natural products are abundantly available on this planet. Some plants are useful for daily needs, and some have medicinal value. Natural products generated from a variety of natural sources, such as plants, animals, and microorganisms, have played an important role in pharmaceutical and traditional medicine development. Natural products refer to secondary metabolites produced by any living organism; they are small molecules that are not necessary for survival, growth, development, or reproduction. They play a crucial role in plant defence against herbivory and other interspecies threats. These bioactive chemicals frequently feature unique structures and complex chemistries that have been optimized by evolution to interact with biological systems, making them invaluable in drug discovery and development. A remarkable number of contemporary medications have been developed from natural sources, with many of them inspired by traditional medicinal applications.

Medicinal plants have a long history of use in traditional medical systems around the world, including Ayurveda, Traditional Chinese medicine, and Native American healing methods. The medicinal properties of these plants are attributed to a wide range of chemical components, such as terpenes, glycosides, alkaloids, and flavonoids. The therapeutic qualities of these plants are still being investigated and verified by modern science, which is producing novel medications and treatments.

39% out of 520 drugs approved from 1983-1994 were of natural products or derived from natural origin. In that, 60-80% were used as antibacterial and anti-cancer agents. Natural products play a crucial role in drug discovery due to their unique chemical structures and "drug-like" qualities. Natural products help in the introduction of new chemical entities with diverse structures that can serve as templates for semi-synthetic and total synthetic modifications [1].

HISTORY AND ROLE OF MEDICINAL PLANTS IN HUMAN DISEASE

The natural products were used in many ways through prehistoric times. There is archeological evidence that the natural products were used as medicine by Neanderthals around 60,000 years ago. In the recent studies by Hardy *et al.*, yarrow and chamomile were found in the samples of dental calculus of Neanderthals [2]. These two plants are bitter and have less nutritional value. It suggests that these plants were used as a self-medication [3]. In Ancient civilizations, clay tablets bearing medical prescriptions were found in numerous Sumerian and Babylonian sites in 1728 BCE. The oldest medical document Papyrus of Ebers, is dated to the 16th century BCE in Egypt. This document contains 877 prescriptions and some remedies, including Myrrh, fennel, and other spices. In Southeast Asian countries like India, traditional folk medicine dates to 1500 BCE. The usefulness of medicine was passed on by word of mouth from father to son, for many generations, until it was in the holy writings known as the Vedas. Treating illness using medicinal plants has continued till today, and the system is known as Ayurveda. Ayurveda is derived from the Sanskrit word, where "*Ayu*" means life and "*Veda*" means science or knowledge. Knowledge of medicinal plants is documented in Charaka Samhitha by the father of Ayurveda, Sage Charaka. Chinese, 5000 years ago, used many herbs in the form of tea. One of the teas that they were consuming was made from a leafless creeper known as Ma-Hung (*Ephedra Sinica*) and was used in the treatment of lung disease, to reduce fever, and to relieve coughing. The phytoconstituent, which is extracted from this plant, is known as ephedrine, which is still used to treat asthma.

Hippocrates, who lived in the fourth century BCE and is regarded as the founder of modern medicine, listed 300 remedies. Theophrastus, the 3rd-century BCE father of botany, presented the details of plant appearance and culture in his work Enquiry into Plants. In his book De Materia Medica, the first-century BCE Greek physician Dioscorides listed 800 treatments made from plant, animal, and mineral sources. He has written about the locations, harvesting schedule, preparation steps, and medical categorization.

The intriguing Doctrine of Signature, which was created in herbal medicine throughout the Middle Ages in Europe, is recorded in works by Archimedes. According to the herbalist, plants are meant to benefit humans and have been used for specific organ-related ailments depending on their shape and color. For instance, kidney-related health conditions were treated with kidney-shaped fruits and pulses, and heart-related issues were treated with fruits and leaves that are in heart shape. In addition to being eaten for their nutritional content, plants are also utilized as medicine to treat several illnesses [4]. One thing we can learn from the history of using plants as medicine is that they can treat illnesses. In more recent history, the use of plants as medicines has involved the isolation of active compounds, beginning with the isolation of morphine from opium in the early 19th century.

Throughout history, human civilization has utilized various plants for food, medicine, clothing, and shelter. Vegetarian foods are rich in "super nutrients," including protective antioxidants, phytochemicals, and micronutrients, which promote health and protect against diseases. Plants have several pharmacological roles, such as antioxidant, antiviral, anti-cancer, antimicrobial, antifungal, and antiparasitic activities. They contain free radical scavenging molecules like flavonoids, phenolics, anthocyanins, and vitamins, which exhibit antioxidant activity. It has been reported that the antioxidant properties of phytochemicals can mitigate oxidative stress in biological systems. Phytochemicals have been shown to reduce the risk of many human diseases, including cardiovascular diseases, hepato-renal diseases, diabetes, cancers, and neurodegenerative disorders. Many current herbal medicines are derived directly or indirectly from plants and are considered important for treating various human diseases [5, 6].

BIOPROSPECTING OF MEDICINAL PLANTS AS A SOURCE OF NEW DRUG

Bioprospecting involves the exploration of plants, animals, and microorganisms for use in various fields such as academia, pharmaceuticals, biotechnology, agriculture, and other industries. This practice aims to commercialize biodiversity, particularly for the development of medicinal products. In 1993, the US National Institutes of Health allocated US $60 million towards research on biodiversity for drug and medical product development from natural sources. The National Cancer Institute (NCI) has amassed over 50,000 samples from plants, microorganisms, and marine organisms from more than 30 tropical countries, with the goal of discovering treatments for cancer and AIDS. These samples are stored in NCI's Natural Product Repository and are accessible to researchers through material transfer agreements [7].

Bioprospecting typically involves the following four phases:

i. ***Phase I:*** Collection of samples on-site
ii. ***Phase II:*** Culturing organisms, isolating, and characterizing specific compounds
iii. ***Phase III:*** Screening compounds for specific applications
iv. ***Phase IV:*** Product development and commercialization, which includes patenting, conducting trials, and engaging in sales and marketing

When well-managed, bioprospecting offers significant advantages to developing countries. It not only facilitates the creation of new products but also generates income and encourages biodiversity conservation. However, improper management can lead to environmental issues, such as over-exploitation and habitat destruction, as well as socioeconomic problems arising from the unfair distribution of benefits.

Herbal medicine is widely practiced around the world. For centuries, people have relied on natural remedies to treat common ailments like colds, allergies, upset stomachs, and toothaches, and this trend is continually growing. This shift from synthetic to herbal medicines is often referred to as a "Return to Nature" for disease prevention and treatment. Nature has always been a rich source of medicinal plants. According to the World Health Organization (WHO), 4 billion people, or 80% of the global population, use herbal medicines for some aspect of primary healthcare [8]. The WHO recognizes herbal medicine as essential for primary healthcare, with approximately 11% of the 252 essential drugs being medicinal plant-derived [9].

PHYTOCHEMICALS AND BIOLOGICAL ACTIVITY OF SOME PROMISING MEDICINAL PLANTS

Medicinal plants have been used for centuries as a source of therapeutic agents. Modern research continues to uncover the vast array of phytochemicals in these plants, which contribute to their diverse biological activities. Below is an overview of the phytochemicals and biological activities of some promising medicinal plants (Fig. **1**). Moreover, the biological sources, their phytochemicals and pharmacological activities of medicinal plants are given in Table **1**.

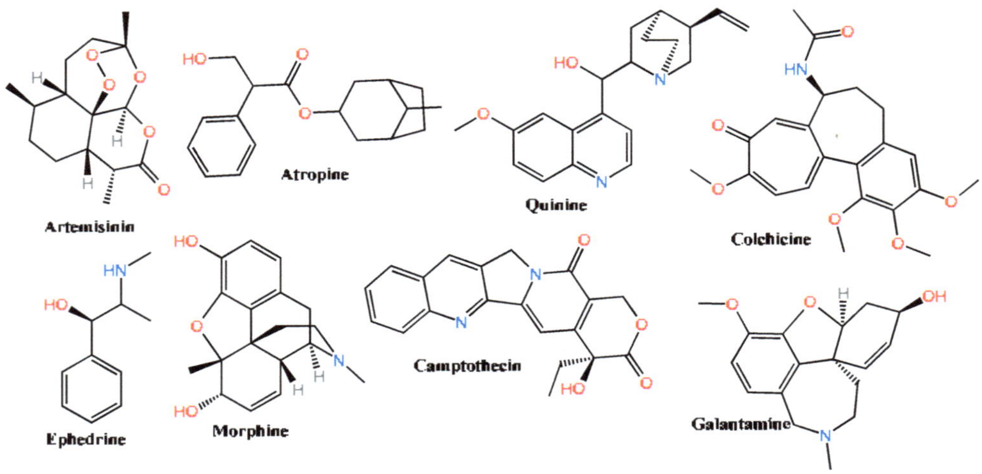

Fig. (1). 2D structure of some promising modern medicines from medicinal plants.

Table 1. Various promising modern phytoconstitutents from the medicinal plants.

SN	Plant biological name	Phytochemicals	Biological activity	Reference
1.	*Artemisia annua*	Artemisinin, Deoxy artemisinin	Antimalarial	[10]
2.	*Atropa belladona*	Atropine, Hyoscyamine, Hyoscine, Homotropine	Parasympatholytic drug, anticholinergic, antidote in opium and chloral hydrate poisoning	[11]
3.	*Catharanthus roseus*	Vincristine, Vinblastine	Anti-cancer, Hodgkin's diseases, leukaemia	[12]

(Table 1) cont.....

SN	Plant biological name	Phytochemicals	Biological activity	Reference
4.	*Cinchona officinalis*	Quinine, Quinidine, Cinchonine, Cupreine, Hydroquinine	Anti-malarial, antipyretics, bitter stomachics	[13]
5.	*Claviceps purpurea*	Ergotamine, Ergocristine, Ergocryptine, Ergosine, Ergocornine, Methysergide	Migraine, oxytocic	[14]
6.	*Colchicum autumnale*	Colchicine, Demecolcine	Used in the treatment of Gout	[15]
7.	*Digitalis purpurea*	Purpurea glycoside A, B, Digitoxin, Digoxin, Lanatosides A, B, and C	Cardiotonic	[16]
8.	*Dioscoreadeltoidea*	Diosgenin, Smilagenin, Epismilagenin, Yamogenin	Rheumatic arthritis, Precursor for synthesis of corticosteroid, sex hormones and oral contraceptives	[17]
9.	*Ephedragerardiana*	Ephedrine, Pseudoephedrine	Sympathomimetic, Antiasthamic	[18]
10.	*Erythroxylumcoca*	Cocaine, Cinnamyl Cocaine, Tropocaine	Local anaesthetic, Stimulant	[19]
11.	*Papaversomniferum*	Morphine, Narcotine, Papaverine	Narcotic analgesic, Antidiarrheal	[20]

DRUGGABILITY OF MEDICINAL PLANT-BASED PHYTOCONSTITUENTS

Challenges in new drug development are primarily found in two main areas: the existing paradigm for drug discovery in large pharmaceutical companies and technical limitations in identifying new compounds with desirable activity. According to Koehn and Carter, compounds isolated from natural products have the following distinctive features [21]:

- A greater number of chiral centers
- Increased steric complexity
- A higher number of oxygen atoms
- A lower ratio of aromatic ring atoms to total heavy atoms
- More solvated hydrogen bond donors and acceptors
- Greater molecular rigidity
- A broader distribution of molecular properties, including molecular mass, octanol-water partition coefficient, and diversity of ring systems

The unique features of natural-origin chemical entities present a series of challenges for medicinal chemists, particularly when developing analogs to improve absorption, reduce toxicity, and enhance efficacy. This often involves the addition or removal of specific functional groups. In China from 1911 to 2000, various bioactive plant compounds were isolated, including alkaloids, steroids, triterpenes, limonoids, diterpenes, sesquiterpenes, monoterpenes, tannins, isoflavonoids, flavonoids, polycyclic aromatics, lignans, coumarins, simple phenolics, and aliphatic compounds. Alkaloids comprised about 20%, flavonoids 15%, triterpenes and simple phenolics around 10%, with other compounds, including limonoids, being less prevalent [22].

Despite the biological activity and favorable ADMET (Absorption, Distribution, metabolism, Excretion, and Toxicity) profiles of many natural products, they often do not meet the "drug-likeness" criteria. The challenge lies in creating a physicochemically-tuned natural products library to facilitate lead generation and fully realize the potential of natural products. Lipinski [23] introduced the "rule of five," a set of calculated properties that many drug candidates reaching Phase II clinical trials adhere to. This rule consists of four criteria, many with cutoff values of five or multiples thereof, which gave rise to its name.

To be considered drug-like, a candidate should meet the following criteria:

- Fewer than five hydrogen bond donors
- Fewer than 10 hydrogen bond acceptors
- A molecular weight of less than 500 Da
- A partition coefficient (log P) of less than 5

The purpose of the "rule of five" is to identify potential bioavailability issues if two or more of these criteria are not met. If Lipinski's rule had been applied, paclitaxel would not have become a drug because it does not comply with the "rule of five." Therefore, a major challenge is to establish alternative druggability criteria for compounds of natural origin.

MEDICINAL PLANT SELECTION APPROACH FOR DRUG DISCOVERY

According to available estimates, there are approximately 250,000 species of higher plants, including angiosperms and gymnosperms. Of these, only about 6% have been screened for biological activity, and around 15% have been screened for phytochemical activity. The initial selection of candidate species for biological activity screening is a significant and essential task. Fabricant and Farnsworth have identified the following approaches currently used by researchers for this purpose [5].

Random Approach

The random approach to selecting medicinal plants for drug discovery involves systematically screening a wide variety of plants without prior knowledge of their traditional uses or chemical compositions. The random approach focuses on the inherent chemical diversity present in the plant kingdom to identify potential therapeutic compounds [24]. Two approaches have been used for screening plants selected randomly for new drug discovery:

i. Screening for specific classes of compounds (*e.g.*, alkaloids, flavonoids): This method is straightforward but does not provide information on biological efficacy. It may still lead to the discovery of novel structures.
ii. Screening randomly selected plants for specific bioassays:

The Central Drug Research Institute and Council of Scientific and Industrial Research in India (CDRICS) and Industrial Research Institute (IRI) employed this approach about three decades ago, screening around 2,000 plants for biological efficacy. However, it did not result in any new drugs. The National Cancer Institute (NCI) of the National Institutes of Health in the USA screened approximately 35,000 plant species for anti-cancer activity from 1960 to 1980, which led to the discovery of paclitaxel and camptothecin. This method has been used for both focused and general screening, showing some success in focused screening. Using target-based bioassays could increase the chances of success. This approach requires an extensive library of extracts, which only a few organizations worldwide possess. Despite its challenges, the random approach remains an important strategy in drug discovery, particularly when used in conjunction with modern analytical and computational techniques. It complements other methods, such as ethnopharmacology and zoo pharmacognosy, by broadening the scope of exploration and enabling the discovery of novel compounds with unique modes of action [24].

Ethnopharmacology Approach

Ethnopharmacology is the scientific study of the medicinal practices of indigenous cultures, particularly the use of plants for therapeutic purposes. This approach bridges traditional knowledge with modern scientific methods, playing a crucial role in the discovery and development of plant-based drugs. By focusing on plants that have been used for centuries by various cultures to treat specific ailments, ethnopharmacology offers a targeted and efficient pathway to identify potential drug candidates [25]. The ethnopharmacology approach relies on empirical experiences related to the use of botanical drugs for discovering biologically active new chemical entities. This process involves:

- Observation, description, and experimental investigation of indigenous drugs.
- Incorporation of various disciplines such as botany, chemistry, biochemistry, pharmacology, anthropology, archaeology, history, and linguistics.

Ethnopharmacology provides a vast amount of information about plants that have been used traditionally for medicinal purposes. This historical and cultural knowledge acts as a valuable starting point for identifying plant species with potential therapeutic effects. Many modern drugs, such as aspirin (derived from willow bark) and quinine (from cinchona bark), have their origins in traditional medicine [26, 27]. Some other examples of successful ethnomedicinal usage include *Andrographis paniculata* (andrographolide used for dysentery), *Papaver somniferum* (source of morphine), *Berberis aristata* (berberine), and *Picrorhiza kurroa* (picroside). Additionally, plants not selected based on ethnomedical use have also led to discoveries, such as *Mucuna pruriens* (source of L-Dopa) and *Taxus brevifolia* (paclitaxel), among others [28].

Traditional System of Medicine Approach

Countries like India, China and Nepal possess a rich heritage of traditional medicine systems that are well-documented. These systems predominantly use botanical sources for medicines but differ from ethnomedicine in several ways. Traditional systems are based on strong conceptual foundations of human physiology and pharmacology, despite using different investigative tools compared to modern methods. Pharmaceutical processes in these systems are more advanced, emphasizing standardization over the crude extraction methods like juices and decoctions used in ethnomedicine. Traditional systems of medicine are extensively documented and institutionalized, whereas ethnomedicinal practices tend to be localized and often controlled by a few families within each community [29].

Ethnomedicinal practices may have a longer historical lineage compared to codified systems of medicine. The discovery of artemisinin from *Artemisia annua* for treating malaria, guggulsterones from *Commiphora mukul* for hyperlipidemia, boswellic acids from *Boswellia serrata* for anti-inflammatory purposes, and bacosides from *Bacopa monnieri* for nootropic and memory-enhancing effects all drew inspiration from these established systems of medicine in China, India, and Nepal. However, this approach to selecting candidates for drug discovery programs has not been widely adopted thus far. Nevertheless, it shows significant promise in terms of success rates. A notable example of this approach is the discovery of reserpine from *Rauwolfia serpentina*, which originated from Unani medicine practices.

Zoo-pharmacognosy Approach

Zoo-pharmacognosy is the study of how animals self-medicate using plants, minerals, and other natural substances in their environment to treat and prevent diseases [30]. This field offers unique insights into the natural selection of medicinal compounds, which animals instinctively utilize to combat various ailments. Understanding these behaviors can significantly impact plant-based drug discovery by identifying new bioactive compounds and therapeutic strategies that have evolved in nature over millions of years. The practice of observing animal behavior to identify potential candidate plants for new drug discovery is not uncommon. For instance, in certain regions of South America, the observation of cattle with straight tails while grazing led to the discovery of a plant called *Cestrum diurnum*, along with three other plants from the Solanaceae family. These plants are likely the only known sources of derivatives of Vitamin D3 from plant origins. This approach requires meticulous observation and monitoring of animal behavior [31]. Moreover, Zoo-pharmacognosy provides direct clues about the medicinal properties of plants that animals use for self-medication. By observing these behaviors, researchers can identify plants and their specific parts that may contain novel bioactive compounds. For instance, certain primates consume specific plants to combat parasitic infections, leading researchers to investigate those plants for potential antiparasitic drugs [32].

Most importantly, animals often use a combination of plants to address specific health issues, suggesting potential synergies between different compounds. Studying these behaviors can provide insights into how different plant compounds interact to produce therapeutic effects, guiding researchers in designing combination therapies or identifying new mechanisms of action. By learning from the self-medicating behaviors of animals, we can identify new bioactive compounds, validate traditional medicinal practices, and develop innovative therapeutic strategies. This approach not only accelerates the drug discovery process but also underscores the importance of conserving biodiversity as a reservoir of natural medicines. As the field of zoo-pharmacognosy continues to grow, its integration into plant-based drug discovery holds the potential to unlock new, effective treatments derived from the wisdom of the natural world [33].

MEDICINAL PLANT-BASED DRUG DISCOVERY AND DEVELOPMENT PROCESS

Traditional Methods of Drug Discovery from Medicinal Plants

In the traditional, more academic approach to drug discovery from natural products, drug targets are exposed to crude extracts. Upon identifying the hit evidence of biological activity, the extract is fractionated, and the active compound is isolated and identified. This process, known as bioassay-guided isolation, relies on bioassays to direct each step of fractionation and isolation. The following scheme outlines the bioassay-guided traditional natural product drug discovery process. Occasionally, a direct natural product isolation approach is employed without considering bioactivity. This method yields various natural compounds, creating a small compound library for subsequent bioactivity screening (Fig. **2**). However, this approach is often slow, inefficient, and labor-intensive, with no assurance that a screened lead will be chemically viable or patentable [25, 34].

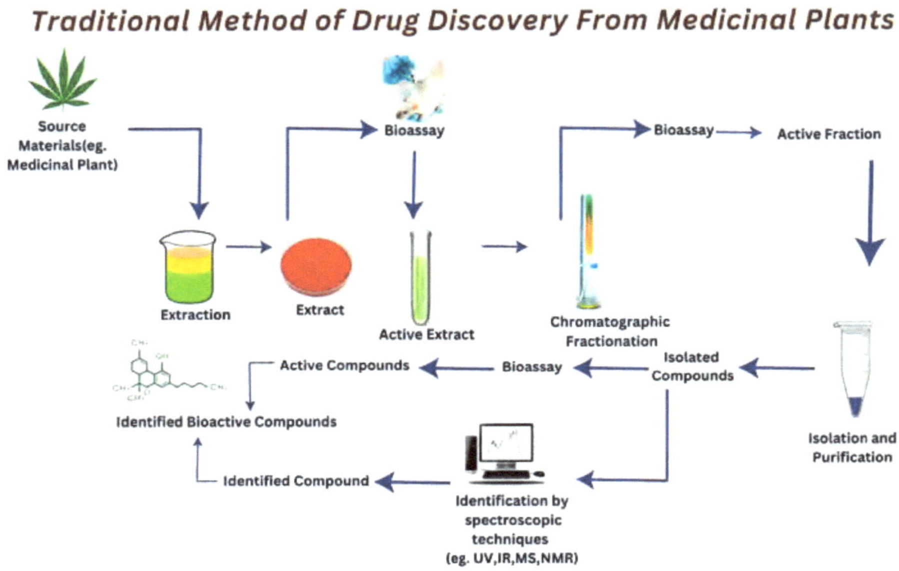

Fig. (2). Traditional method of drug discovery from medicinal plants.

Traditional methods of drug discovery from medicinal plants involve leveraging the extensive knowledge accumulated over generations regarding the therapeutic uses of plants. These methods are deeply rooted in cultural practices, folklore, and historical documentation, often guiding researchers toward plants with known medicinal properties [35]. Traditional methods play a crucial role in drug discovery by:

- Guiding Plant Selection: Traditional knowledge helps identify specific plants or plant parts used in folk medicine to treat various ailments, reducing the need for random screening and increasing the efficiency of the drug discovery process [36].

- Providing Ethnobotanical Evidence: Ethnobotanical studies document the medicinal uses of plants in different cultures, offering valuable insights into potential pharmacological activities. This evidence forms the basis for selecting plants for further scientific investigation [37].
- Facilitating the Identification of Bioactive Compounds: Plants used traditionally for specific health conditions are more likely to contain bioactive compounds relevant to those conditions. This traditional use can guide researchers in identifying and isolating these compounds [38].

Modern Methods of Drug Discovery from Medicinal Plants

Modern drug discovery approaches utilize High-Throughput Screening (HTS), where full automation and robotics enable the rapid screening of hundreds of molecules using various assays with minimal compound amounts (Table **2**). To integrate medicinal plants into modern HTS programs, a natural product library composed of dereplicated natural products must be created. Dereplication involves eliminating the recurrence or re-isolation of the same or similar compounds from different extracts. Several hyphenated techniques, such as LC-PDA (Liquid Chromatography-Photo-Diode-Array detector), LC-MS (Liquid Chromatography-Mass Spectrometry), and LC-NMR (Liquid Chromatography-Nuclear Magnetic Resonance Spectroscopy), are employed for dereplication (Fig. **3**).

Table 2. Example of drugs discovered through modern methods.

Name of compound	Origin	Method of discovery
Paclitaxel	From Pacific Yew Tree, *Taxus brevifolia.*	Paclitaxel, initially discovered through traditional methods, was further developed using modern techniques, including bioassay-guided fractionation and advanced chemical synthesis. High-throughput screening played a role in identifying its anti-cancer properties [47].
Camptothecin Derivatives	From *Camptotheca acuminata.*	Camptothecin was initially isolated through traditional methods, but its development into effective drugs like topotecan and irinotecan involved modern techniques such as semi-synthetic modification and molecular modeling [48].
Galantamine	From *Galanthus spp.*	The development of galantamine as a treatment for Alzheimer's disease involved high-throughput screening and bioassay-guided fractionation. These modern methods were essential in confirming its effectiveness as an acetylcholinesterase inhibitor [49].
Etoposide	From *Podophyllum peltatum.*	Etoposide was developed from the compound podophyllotoxin using bioassay-guided fractionation and chemical modification techniques. Modern synthetic chemistry played a crucial role in enhancing its therapeutic properties [50].

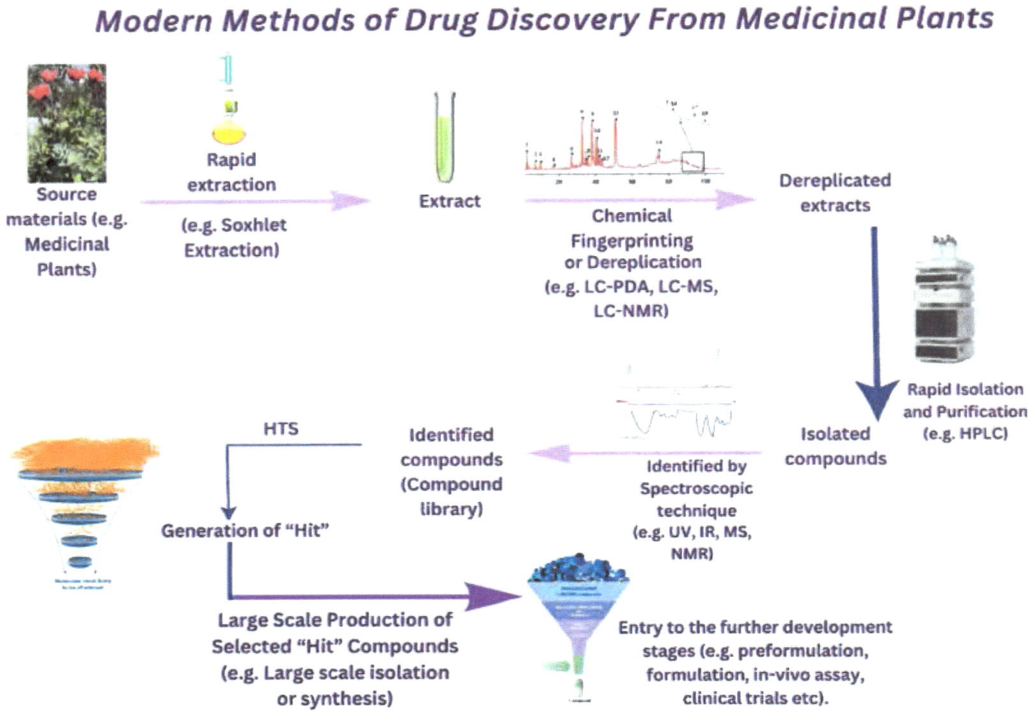

Fig. (3). Modern methods of drug discovery from medicinal plants.

Building such a library from purified natural products was once extremely difficult, time-consuming, and labor-intensive. However, advancements in separation, isolation, and identification technologies have significantly improved the process. It is now feasible to create high-quality, chemically diverse natural product libraries. These libraries can consist of crude extracts, chromatographic fractions, or semi-purified compounds; however, the most effective results are obtained from a fully identified, pure natural product library. This allows scientists to rapidly handle the lead compound for further development, including total or partial synthesis, addressing formulation factors, conducting *in vivo* assays, and progressing to clinical trials. To continue leveraging natural sources for drug candidates, the focus must shift to newer approaches in natural product drug discovery. These approaches include applying genomic tools, exploring novel sources of organisms from the environment, implementing new screening technologies, and improving sample preparation processes for screening. Additionally, the recent emphasis on synthesizing diversity-oriented combinatorial libraries based on natural product-like compounds aims to enhance the productivity of synthetic chemical libraries [25, 34].

The modern method of drug discovery fastens the process by:

1. High-Throughput Screening (HTS): HTS allows for the rapid testing of thousands of plant extracts or compounds to identify those with potential biological activity. This method significantly accelerates the drug discovery process by quickly narrowing down the candidates for further study [39].
2. Bioassay-Guided Fractionation: This method involves systematically separating plant extracts into smaller fractions and testing each for biological activity. It helps in identifying and isolating the active compounds responsible for the therapeutic effects [40].
3. Metabolomics and Chemoinformatics: These techniques involve the comprehensive analysis of metabolites within a plant to understand its chemical profile. Chemoinformatics, coupled with computational modeling, can predict the biological activity of compounds, aiding in the identification of new drug leads [41, 42].
4. Genomics and Proteomics: Genomic and proteomic analyses provide insights into the genes and proteins involved in the biosynthesis of medicinal compounds in plants. This information can be used to enhance the production of bioactive compounds through genetic engineering or synthetic biology [43].
5. Nanotechnology: Nanotechnology is used to enhance the delivery and efficacy of plant-derived compounds. For example, nanoparticles can be employed to improve the solubility, stability, and bioavailability of plant-based drugs [44].
6. Molecular Docking and Virtual Screening: These computational techniques simulate the interaction between plant-derived compounds and target proteins. They help in predicting the binding affinity and efficacy of compounds, thus guiding the selection of promising drug candidates [45, 46].

MEDICINAL PLANT-BASED DATABASE USED IN DRUG DISCOVERY

Plant-based databases are crucial for lead identification in the drug discovery process. It is important to note that more beneficial information could be available in medicinal herbs databases from different sources. These databases provide information on natural products, biological sources, 2D and 3D structural representation, molecular descriptors, drug likeness properties, and many more. These databases store the information and are arranged systematically so that we can extract it in a faster way. The following are some important databases used to search natural product-based leads (Table **3**).

DRUG DISCOVERY FROM MEDICINAL PLANTS: ADVANTAGES AND DISADVANTAGES

Using medicinal plant sources as a starting point in drug development offers specific advantages:

- The selection of candidate species often relies on their long-term use in human ethnomedicine. This approach assumes that active compounds isolated from such plants are likely safer compared to those from plants without a human use history. Past drug developments from plants like *Rauwolfia serpentina* and *Digitalis purpurea* exemplify this strategy [51].
- Sometimes, this approach leads to the development of novel molecules derived from natural sources, addressing the inherent limitations of the original molecule. For instance, podophyllin from *Podophyllum hexandrum* faced dose-limiting toxicities, which were largely overcome by semi-synthesis into etoposide, a key cancer therapy drug today. Likewise, Camptothecin initially from *Camptotheca sp.* and later from *Mappia sp.*, similarly led to novel anti-cancer drugs like topotecan and irinotecan.
- Starting with natural resources holds the dual promise of either delivering the original isolate as a candidate or advancing to semi-synthetic molecule development to overcome inherent limitations.

Table 3. Natural products-based free access database for lead identification in drug discovery process.

SN	Name of databases	Year	Characteristics of database	URL
1.	COCONUT	2022	The COlleCtion of Open Natural ProdUcTs (COCONUT) is a vast database designed for the archiving, exploration, and evaluation of natural products. The database contains 407,270 distinct natural products. Starting with the best annotated, they are arranged according to their level of annotation.	https://coconut.naturalproducts.net/
2.	IMPPAT 2.0	2022	The 2D and 3D chemical structures, physicochemical characteristics, drug-likeness, chemical similarity, and ADMET attributes are all included in the manually curated database Indian Medicinal Plants, Phytochemistry and Therapeutics 2.0 (IMPPAT 2.0). About 4010 Indian medicinal plants, 17967 phytochemicals, and 1095 therapeutic applications are captured in the database.	https://cb.imsc.res.in/imppat/

(Table 3) cont.....

SN	Name of databases	Year	Characteristics of database	URL
3.	Phytochemdb	2022	This platform facilitates computer-aided drug design using natural products and virtual screening. With the goal of incorporating the activities of phytochemicals from medicinal plants, Phytochemdb is a manually maintained database that gathers 525 plants and the 8093 phytochemicals that connect with them.	https://phytochemdb.com/
4.	TCMPG	2021	Traditional Chinese Medicine Plant Genome (TCMPG) offers scholars a range of computer tools to enable systematic analysis in addition to depositing the genome data of traditional Chinese medicinal plants. TCMPG now has information on 160 plant species, 195 associated genomes, and 255 herbs (various portions of the same plant), as well as relevant data on plant species, genomes, and herbal medications.	http://cbcb.cdutcm.edu.cn/TCMPG/
5.	SuperTCM	2020	SuperTCM is a biocultural database that integrates historical language information with biological routes for medication creation. Information on 6516 TCM medications (often referred to as "herbs") with 5372 botanical species, 55,772 active components, and 543 targets in 254 KEGG pathways linked to 8634 disorders is provided.	https://bioinf-applied.charite.de/supertcm/
6.	PMhub	2024	A comprehensive library of plant metabolites that is openly accessible and includes specific information about small-molecule metabolites found in nature is the Plant Metabolite Hub (PMhub). Data on reactions, mass spectra, and chemicals are all intended to be included in the database.	https://pmhub.org.cn/#/

(Table 3) cont.....

SN	Name of databases	Year	Characteristics of database	URL
7.	PMDB	2021	With 6156 spectra of 1026 plant metabolites and 72308 electrospray ionisation (ESI)-MSn spectra from public mass spectrometry libraries (such as Mass Bank, LipidBlast, and HMDB), the Plant Metabolites DataBase (PMDB) is a publicly accessible database. One of PMDB's most notable advantages is its ability to quickly and easily do data analysis tasks such as removing duplicate features, finding isotope, adduct, and neutral loss ions, executing statistical analyses like principal component analysis, and screening important features. Additionally, users can easily download all collected information, and the analyzed results can be used directly for metabolite identification on the web.	http://www.pmdb.org.cn/home

However, drug development from natural resources also presents certain disadvantages:

- Often, the process of drug discovery and commercialization puts substantial pressure on natural resources, raising environmental concerns. While synthesis is an option for some molecules, such as etoposide, paclitaxel, and others, still heavily rely on vulnerable plant resources due to challenges in complete synthesis. It's estimated that around 25,000 plant species could disappear by the end of the century [52].
- Intellectual property rights related to natural products are increasingly complex. Leads often stem from traditional usage, and with more countries adhering to the Convention on Biological Diversity, accessing and benefit-sharing from basic resources during commercial phases has become intricate. These processes can significantly hinder the pace of discovery across various phases, regardless of the concerns prompting their implementation.

Role of Metabolomic in Plant-Based Drug Discovery

Metabolomics, the comprehensive study of metabolites within a biological system, plays a pivotal role in advancing plant-based drug design. As plants are rich sources of bioactive compounds, they have historically served as the foundation for many therapeutic agents. However, the complexity of plant metabolomes, with their vast array of primary and secondary metabolites, presents challenges and opportunities in the identification and development of new drugs. Metabolomics, by enabling the profiling, quantification, and understanding of these metabolites, offers a powerful approach to unraveling this complexity and accelerating the drug discovery process [53, 54]. The integration of metabolomics in plant-based drug design involves several key steps:

1. Metabolite Profiling: By employing techniques such as Mass Spectrometry (MS) and Nuclear Magnetic Resonance (NMR) spectroscopy, metabolomics facilitates the comprehensive profiling of plant metabolites. This allows researchers to identify bioactive compounds that may have therapeutic potential.
2. Identification of Bioactive Compounds: Metabolomics enables the identification of specific metabolites responsible for observed biological activities. Through bioassay-guided fractionation, researchers can pinpoint compounds that exhibit desirable pharmacological properties, such as anti-inflammatory, hepatoprotective, anti-cancer, or antimicrobial activities [55 - 57].
3. Pathway Elucidation: Understanding the biosynthetic pathways of bioactive compounds is crucial for optimizing their production and yield. Metabolomics provides insights into these pathways, enabling the manipulation of metabolic networks to enhance the yield of target compounds or to engineer plants to produce novel derivatives with improved therapeutic properties.
4. Biomarker Discovery: In the context of drug development, metabolomics aids in the identification of biomarkers that can predict the efficacy and safety of plant-derived drugs. These biomarkers can be used in both preclinical and clinical studies to monitor therapeutic response and potential side effects [58].
5. Quality Control and Standardization: The consistency and efficacy of plant-based drugs depend on the quality of the raw material. Metabolomics supports the standardization of plant extracts by ensuring the presence and concentration of active metabolites, thus maintaining the therapeutic potency of the final product [59].

CHALLENGES IN DRUG DISCOVERY FROM MEDICINAL PLANTS

Despite the notable successes in drug discovery from medicinal plants, future efforts are fraught with numerous challenges. Natural product chemist, phyto chemists, and other pharmacognosy scientists must enhance both the quality and quantity of compounds entering drug development to compete with other discovery methods [60]. The drug discovery process is lengthy, averaging over 10 years and costing upwards of 800 million dollars [61]. Much time and resources are expended on the vast number of leads discarded during this process, with only approximately one in 5000 lead compounds progressing successfully through clinical trials for approval. Lead identification is the initial step, followed by optimization (involving medicinal and combinatorial chemistry), development, including pharmacology, toxicology, pharmacokinetics, ADME, and drug delivery, as well as clinical trials, all of which are time-consuming [62].

Traditionally, drug discovery from medicinal plants has been more complex and prolonged compared to other methods, prompting many pharmaceutical companies to reduce or eliminate natural product research [21]. Moreover, academic pharmacy departments, focusing increasingly on clinical and community pharmacy, are scaling back their emphasis on pharmaceutical research and development related to medicinal plants and natural products. This shift has led to a decline in teaching and research positions in pharmacognosy and natural product chemistry, posing another challenge in drug discovery from medicinal plants [62].

Pharmacognosists and natural product scientists may seek employment in alternative academic departments such as biology, chemistry, ecology, and nutrition to sustain research on medicinal plants. To address the historically slow pace of drug discovery from medicinal plants, improved methodologies are essential for plant collection, bioassay screening, compound isolation, and development [21]. Innovative strategies are needed for efficient plant collection, especially given the legal and political complexities surrounding benefit-sharing agreements [63].

Developing suitable, clinically relevant, high-throughput bioassays is a formidable challenge across all drug discovery programs. While designing these assays is challenging, once established, they enable testing of compounds and extract libraries for biological activity. Screening these libraries poses challenges, but techniques such as pre-fractionation of extracts can mitigate some of these issues. Challenges in bioassay screening remain critical in the future of drug discovery from medicinal plants [21, 64].

Accelerating the isolation of active compounds requires the adoption of new technologies. Although Nuclear Magnetic Resonance (NMR) and Mass Spectrometry (MS) are standard for compound identification, novel applications of these technologies could expedite compound isolation in medicinal plant drug discovery. High-throughput X-ray crystallography offers another potential avenue for lead discovery from medicinal plants [65, 66].

Developing drugs from natural products have unique consequences. Natural products are typically isolated in limited quantities, unsuitable for subsequent optimization, development, and clinical trials. Collaboration with synthetic and medicinal chemists is crucial to explore options for synthesis or semi-synthesis. Creating libraries of natural products and natural-product-like compounds, blending natural product features with combinatorial chemistry, may offer a pathway to enhance compound development [67].

FUTURE PERSPECTIVE AND CONCLUSION

There is a pressing need to reignite scientific interest in natural products for inclusion in drug discovery programs. A significant concern has been the unpredictability of success rates at various stages of drug development when dealing with natural products. This unpredictability is particularly pronounced when candidate species are selected randomly, given the intricate nature of botanical sources for New Chemical Entities (NCE). To improve predictability, it is essential to select and shortlist candidate species strategically. Drawing on documented clinical experience with botanical medicines codified in traditional systems of medicine could streamline issues linked to unpredictable outcomes. Discovering new functional leads from traditional knowledge and experiential databases holds promise for reducing the time, costs, and toxicities associated with drug development processes [68].

An integrated approach that combines diverse discovery tools and incorporates the emerging field of integrative biology will be crucial for the success of natural product drug discovery and development. Since plant selection is a critical initial step, it requires a well-conceived strategy.

Plants have historically served and are likely to continue serving as vital sources of new therapeutic agents, including semi-synthetic derivatives designed to enhance the pharmacokinetic profiles of developed compounds. While the pathway from drug development to market approval is complex, expensive, and daunting, it provides essential assurances of safety and efficacy necessary for these agents to enter widespread clinical use.

Recent research by B. Pandey's team exemplifying the effectiveness of nine promising hepatoprotective agents derived from medicinal plants in alleviating various forms of liver injury highlights the potential of plant-derived medicines to become mainstream in medical practice [69]. Such successes underscore the substantial potential for further advancements in drug development from plants. However, significant challenges, including time constraints and financial pressures in the current drug development landscape, necessitate innovation and reform to ensure a consistent flow of new therapeutic products.

LIST OF ABBREVIATIONS

ADMET	Absorption, Distribution, Metabolism, Excretion, and Toxicity
AIDS	Acquired Immunodeficiency Syndrome
BCE	Before the Common Era
COCONUT	The Collection of Open Natural Products
HPLC	High Performance Liquid Chromatography
HTS	High Throughput Screening
IMPPAT	Indian Medicinal Plant, Phytochemistry and Therapeutics
IR	Infrared
LC-MS	Liquid Chromatography-Mass Spectrometry
LC-NMR	Liquid Chromatography-Nuclear Magnetic Resonance
LC-PDA	Liquid Chromatography-Photodiode Array Detector
MS	Mass Spectrometry
NCI	National Cancer Institute
NMR	Nuclear magnetic resonance
PMDD	Plant Metabolite Database
PMhub	Plant Metabolite Hub
TCMPG	Traditional Chinese Medicinal Plant Genome
UV	Ultraviolet
WHO	World Health Organization

CONSENT FOR PUBLICATION

All authors agreed for publication.

CONFLICT OF INTEREST

No conflict of interest.

ACKNOWLEDGEMENT

We thank the Madan Bhandari Academy of Health Sciences, Hetauda, Nepal.

REFERENCES

[1] Sarker SD, Nahar L. An introduction to natural products isolation. Springer 2012. [http://dx.doi.org/10.1007/978-1-61779-624-1_1]

[2] Hardy K, Buckley S, Collins MJ, *et al.* Neanderthal medics? Evidence for food, cooking, and medicinal plants entrapped in dental calculus. Naturwissenschaften 2012; 99(8): 617-26. [http://dx.doi.org/10.1007/s00114-012-0942-0] [PMID: 22806252]

[3] Hardy K. The use of plants by Neanderthals as food, medicine, and raw materials Updating Neanderthals. Elsevier 2022; pp. 145-61.

[http://dx.doi.org/10.1016/B978-0-12-821428-2.00004-4]

[4] Yaniv Z. Introduction: Medicinal plants in ancient traditions. Medicinal and Aromatic Plants of the Middle-East 2014; pp. 1-7.
[http://dx.doi.org/10.1007/978-94-017-9276-9_1]

[5] Fabricant DS, Farnsworth NR. The value of plants used in traditional medicine for drug discovery. Environ Health Perspect 2001; 109(Suppl 1) (Suppl. 1): 69-75.
[http://dx.doi.org/10.1289/ehp.01109s169] [PMID: 11250806]

[6] Berdigaliyev N, Aljofan M. An overview of drug discovery and development. Future Med Chem 2020; 12(10): 939-47.
[http://dx.doi.org/10.4155/fmc-2019-0307] [PMID: 32270704]

[7] Upadhyay SK, Singh SP. Bioprospecting of plant biodiversity for industrial molecules. Wiley Online Library 2021.
[http://dx.doi.org/10.1002/9781119718017]

[8] Organization WH. WHO global report on traditional and complementary medicine 2019. World Health Organization 2019.

[9] Qadir SU, Raja V. Herbal medicine: Old practice and modern perspectives Phytomedicine. Elsevier 2021; pp. 149-80.
[http://dx.doi.org/10.1016/B978-0-12-824109-7.00001-7]

[10] Zhang D, Sun W, Shi Y, Wu L, Zhang T, Xiang L. Red and blue light promote the accumulation of artemisinin in *Artemisia annua L.* Molecules 2018; 23(6): 1329.
[http://dx.doi.org/10.3390/molecules23061329] [PMID: 29857558]

[11] Li F, Ye X, Li M, *et al.* Enhanced ophthalmic bioavailability and stability of atropine sulfate *via* sustained release particles using polystyrene sulfonate resin. Int J Pharm 2024; 660: 124294.
[http://dx.doi.org/10.1016/j.ijpharm.2024.124294] [PMID: 38823467]

[12] Potbhare AK, Yerpude S, Daddemal-Chaudhary AR, *et al.* Catharanthus roseus-mediated $CuAl_2O_4$ nanocomposites for evaluation of killing kinetics. Chemosphere 2024; 359: 142369.
[http://dx.doi.org/10.1016/j.chemosphere.2024.142369] [PMID: 38761825]

[13] Hariyanti H, Mauludin R, Sumirtapura YC, Kurniati NF. A review: Pharmacological activities of quinoline alkaloid of Cinchona sp. Biointerface Res Appl Chem 2022; 13(4): 3.
[http://dx.doi.org/10.33263/BRIAC134.319]

[14] Smakosz A, Kurzyna W, Rudko M, Dąsal M. The usage of ergot (*Claviceps purpurea* (fr.) Tul.) in obstetrics and gynecology: A historical perspective. Toxins (Basel) 2021; 13(7): 492.
[http://dx.doi.org/10.3390/toxins13070492] [PMID: 34357964]

[15] Thakur S, Chaudhary G, Kaurav H. Colchicum autumnale (suranjan): A cytotoxic plant with anti-arthritis properties. Advance Pharmaceutical Journal 2021; 6(3): 80-6.
[http://dx.doi.org/10.31024/apj.2021.6.3.4]

[16] Whayne TF Jr. Clinical use of digitalis: a state of the art review. Am J Cardiovasc Drugs 2018; 18(6): 427-40.
[http://dx.doi.org/10.1007/s40256-018-0292-1] [PMID: 30066080]

[17] Semwal P, Painuli S, Cruz-Martins N. Dioscorea deltoidea wall. Ex Griseb: A review of traditional uses, bioactive compounds and biological activities. Food Biosci 2021; 41: 100969.
[http://dx.doi.org/10.1016/j.fbio.2021.100969]

[18] Minami M, Mori T, Honda Y, *et al.* Relationship between ephedrine alkaloid profile in Ephedra gerardiana and soil characteristics of glacial landforms in southeastern Tibetan Plateau, China. J Nat Med 2022; 76(3): 703-14.
[http://dx.doi.org/10.1007/s11418-022-01628-z] [PMID: 35461469]

[19] Docimo T, Reichelt M, Schneider B, *et al.* The first step in the biosynthesis of cocaine in

Erythroxylum coca: the characterization of arginine and ornithine decarboxylases. Plant Mol Biol 2012; 78(6): 599-615.
[http://dx.doi.org/10.1007/s11103-012-9886-1] [PMID: 22311164]

[20] Labanca F, Ovesnà J, Milella L. *Papaver somniferum L.* taxonomy, uses and new insight in poppy alkaloid pathways. Phytochem Rev 2018; 17(4): 853-71.
[http://dx.doi.org/10.1007/s11101-018-9563-3]

[21] Koehn FE, Carter GT. The evolving role of natural products in drug discovery. Nat Rev Drug Discov 2005; 4(3): 206-20.
[http://dx.doi.org/10.1038/nrd1657] [PMID: 15729362]

[22] Ehrman TM, Barlow DJ, Hylands PJ. Phytochemical databases of Chinese herbal constituents and bioactive plant compounds with known target specificities. J Chem Inf Model 2007; 47(2): 254-63.
[http://dx.doi.org/10.1021/ci600288m] [PMID: 17381164]

[23] Lipinski CA, Lombardo F, Dominy BW, Feeney PJ. Experimental and computational approaches to estimate solubility and permeability in drug discovery and development settings 1PII of original article: S0169-409X(96)00423-1. The article was originally published in Advanced Drug Delivery Reviews 23 (1997) 3–25. 1. Adv Drug Deliv Rev 2001; 46(1-3): 3-26.
[http://dx.doi.org/10.1016/S0169-409X(00)00129-0] [PMID: 11259830]

[24] Katiyar C, Kanjilal S, Gupta A, Katiyar S. Drug discovery from plant sources: An integrated approach. Ayu 2012; 33(1): 10-9.
[http://dx.doi.org/10.4103/0974-8520.100295] [PMID: 23049178]

[25] Süntar I. Importance of ethnopharmacological studies in drug discovery: role of medicinal plants. Phytochem Rev 2020; 19(5): 1199-209.
[http://dx.doi.org/10.1007/s11101-019-09629-9]

[26] Mahdi JG, Mahdi AJ, Mahdi AJ, Bowen ID. The historical analysis of aspirin discovery, its relation to the willow tree and antiproliferative and anticancer potential. Cell Prolif 2006; 39(2): 147-55.
[http://dx.doi.org/10.1111/j.1365-2184.2006.00377.x] [PMID: 16542349]

[27] Achan J, Talisuna AO, Erhart A, *et al.* Quinine, an old anti-malarial drug in a modern world: role in the treatment of malaria. Malar J 2011; 10(1): 144.
[http://dx.doi.org/10.1186/1475-2875-10-144] [PMID: 21609473]

[28] Ganesan A. The impact of natural products upon modern drug discovery. Curr Opin Chem Biol 2008; 12(3): 306-17.
[http://dx.doi.org/10.1016/j.cbpa.2008.03.016] [PMID: 18423384]

[29] Huang N, Huang W, Wu J, Long S, Luo Y, Huang J. Possible opportunities and challenges for traditional Chinese medicine research in 2035. Front Pharmacol 2024; 15: 1426300.
[http://dx.doi.org/10.3389/fphar.2024.1426300] [PMID: 38974044]

[30] Chamberlin B. What is Zoopharmacognosy. Academia Letters 2021; p. 2.

[31] Voltura EV, Brightsmith DJ, Cornejo J, Tizard I, Bailey CA, Heatley JJ. Parrot dietary habits and consumption of alternate foodstuffs. J Avian Med Surg 2024; 37(4): 297-313.
[http://dx.doi.org/10.1647/20-00028] [PMID: 38363162]

[32] Krishnaswamy S. Bioprospecting, botany, biodiversity, and their impact on botanical drug development Botanical Drug Products. CRC Press 2018; pp. 39-60.

[33] Streams A. Method of Drug Discovery in the Classical Tradition of Ayurveda as a Preliminary Tool for Refinement of Folklore Knowledge of Medicinal Plants

[34] Anmol , Aggarwal G, Sharma M, Singh R, Shivani , Sharma U. Plant-based natural product chemistry: An overview of the multistep journey involved in scientific validation of traditional knowledge. Studies in Natural Products Chemistry 2024; 80: 327-77.
[http://dx.doi.org/10.1016/B978-0-443-15589-5.00010-4]

[35] Ji HF, Li XJ, Zhang HY. Natural products and drug discovery. EMBO Rep 2009; 10(3): 194-200. [http://dx.doi.org/10.1038/embor.2009.12] [PMID: 19229284]

[36] Balunas MJ, Kinghorn AD. Drug discovery from medicinal plants. Life Sci 2005; 78(5): 431-41. [http://dx.doi.org/10.1016/j.lfs.2005.09.012] [PMID: 16198377]

[37] Rijal A. Surviving on Knowledge: Ethnobotany of Chepang community from mid-hills of Nepal. Ethnobot Res Appl 2011; 9: 181-215. [http://dx.doi.org/10.17348/era.9.0.181-215]

[38] Cieśla Ł, Moaddel R. Comparison of analytical techniques for the identification of bioactive compounds from natural products. Nat Prod Rep 2016; 33(10): 1131-45. [http://dx.doi.org/10.1039/C6NP00016A] [PMID: 27367973]

[39] Szymański P, Markowicz M, Mikiciuk-Olasik E. Adaptation of high-throughput screening in drug discovery-toxicological screening tests. Int J Mol Sci 2011; 13(1): 427-52. [http://dx.doi.org/10.3390/ijms13010427] [PMID: 22312262]

[40] Nothias LF, Nothias-Esposito M, da Silva R, *et al.* Bioactivity-based molecular networking for the discovery of drug leads in natural product bioassay-guided fractionation. J Nat Prod 2018; 81(4): 758-67. [http://dx.doi.org/10.1021/acs.jnatprod.7b00737] [PMID: 29498278]

[41] Gote S, Thapa S, Dubey S, Nargund SL, Biradar MS. Computational investigation of quinazoline derivatives as Keap1 inhibitors for Alzheimer's disease. Informatics in Medicine Unlocked 2023; 41: 101334. [http://dx.doi.org/10.1016/j.imu.2023.101334]

[42] Shyur LF, Yang NS. Metabolomics for phytomedicine research and drug development. Curr Opin Chem Biol 2008; 12(1): 66-71. [http://dx.doi.org/10.1016/j.cbpa.2008.01.032] [PMID: 18258212]

[43] Rastogi S, Rastogi P. Bioinformatics: methods and applications-genomics, proteomics and drug discovery. PHI Learn Pvt Ltd 2022.

[44] George R, Hehlgans S, Fleischmann M, Rödel C, Fokas E, Rödel F. Advances in nanotechnology-based platforms for survivin-targeted drug discovery. Expert Opin Drug Discov 2022; 17(7): 733-54. [http://dx.doi.org/10.1080/17460441.2022.2077329] [PMID: 35593177]

[45] Thapa S, Biradar MS, Banerjee J, Karati D. *In-silico* approach for predicting the inhibitory fffect of home remedies on severe acute respiratory syndrome coronavirus-2. Makara J Sci 2023; 27(3): 5. [http://dx.doi.org/10.7454/mss.v27i3.1609]

[46] Thapa S, Nargund SL, Biradar MS. Molecular design and *in-silico* analysis of trisubstituted benzimidazole derivatives as ftsz inhibitor. J Chem 2023. [http://dx.doi.org/10.1155/2023/9307613]

[47] Cech NB, Oberlies NH. From plant to cancer drug: lessons learned from the discovery of taxol. Nat Prod Rep 2023; 40(7): 1153-7. [http://dx.doi.org/10.1039/D3NP00017F] [PMID: 37449327]

[48] Fan X, Lin X, Ruan Q, *et al.* Research progress on the biosynthesis and metabolic engineering of the anti-cancer drug camptothecin in Camptotheca acuminate. Ind Crops Prod 2022; 186: 115270. [http://dx.doi.org/10.1016/j.indcrop.2022.115270]

[49] Heinrich M, Lee Teoh H. Galanthamine from snowdrop—the development of a modern drug against Alzheimer's disease from local Caucasian knowledge. J Ethnopharmacol 2004; 92(2-3): 147-62. [http://dx.doi.org/10.1016/j.jep.2004.02.012] [PMID: 15137996]

[50] Kluska M, Woźniak K. Natural polyphenols as modulators of etoposide anti-cancer activity. Int J Mol Sci 2021; 22(12): 6602. [http://dx.doi.org/10.3390/ijms22126602] [PMID: 34202987]

[51] Ndung'u JK, Nguta JM, Mapenay IM, Moriasi GA. A comprehensive review of ethnomedicinal uses, phytochemistry, pharmacology, and toxicity of *Prunus africana* (Hook. F.) kalkman from Africa. Scientifica (Cairo) 2024; 2024(1): 1-17.
[http://dx.doi.org/10.1155/2024/8862996] [PMID: 38654751]

[52] Bonanno G, Veneziano V. Seed dormancy, climate changes, desertification and soil use transformation threaten the Mediterranean endemic monospecific plant Petagnaea gussonei. Sci Rep 2024; 14(1): 8235.
[http://dx.doi.org/10.1038/s41598-024-58948-1] [PMID: 38589665]

[53] Pandohee J, Kyereh E, Kulshrestha S, Xu B, Mahomoodally MF. Review of the recent developments in metabolomics-based phytochemical research. Crit Rev Food Sci Nutr 2023; 63(19): 3734-49.
[http://dx.doi.org/10.1080/10408398.2021.1993127] [PMID: 34672234]

[54] Rangel-Huerta O, Gil A. Nutrimetabolomics: an update on analytical approaches to investigate the role of plant-based foods and their bioactive compounds in non-communicable chronic diseases. Int J Mol Sci 2016; 17(12): 2072.
[http://dx.doi.org/10.3390/ijms17122072] [PMID: 27941699]

[55] Sieniawska E, Georgiev MI. Metabolomics: towards acceleration of antibacterial plant-based leads discovery. Phytochem Rev 2022; 21(3): 765-81.
[http://dx.doi.org/10.1007/s11101-021-09762-4]

[56] Kc S, Pandey B, Kc S, Gurung S, Gautam A. Anti-inflammatory, analgesic, and acute toxicity evaluation of Litchi chinensis seed extract in albino rat. Natural Resources for Human Health 2021; 1(1): 30-5.
[http://dx.doi.org/10.53365/nrfhh/141230]

[57] Pandey B, Thapa S, Kaundinnyayana A, Panta S. Hepatoprotective effects of *Juglans regia* on carbon tetrachloride-induced hepatotoxicity: In silico/in vivo approach. Food Sci Nutr 2024; 12(9): 6482-97.
[http://dx.doi.org/10.1002/fsn3.4288] [PMID: 39554326]

[58] Manickavasagam G, Mahendran TR, Lim V. Metabolomics and cancer: Identification of biomarkers from plant-based pharmaceuticals using an integrated approach. Springer 2024.
[http://dx.doi.org/10.1007/16833_2024_223]

[59] Mukherjee PK, Harwansh RK, Bahadur S, *et al.* Metabolomics of medicinal plants–a versatile tool for standardization of herbal products and quality evaluation of ayurvedic formulations. Curr Sci 2016; 111(10): 1624-30.
[http://dx.doi.org/10.18520/cs/v111/i10/1624-1630]

[60] Cahlíková L, Šafratová M, Hošťálková A, Chlebek J, Hulcová D, Breiterová K, *et al.* Pharmacognosy and its role in the system of profile disciplines in pharmacy. Nat Prod Commun 2020; 15(9)
[http://dx.doi.org/10.1177/1934578X20945450]

[61] Amir-Aslani A. Toxicogenomic predictive modeling: Emerging opportunities for more efficient drug discovery and development. Technol Forecast Soc Change 2008; 75(7): 905-32.
[http://dx.doi.org/10.1016/j.techfore.2007.10.002]

[62] Bano I, Butt UD, Mohsan SAH. New challenges in drug discovery Novel platforms for drug delivery applications. Elsevier 2023; pp. 619-43.
[http://dx.doi.org/10.1016/B978-0-323-91376-8.00021-5]

[63] Kramer JA, Sagartz JE, Morris DL. The application of discovery toxicology and pathology towards the design of safer pharmaceutical lead candidates. Nat Rev Drug Discov 2007; 6(8): 636-49.
[http://dx.doi.org/10.1038/nrd2378] [PMID: 17643090]

[64] Inglese J, Johnson RL, Simeonov A, *et al.* High-throughput screening assays for the identification of chemical probes. Nat Chem Biol 2007; 3(8): 466-79.
[http://dx.doi.org/10.1038/nchembio.2007.17] [PMID: 17637779]

[65] Gomes NGM, Pereira DM, Valentão P, Andrade PB. Hybrid MS/NMR methods on the prioritization

of natural products: Applications in drug discovery. J Pharm Biomed Anal 2018; 147: 234-49. [http://dx.doi.org/10.1016/j.jpba.2017.07.035] [PMID: 28826951]

[66] Koparde AA, Doijad RC, Magdum CS. Natural products in drug discovery. Pharmacogn Med Plants 2019. [http://dx.doi.org/10.5772/intechopen.82860]

[67] Sayed N, Khurana A, Godugu C. Pharmaceutical perspective on the translational hurdles of phytoconstituents and strategies to overcome. J Drug Deliv Sci Technol 2019; 53: 101201. [http://dx.doi.org/10.1016/j.jddst.2019.101201]

[68] Patwardhan B, Vaidya AD, Chorghade M. Ayurveda and natural products drug discovery. Curr Sci 2004; 789-99.

[69] Pandey B, Baral R, Kaundinnyayana A, Panta S. Promising hepatoprotective agents from the natural sources: a study of scientific evidence. Egyptian Liver Journal 2023; 13(1): 14. [http://dx.doi.org/10.1186/s43066-023-00248-w]

CHAPTER 3

Secondary Metabolites: Nature's Gift for Holistic Health Management

Manisha Bhatia[1], **Divya Dhawal Bhandari**[2] and **Prerna Sarup**[3,*]

[1] *Department of Pharmacognosy, MM College of Pharmacy, Maharishi Markandeshwar (Deemed to be University), Mullana, Ambala 133203, Haryana, India*

[2] *Department of Pharmaceutical Chemistry, University Institute of Pharmaceutical Sciences, Panjab University, Chandigarh, Punjab, India*

[3] *Department of Pharmacognosy, University Institute of Pharmaceutical Sciences, Panjab University, Chandigarh, Punjab, India*

Abstract: Plant Secondary Metabolites (PSM) are compounds vital for plant survival that play a pivotal role in their mechanisms of action, and possess various medicinal properties that can enhance human health. These bioactive substances, generated by plants as defense mechanisms against predators and to attract pollinating insects, are garnering increased attention for their potential pharmacological benefits. PSM encompassing alkaloids, flavonoids, terpenes, saponins, and more, exhibit diverse pharmacological activities such as antihypertensive, anticancer, and antimicrobial effects. Ancient civilizations practiced medicinal plant usage, with secondary metabolites primarily responsible for their therapeutic efficacy. Classified based on structure and biosynthetic derivation into primary and secondary metabolites, the latter category includes terpenoids, phenolics, alkaloids, and glycosides. They serve as crucial sources of bioactive ingredients in both nutraceuticals and modern pharmaceuticals. Secondary metabolites display diverse pharmacological activities, interacting with receptors, cell membranes, and nucleic acids. This comprehensive book chapter delves into their classification, phytochemistry, and pharmacological activities, shedding light on their application in modern medicine for human health enhancement and drug innovation. Understanding these compounds aids in identifying and isolating pharmacologically active lead compounds for drug discovery.

Keywords: Alkaloids, Biological activity, Drug discovery, Flavonoids, Plant secondary metabolites, Polyphenols, Saponins, Terpenes.

* **Corresponding author Prerna Sarup:** Department of Pharmacognosy, University Institute of Pharmaceutical Sciences, Panjab University, Chandigarh, Punjab, India; E-mail: psarup_pu@hotmail.com

M.S. Ashawat, Aditi Kaushik, Akash Jain, Jasmine Chaudhary & Manish Kaushik (Eds.)
All rights reserved-© 2025 Bentham Science Publishers

INTRODUCTION

Plant chemistry is mainly attributed to the therapeutic potential of herbs. In other words, an in-depth understanding of the chemical composition of plants enriches our comprehension of their potential curative value. Modern chemistry has explained the role of primary plant metabolites in fundamental life functions such as cell division, growth, respiration, storage, and reproduction. These metabolites include small molecules like sugars, amino acids, tricarboxylic acids (Krebs cycle intermediates), proteins, nucleic acids, and polysaccharides, involved in processes like glycolysis, the citric acid cycle, and photosynthesis.

Secondary plant metabolites are organic compounds that are not directly involved in the basic processes of growth, development, or reproduction. Unlike primary metabolites, which include carbohydrates, proteins, and nucleic acids, secondary metabolites often play a role in defense against herbivores and pathogens, as well as in interactions with pollinators and seed dispersers. These compounds can also have significant pharmacological or toxicological effects on other organisms [1]. Secondary plant metabolites are diverse compounds produced by plant cells using precursors from primary metabolism *via* various metabolic pathways such as shikimic acid, acetate, and amino acid pathways. This concept, first introduced by Nobel laureate Albrecht Kossel in 1910, was later expanded by Czapek, who described these compounds as end-products of nitrogen metabolism involving secondary modifications [2].

These secondary metabolites exhibit various biological effects, providing a scientific basis for the use of herbs in traditional medicine across many cultures. They have been identified as antibiotics, antifungals, antivirals, and UV protectants, defending plants from pathogens and environmental damage. Some herbs, like clover or alfalfa, exhibit estrogenic properties, affecting animal fertility.

Secondary plant metabolites are categorized into various classes. The current chapter explores these categories, highlighting their phytochemical structures and pharmacological potential. The main categories, as given in Fig. (**1**), include:

i. Alkaloids
ii. Phenolics
iii. Saponins
iv. Terpenes

Alkaloids

Alkaloids often contain one or more rings of carbon atoms, usually with a nitrogen atom in the heterocyclic ring. The position of the nitrogen atom in the ring varies with different alkaloids and different plant families. These compounds are renowned for their pharmacological properties and have been utilized in traditional systems of medicine and modern pharmaceuticals for centuries. Alkaloids are produced through a complex biosynthesis process regulated by environmental factors, providing plants with adaptive advantages. Many well-known drugs, like quinine and morphine, are derived from natural alkaloids. A particularly fascinating feature of alkaloids is their structural diversity. Alkaloids have a crucial part to play in the development of clinical medicine, along with providing natural defense to organisms. Around 20% of known plant secondary metabolites are alkaloids [3]. These compounds can vary from simple molecules like nicotine to more complex structures such as morphine. This diversity in structure is reflected in their wide range of biological activities. Depending on their specific makeup and the organisms they interact with, alkaloids can function as stimulants, sedatives, analgesics, and even poisons [4, 5]. Alkaloids are categorized based on their chemical structure, biological origin, and biosynthetic pathways. However, the most common classification out of all is based on a chemical structure, which is given below along with a few examples from the particular category [1]:

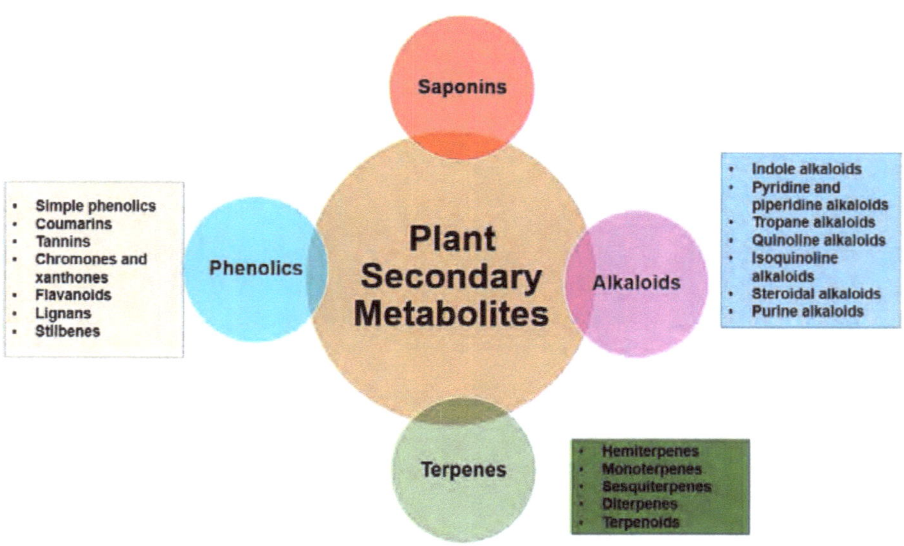

Fig. (1). Types of plant secondary metabolites.

- **Indole Alkaloids**: strychnine and reserpine.
- **Pyridine and Piperidine Alkaloids**: nicotine and coniine.
- **Tropane Alkaloids**: atropine and cocaine.
- **Quinoline Alkaloids**: quinine and quinidine.
- **Isoquinoline Alkaloids**: morphine and codeine.
- **Steroidal Alkaloids**: solanine and tomatine.
- **Purine Alkaloids**: caffeine and theobromine.

Phenolics

Phenolics, the most extensive group of plant secondary metabolites, are defined by the presence of one or more phenol groups. Their structures vary from simple molecules with a single aromatic ring to complex polymers. They significantly influence the color, taste, and flavor of many herbs, foods, and beverages. Silybin and Quercetin are phenolic compounds known for their hepatoprotective and anti-inflammatory potential, respectively. Compounds like genistein and daidzein act as phytoestrogens, while naringenin serves as an insecticide. Many phenolics, especially flavonoids, are free radical scavengers and potent antioxidants. These compounds play a crucial role in shielding plants from ultraviolet radiation, pathogens, and herbivores, and they also have structural roles, such as in the formation of lignin in plant cell walls [6].

Phenolics can be categorized based on their biosynthetic origin or chemical structure into:

i. Simple Phenolics
ii. Coumarins
iii. Tannins
iv. Chromones and xanthones
v. Flavonoids
vi. Lignans
vii. Stilbenes

Simple Phenolics

Phenolic acids are abundant in plants, whereas free phenols are rare. The most common compound, gallic acid, is widespread and known for its astringent properties, along with other activities such as antibacterial, antiviral, antifungal, anti-inflammatory, and antitumor actions [7]. Phenolic compounds vary according to their functional groups, including hydroxyl, aldehydic, or carboxylic groups. Compounds like eugenol, vanillin, and salicylic acid are notable examples [8, 9].

Coumarins

Coumarins (derived from benzo-α-pyrone) are a group of natural compounds found in about 150 species across more than 30 families. More than a thousand natural coumarins have been identified so far. The main source of coumarins includes tonka bean, sweet clover, and sweet woodruff [9]. Umbelliferone, aesculetin, and scopoletin are the most common coumarins present in plants in their free or glycosidic form. The most notable pharmacological activities of

coumarins include anti-Alzheimer's, anticancer, anti-inflammatory, and anticoagulant activity [10].

Tannins

Tannins are polyphenols capable of precipitating proteins, historically used in leather production. Two major types exist: hydrolyzable tannins (composed of phenolic acids like gallic acid) and condensed tannins [1] (based on oligomeric flavonoid precursors). Tannin-containing drugs act as antidiarrheals and antidotes for heavy metal and alkaloid poisoning. Epigallocatechin-3-gallate from tea exhibits antiangiogenic properties [11], while cranberry juice acts as a urinary antiseptic [12].

Chromones and Xanthones

Chromones and xanthones, derivatives of benzo-γ-pyrone, have limited pharmaceutical importance but include compounds like eugenin and khellin with notable activities. Xanthones from plants like Polygala exert antifungal activity [13].

Flavonoids

One of the major groups of naturally occurring phenols is the flavonoids, which constitute over 2000 identified compounds. They possess an aromatic ring with a chroman ring and are classified based on the level of oxidation of the central ring. Common classes of flavonoids are anthocyanins, flavones, and flavonols. Flavonoids are known for their potential role as antiallergic, anti-inflammatory, antithrombotic, and vasoprotective agents [14, 15].

Lignans

Dimeric compounds formed from phenylpropene derivatives are called lignans, found in Asteraceae, Pinaceae, and Rutaceae. They exhibit antimicrobial, antifungal, and cytotoxic activities [16, 17].

Stilbenes

Stilbenes are a very small group of secondary metabolites found mainly in heartwood. The most significant compound of this class, which exhibits estrogen-like activity, is Resveratrol, which is also widely distributed across various genera like Eucalyptus, Pinus, and Vitaceae [18].

Saponins

Saponins are compounds with a steroid or triterpenoid aglycone attached to a carbohydrate unit. They cause hemolysis of blood erythrocytes and exhibit soap-like properties. Saponins have diverse pharmacological properties, including antitumor, sedative, and anti-inflammatory effects [19].

Terpenes

Terpenes also form the largest and most diverse group of chemical compounds, derived from 5-carbon isoprene units. They are classified based on the number of isoprene units present in them. Terpenoids are crucial for plant defense, pigmentation, growth regulation, and attracting pollinators. Terpenes are known to be pharmacologically active compounds as they have a significant role as anticancer, anti-inflammatory, analgesic, and antimicrobial agents [9, 20, 21]. The primary plant metabolites also play significant roles in medicine. Unlike secondary metabolites, which are specialized compounds often involved in the plant's defense mechanisms, primary metabolites are essential for the basic physiological functions of plants. These include carbohydrates, lipids, proteins, and nucleic acids.

Types of Terpenes

- *Hemiterpenes*: Single isoprene unit, like angelic acid.
- *Monoterpenes*: Two isoprene units, components of essential oils with medicinal uses.
- *Sesquiterpenes*: Three isoprene units, with antibacterial and antiprotozoal activities.
- *Diterpenes*: Four isoprene units, including compounds like Vitamin K1 and Vitamin A.

Carbohydrates

Carbohydrates are found in all living organisms and are the primary products of photosynthesis, serving as the foundation for all phytochemicals and animal biochemicals. Cellulose, a polymer of glucose, is the most abundant organic material on Earth and the main structural component of plants. While primarily metabolites, carbohydrates are often incorporated into secondary metabolites through glycosidic bonds, forming substances like gums and mucilages. Carbohydrates are organic compounds consisting of carbon, hydrogen, and oxygen, characteristically in the same ratio as in water. They can be classified into four different groups: monosaccharides, disaccharides, oligosaccharides, and polysaccharides. The building blocks for the other types are the monosaccharides, which contain three to nine carbon atoms. In addition to their structural and biological roles, some carbohydrates have medicinal properties. For instance, mucilage—a sticky, viscous substance produced by plants—acts as a demulcent, soothing, and protecting mucous membranes and skin. Significant sources of mucilage include marshmallow plants, flax seeds, and cactus. Mucilage is particularly beneficial for protecting inflamed gastrointestinal surfaces and treating inflammatory digestive disorders [22, 23].

Lipids

Lipids encompass a broad category of naturally occurring compounds, including waxes, fixed and essential oils, phospholipids, sterols, and various fat-soluble vitamins. All these play vital roles as hormones, vitamins, energy reserves, and structural components of cell membranes. Although traditionally regarded as primary metabolites, recent studies have highlighted the pharmacological activities of various lipids [24].

Fixed Oils

Various aliphatic long-chain fatty acids like stearic, oleic, and palmitic acids esterified with glycerol form the composition of fixed oils. These oils are rich in liquid (polyunsaturated) glycerides like glycerinoleate, whereas fats contain more solid glycerides like glycerin stearate. Flaxseed oil, sourced from Linumusitatissimum, is notable for its polyunsaturated fatty acids, which are potent antioxidants and anti-inflammatory agents that help in reducing lipid peroxidation which further reduces the lowering the threat of cardiovascular disorders [25].

Waxes

Waxes are compounds that are primarily composed of long aliphatic chains that often include functional groups such as amides, carboxylic acids, hydroxyls, esters, unsaturated bonds, and aromatic systems. Synthetic waxes, in contrast, are long-chain hydrocarbons without functional groups. Jojoba wax, extracted from the seeds of Simmondsia chinensis, consists of straight-chain alcohol and fatty acid esters. Jojoba wax is used in topical treatments, cosmetics such as moisturizers and sunscreens, and other skin care products due to its well-known wound-healing properties. It also possesses promising anti-aging and anti-inflammatory properties [25].

Essential Oils

Essential/volatile oils are aromatic mixtures of low molecular weight compounds that contain two or three major constituents present in high concentrations (20-70%), while other constituents are in trace quantities. For example, Oil of *Origanum compactum* is rich in thymol (27%) and carvacrol (30%), while *Mentha piperita* oil contains high levels of menthol (59%) and menthone (19%). These major constituents determine the biological properties of essential oils, which are used for a variety of therapeutic purposes, including antiseptic, anti-inflammatory, spasmolytic, analgesic, antibacterial, sedative, and anesthetic treatments. Volatile oils are also used in perfumes, embalming, and food preservation [26].

Proteins

Legumes and soy are good sources of plant-derived proteins, which are also useful in nutritional therapies and as protein supplements for people with special dietary demands or inadequacies. Because of their ability to aid in digestion and reduce inflammation, plant-based enzymes such as papain from papaya and bromelain from pineapple are utilized in medicine.

Nucleic Acids

Plant-derived nucleic acids, such as those used in genetic studies or as part of certain therapeutic approaches, contribute to advancements in biotechnology and medicine. Overall, while secondary metabolites often provide direct therapeutic effects, primary metabolites are essential for their roles in nutrition, energy provision, and support of overall health.

ROLE OF SECONDARY METABOLITES IN PLANTS

Secondary metabolites perform various critical functions that aid in the survival and fitness of plants [27, 28].

- Defense Mechanisms against herbivores and pathogens: Compounds like alkaloids and terpenoids are often toxic, deterring herbivory. Phenolic compounds and saponins possess antimicrobial properties that protect plants from infections.
- Pollinator Attraction: Terpenoids and phenolics contribute to the production of essential oils and pigments, which attract pollinators.
- Seed Dispersal: Some secondary metabolites influence the flavor and color of fruits, making them attractive to animals that disperse seeds.
- Allelopathy: Certain secondary metabolites can suppress the growth of neighboring plants, reducing competition for resources.
- Protection from UV Radiation: Phenolic compounds like flavonoids absorb harmful UV radiation, protecting plant tissues from damage.
- Symbiotic Relationships: Secondary metabolites can facilitate symbiotic relationships with beneficial microorganisms, enhancing nutrient uptake and overall plant health.

PHYTOCHEMISTRY OF SECONDARY METABOLITES

Phytochemistry of secondary metabolites aims towards the study of plant based compounds obtained from secondary metabolites which includes a long process from identification followed by preparation and finally towards the use of sophisticated analytical techniques for elucidation of the structure. Today's era of emerging diseases demands the search for newer entities in various pharmaceutical and agrochemical industries and also their continual optimization.

The pharmacological properties of medicinal plants are attributed to the various phytoconstituents present in them. The secondary metabolites of plants such as phenolics, alkaloids, and terpenes include a large number of phytoconstitutents [29] which are used to treat different diseases, some of these compounds are-atropine, codeine, morphine, and nicotine, coming under alkaloids; linalool, ginsenosides, artemisinin, morgroside comes under terpenoids, while flavonoids, coumarins, xanthoneslignans and proanthocyanidins are categorized as phenolics as given in Fig. (**2**) [30, 31].

A number of such phytoconstituents have been isolated with the help of various solvents as extracts and further characterized with the help of various analytical techniques for drug design and discovery [32, 33]. The pharmacological activities of some secondary metabolites that have been used to treat various diseases are listed below. (Table **1**).

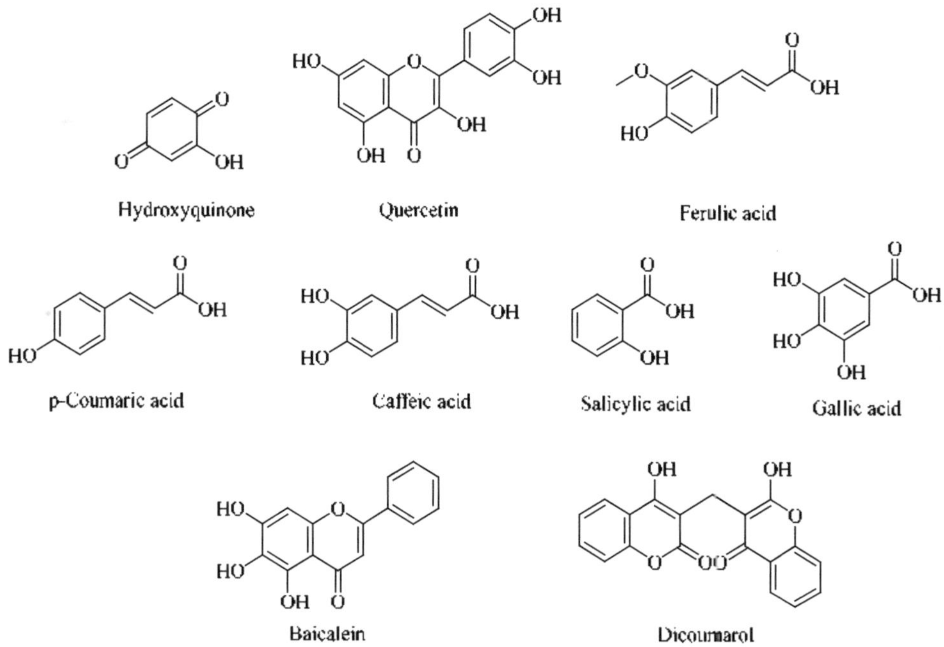

Phytoconstituents present as Phenolics

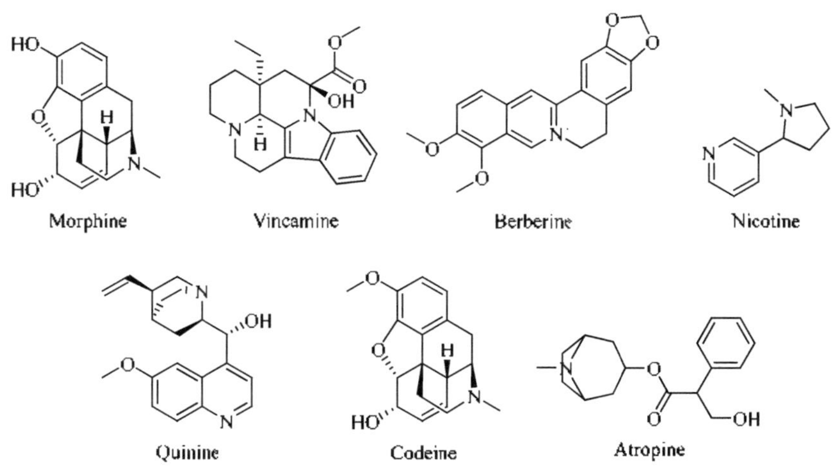

Phytoconstituents present in Alkaloids

(Fig. 2) contd.....

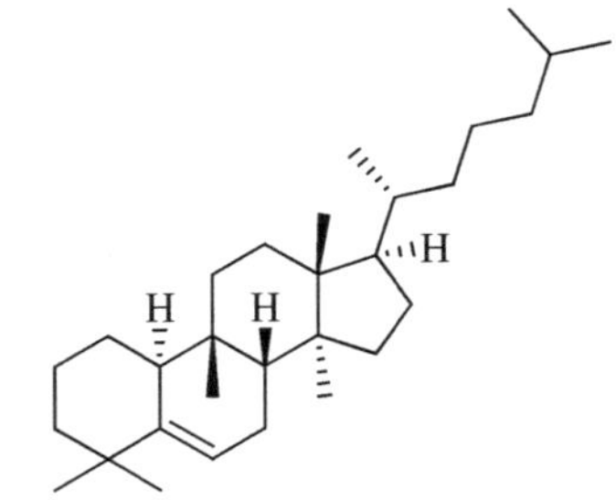

Cucurbitacin

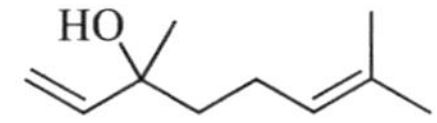

Linalool

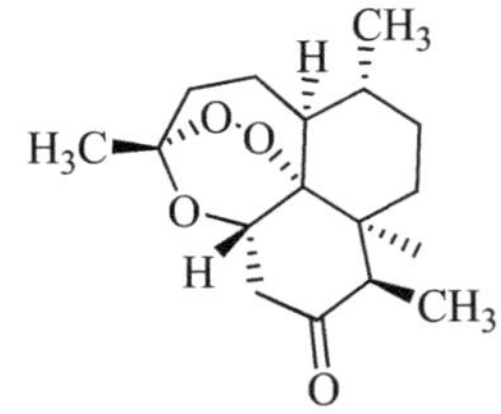

Artemisinin

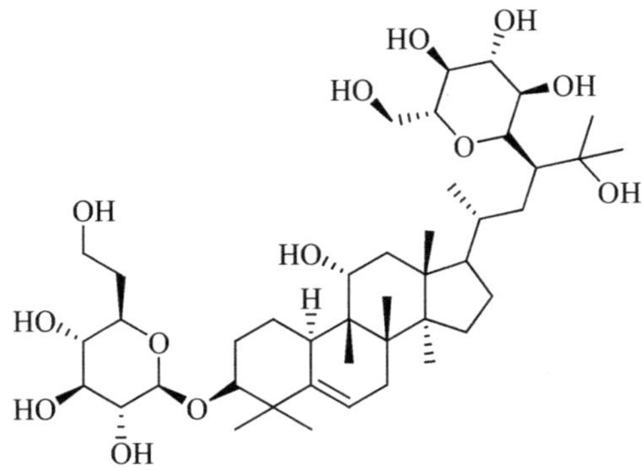

Morgroside

Phytoconstituents present as Terpenes

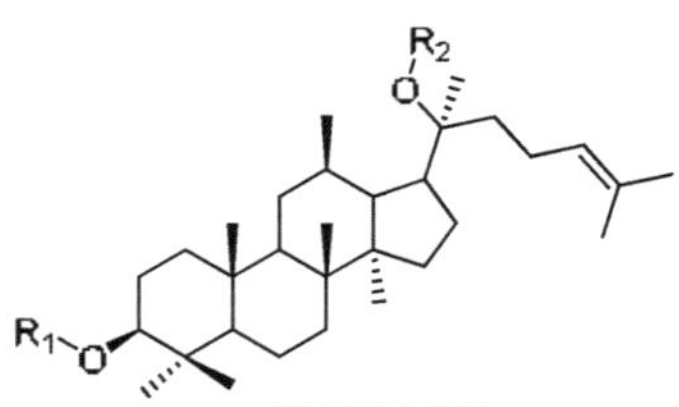

Ginsenoside

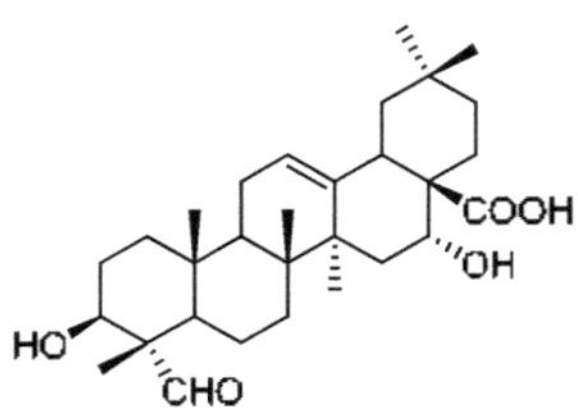

Quillaic acid

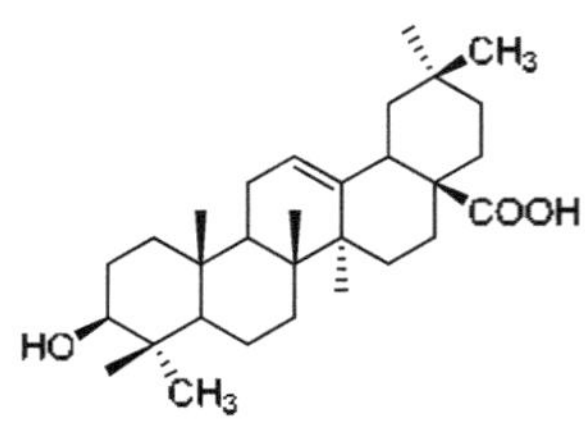

Oleanolic acid

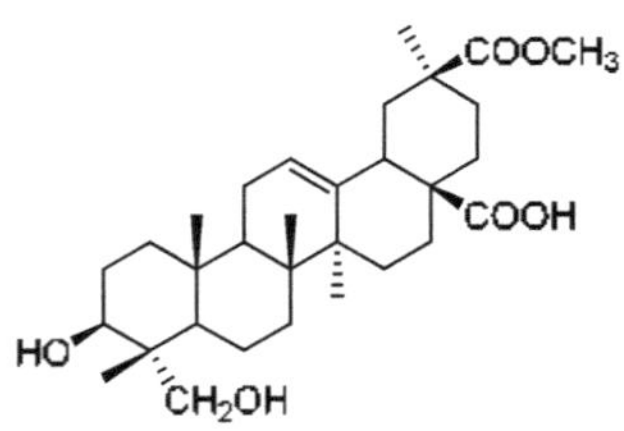

Phytolaccagenic

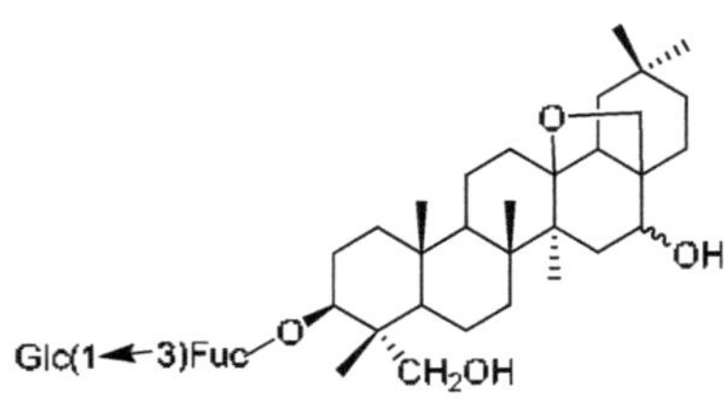

Saikosaponin a

Fig. (2). Various phytoconstituents present in secondary metabolites.

Table 1. Phytoconstitutents of secondary metabolites and their pharmacological activities.

Class of Secondary metabolites	Plant species and part from which phytoconstituent can be extracted	Pharmacological activities	Reference
PHENOLICS			
Gallic acid	Fruits of *O. Sativa* and *C. sativus*	• Antibacterial • Antiviral • Antifungal • Anti-inflammatory • Antitumor • Bronchodilator • Muscle relaxant	[34]
Hydroquinone	Leaves of *Arbutus unedo L.*	• Antimicrobial • Antiseptic	[35]
Xanthohumol	Female inflorescences of *Humuluslupulus*	• Anticancer	[36]
Salvianolic acid	*Salvia miltiorrhiza*	• CVS diseases • CNS diseases	[36]
Hydrolyzable tannins	Fruits of *Castaneasativa* and leaves of *Quercusrobur, Quercuspetraea*, and *Quercus alba*	• Anti-diarrhoeal • Antidotes in heavy metals poisoning • Antiangiogenic	[37]
Scutellarin	Flowers of *Scutellariabarbata* and *S. lateriflora*	• Anti-cancer • Diabetic retinopathy	[36]
Baicalein	Flowers of *Scutellariabarbata* and *S. lateriflora*	• Anti-bacterial • Anti-fungal • Apoptosis inducer	[36]
Coumarins	Extracts of the solid residue of *L. angustifolia* and *L. x intermedia*	• Anti-inflammatory • Anticoagulant • Anticancer • Anti-Alzheimer's	[38]
Caffeic acid	*V. faba* *L. sativa*	• Reverses growth inhibition by Abscisic acid (ABA)	[39]
Ferulic acid	*Malus' Jork 9'* *Zea mays* *Oryzasativa* *L. sativa* *V. faba*	• Increases rooting • Inhibits the decarboxylation of IAA • Increases the activity of IAA oxidase in seedlings	[40]
Cinnamic acid	*G. max* *Pisumsativum*	• Increases the activity of IAA oxidase in roots • Antagonizes the growth-promoting effects of IAA	[41]
p-Coumaric acid	*L. sativa*	• Inhibitory effect on growth along with ABA	[39]

(Table 1) cont.....

Class of Secondary metabolites	Plant species and part from which phytoconstituent can be extracted	Pharmacological activities	Reference
ALKALOIDS			
Codeine	Unripe seeds of *Opium poppy*	• Antitussive • Antidepressant • Analgesic • Sedative	[42]
Morphine	Unripe seeds of *Opium poppy*	• Acute pulmonary edam • Reduces shortness of breath	[43]
Quinine	Bark of the cinchona (*QuinaQuina*) tree	• Antipyretic • Antimalarial • Analgesic	[34]
Atropine	Leaves and roots of *Atropa belladonna*	• Anti-cholinergic • Antagonist at muscarine acetylcholine receptors	[44]
Nicotine	Stems and leaves of *Nicotianatabacum*	• Insecticide • Anti-inflammatory • Antiherbivore	[45]
Berberine	Root, stem bark, and rhizome of *B. vulgaris, B. aristata, B. aquifolium, C. chinensis*	• Antiviral • Antibacterial • Anticancer • Antidiabetic • Anti-inflammatory	[34]
TERPENES			
Linalool	Essential oils of seeds of *C. sativum, C. martini*, *C. sinensis* and flowers of *Lavandulaofficinalis, Laurusnobilis,* and *Ocimumbasilicum*	• Antibacterial • CNS stimulant	[46]
Ginsenosides	Root, fruits, stems and leaves of *P. ginseng*	In treatment of • Insomnia • Anorexia • Impotence • Diabetes	[47]
Cucurbitacin	Fruits of about 30 genera of *Cucurbitaceae* families	• Anti-cancer • Anti-inflammatory • Hepatoprotective • Anti-viral	[48]
Artemisinin	*Artemisia annua*	• Anti-malarial • Anti-pyretic	[49]
Morgroside	Fruits of *Siraitiagrosvenorii*	• Antidiabetic • Anti-obestic • Anti-hyperlipidemic	[50]
SAPONINS			
Ginsenosides	Roots of *Panaxquinquefolius*	• Anti-fungal	[51]

(Table 1) cont.....

Class of Secondary metabolites	Plant species and part from which phytoconstituent can be extracted	Pharmacological activities	Reference
Oleanolic acid, Phytolaccagenic acid	Seeds of *Chinopodium quinoa* and fruit of *Phytolaccadodecandra*	• Anti-viral • Cytotoxicity	[51]
Shatavarin	Roots of *Asparagus racemosus*	• Anti-bacterial	[51]

APPLICATIONS OF SECONDARY METABOLITES IN MODERN MEDICINE

From time immemorial, man has been dependent on the indispensable plant products, besides being a good source of food. These plant products, termed as secondary metabolites, possess a plethora of applications as pharmaceutical, and flavoring agents, in food industries, perfumery, agrochemicals, insecticides, cosmetics production, and raw materials for industries.

Also known by varied names as phytoconstituents, specialized metabolites, bioactive moiety, and secondary products, this unique biochemical category of substances is produced through complex secondary metabolic pathways. These novel metabolic products have high pharmaceutical value, exhibiting enormous impact in plant defence and human healthcare. Secondary metabolites with remarkable therapeutic activity are a potential substitute for the majority of the commercially valuable synthetic medicines [52]. They represent an interesting collection of assorted bioactive drugs for medicinal and therapeutic purposes meant for humans, bacteria, fungi, and parasites [53]. They have captured significant interest nowadays due to their dramatic implications for pharmaceutical, nutritional, and industrial purposes [54]. Because of their diverse role as pharmaceuticals, agrochemicals, and flavours, secondary metabolites have widespread demand, and a range of commercial formulations are readily available in the pharmaceutical market. Their evolving commercial importance has increased manifold in recent years.

Secondary metabolites also serve crucial ecological functions for the plants producing them. They confer adaptive roles by serving as weapons to defend themselves against herbivores, bacteria, fungi and viruses, amoebae, plants, insects, and large animals due to their toxic or repellent effects, symbiosis, in metal transport, reproductive agent, as signaling compounds in attracting seed-dispersing animals, as sexual hormones and as differentiation effectors [55]. They facilitate pollination and can inhibit the growth of nearby competing plants by a phenomenon termed allelopathy. They help plants cope with stress, including UV radiation and drought, through the activation of plant defense mechanisms by the recognition of foreign agents, act as protective agents, and regulate various vital physiological functions such as growth, development, and responses to environmental stimuli. They are enriched with a complete array of bioactive compounds, with great medicinal and therapeutic value in plenty of health issues, and also possess a diverse role as a spice, perfume, poison, toxins and pesticides [56]. Their economic impact is immense due to their significant medicinal value as an anti-diabetic agent, antibiotic, cancer treatment, anti-viral, anti-inflammatory, cardioprotective, anti-fertility, analgesic, and growth regulator. They serve as the basis for many pharmaceutical drugs for the treatment of diseases, and management of health conditions [57].

To alleviate the challenge of insects, restricting the usage of toxic synthetic pesticides and promoting environment-friendly, plant-based pesticides is the need of the hour. Secondary plant metabolites provide sustainable pest management solutions in replacement of synthetic pesticides, herbicides, insecticides, and preservatives, thereby enhancing agricultural productivity [58, 59]. Thus, they impart wide applications as biopesticides, bioinsecticides, bioherbicides and antihelmintics against worms, lice, ticks, and mites, growth promoters, and regulators [60]. Terpenoids and flavonoids have noteworthy contributions to the flavor, aroma, and color, thereby being used as natural flavoring agents and colorants in the food and beverage industry [61]. A variety of drugs, fragrances, flavors, dyes, pesticides, and insecticides are manufactured in the market by using secondary metabolites owing to their high economic value.

Essential oils and fragrant compounds serve as key ingredients and are widely incorporated into cosmetics and perfumes due to their pleasant properties [62]. The cosmetics industry uses alkaloids for lightening discoloration, reducing cellulite, fine lines, and wrinkles, reducing irritation, soothing effect, emollient and protecting against harmful ultraviolet radiations. These compounds are utilized by cosmetologists in the production of tonics, creams, lotions, face and hair masks, skincare, and anti-aging products [63]. Tannins have applications in wastewater treatment because of their tendency to remove pollutants, thereby being used as natural antioxidants in environmentally friendly products [64]. The plant-derived secondary metabolites are valuable sources of pharmaceuticals with nutritional elements endowed with healing potential and betterment of human life. These nutritional phytochemicals are termed nutraceuticals and are encapsulated in diverse dosage forms for health benefits [65]. Natural plant diets in the form of unique nutraceuticals have drawn a lot of interest to promote good health, and treat chronic illnesses and pathological ailments [66].

Thus, secondary metabolites are meant to improve health in the form of antibiotics, analgesics, enzyme inhibitors, immunomodulators, antitumors, and growth promoters, broaden the sphere of healthy nutrition as nutraceuticals, sources of medicinal compounds, enhance agricultural productivity using pesticides, insecticides, and pheromones. They have an important impact on ecology and serve diverse survival functions for the improvement of health, nutrition, and economics in a positive way.

They have various properties that make them effective in mitigating and preventing chronic diseases. Numerous plants possess different phytochemicals such as alkaloids, flavonoids, glycosides, phenolic acids, isothiocyanates, isoflavones, carotenoids, tannins, resins, essential oils, volatile oils, proteins, amino acids, enzymes [67, 68] which have anticancer, anti-inflammatory, antidiabetic, cardioprotective, anti-obesity, antioxidants and antirheumatic activities. Additionally, they have the potential to manage cancer, chronic inflammation, chronic heart failure, Alzheimer's disease, chronic neuropathy, epilepsy, seizures, asthma, Parkinson's disease, renal impairment, diabetes, and polycystic ovarian syndrome [69].

Secondary metabolites have gained importance recently owing to their curative effects in ancient as well as modern communities. The well-established role of these potent compounds in improving overall health has increased their importance as a potential alternative to synthetic medicines. Being completely crude in origin, with almost insignificant reported side effects, has been the main factor for their market demand and popularity among the population.

PHARMACOLOGICAL ACTIVITIES OF SECONDARY METABOLITES

Terrestrial plants, along with fungi, bacteria, and marine organisms, synthesize a huge range of imperative biologically active compounds with unique diversity in structure as well as functions [70]. This natural reservoir of metabolites from natural reservoirs is a potential approach for discovering novel lead compounds for future drug discovery and development. These distinct intermediate products procured from different parts of plants have varied biological actions against numerous ailments. These phytoconstitutents display a promising curative effect in the treatment of chronic ailments with negligible side effects. The plant-based drug discovery has a broad range of utilization in the diseases which pose enormous challenge to the modern healthcare system and creates enormous scope in the field of natural products research for isolation of novel bioactive compounds.

Antibacterial Activity

Antibiotics are a very potent category of secondary metabolites produced by microorganisms that have the capacity to reduce the growth of bacteria by inhibiting essential cellular processes such as cell wall synthesis, disruption of the cytoplasmic membrane, interaction amongst membrane proteins, disturbance in

DNA synthesis, destabilization, leakage, preventing synthesis of enzymes, coagulation of constituents, and interruption of communication [71]. Out of the 30 antibiotics launched, 16 belong to natural products, which include the lipopeptide daptomycin and fidaxomicin and a fungal product retapamulin, for topical use [72]. Numerous natural metabolites such as anthrasil, dalbavacin, ceftarolinefasamil acetate, lefamulin, sarecycline, plazomicin, eravacycline and imi-cilast-relebactam have proven potent antibacterial activity [73].

Due to an increase in resistance of hazardous pathogens to current antibiotics at an alarming rate, the search for new potent antibacterial medicines is the need of the hour. During the last two decades, the secondary metabolites procured from plants appear to be an unlimited reservoir of potent antimicrobial agents by overcoming antibiotic resistance. The enormous variety of plant-derived natural compounds possess the additional benefit of being readily available, cheap, broad-spectrum, novel mechanisms against pathogens, diverse chemical structures, few adverse effects, and quite safe. Ongoing research proves that some secondary metabolites possess intrinsic strong antiseptic effects and a new approach is to combine them with conventional antibiotics in case of non-susceptible bacteria, which may develop resistance. Currently, combinations of antibiotics with plant-based extracts result in enhanced biological effects, high levels of efficacy, and a reduction in the toxicity caused by synthetic chemicals [74].

Among different plant lineages, non-vascular plants or Bryophytes, particularly mosses, namely *Physcomitrium patens* and *Sphagnum fallaxis*, are of great interest owing to miscellaneous unique active compounds with promising antibacterial properties [75]. Highly stable antibacterial activity was detected, highlighting their biotechnological potential in the field of medicine. An important category of phenols primarily aids in the treatment of microbial contamination in the urinary bladder, dental, and urinary tract regions. Clove and cinnamon oils are used as powerful inhibitors of bacterial and fungal growth on the surface of food materials.

Anti-inflammatory Activity

Inflammation appears as a natural biological reaction to microbial attack, irritation, or tissue damage by migration of inflammatory cells, release of reactive oxygen species, and pro-inflammatory cytokines at the site of injury to fight the foreign pathogens. A large number of natural secondary products with anti-inflammatory potential have been reported including moupinamide, capsaicin, and hypaphorine by Aswad and coworkers. Mona *et al.* also reported numerous herbs such as *Curcuma longa*, *Zingiber officinale*, *Rosmarinus officinalis*, and *Borago officinalis* with strong anti-inflammatory effects [76]. The phytoconstituents procured from *Cinnamomum osmophloeum*, in particular lipopolysaccharides, exhibit a strong effect by reducing the development of inflammation-causing factors by stimulating the production of macrophages [77].

Anticancer Activity

Cancer is the second most common reason for mortality, with an estimated burden as reported by the WHO of 18.1 million emerging cases, causing approximately 9.6 million deaths. It is presently becoming a high-profile disease presenting a major struggle in its treatment regimen, mainly due to its lethal effects. This leads to increasing demand for alternatives, and natural products with anticancer potential are considered the best choice. Quite a lot of metabolites can prevent oxidative stress along with inflammation, thereby preventing carcinogenesis [78]. They are excellent compounds with enhanced pharmacological potential for cancer therapeutic purposes using nanotech approaches such as irinotecan, vincristine, vinblastine, etoposide, actinomycin D, mitomycin C, and bleomycin [79]. The abundant natural compounds present in fruits and leafy vegetables such as vitamins, minerals, sterols, anthocyanins, folate, carotenoids, flavonoids, and polyphenols have proven ability to reduce cancer mortality [80]. The critical relationship elucidates that cancer prevention can be prevented to an extent by considering regular consumption of fruits and vegetables.

Antioxidants and phenolic compounds in herbs such as ginger, sage, rosemary, capsicum, curcumin, clove, oregano, and cinnamon can neutralize damage caused by reactive oxygen species in various cancers [81]. Numerous categories of cyclic peptides procured from marine species possess anticancer properties. In addition, lactoferrin, a multifunctional protein from bovine and camel milk, has also proven anticancer properties. Vincristine, a two-indole-type nucleus, the vindoline and the catharanthine type portion possess a non-symmetrical dimeric structure with approved clinical use in cancer. This natural alkaloid from *Catharanthusroseus* (L.) leaves has been used against acute lymphoblastic leukemia, rhabdomyosarcoma, neuroblastoma, lymphomas and nephroblastoma [82, 83]. Paclitaxel, obtained from the bark of *Taxus brevifolia Nutt.*, is a complex tricyclic diterpenoid, belonging to the category of pseudo alkaloid, with a complex 6,8,6-tricycle-fused skeleton with a four-member oxetane ring along with alcohol, ester, ketone and amide groups. It is amongst the most potent and effective chemotherapeutic drugs known in cancer therapy [84]. Homoharringtonine, an alkaloid isolated from *Cephalotaxusharringtonii* bark were initially utilized in Chinese traditional medicine for the treatment of cancer [85].

Antiviral Activity

Natural phytocompounds serve as a significant supply for developing novel antiviral medicaments owing to their easy availability, low side effects, and safe usage, but the extensive search for more effective drugs is the need of the hour. The mode of action of these antiviral moieties involves the inhibition of associated enzymes required for the life cycle of viruses. Strong structure and function association amongst miscellaneous secondary metabolites and HIV enzyme inhibition have already been ascertained.

Hepatoprotective Activity

According to an estimate by the WHO, an average of 500 million people are suffering from chronic hepatitis, thereby making it a significant concern in the healthcare system. Constant exposure to infectious agents that include drugs, viruses, parasites, and toxins results in degeneration, inflammation, fibrosis, and cirrhosis of the liver and hepatic clinical manifestations [86].

The Flavonoids class of secondary metabolites, including catechin, apigenin, quercetin, naringenin, rutin, and venoruton, possess strong hepatoprotective activities. Muhammad, Meng *et al.* and coworkers listed the composition, mechanism of action and pharmacology of certain plants in the prevention of liver damage induced by certain chemicals [87].

Antifungal Activity

According to the latest research conducted, plant secondary metabolites show antifungal mechanisms against various pathogenic fungi. Their mechanism of action includes inhibition of mycotoxin synthesis, preventing the formation of biofilm, causing destruction of the established biofilm, a significant decrease in spore formation, inhibiting hyphal growth, ergosterol synthesis, disrupting cell membrane permeability, causing lysis, and altering DNA replication [88]. Tissue inflammation was also reduced and had a potent antifungal effect by reducing the release of pro-inflammatory factors. These secondary metabolites have been used in clinical therapy either alone or in combination with existing antifungal drugs. Thus, we can conclude that they possess broad prospects for the development of unique antifungal drugs.

Antiulcer Activity

Secondary metabolites derived from plant sources are highly effective in treating infections caused by Helicobacter pylori, and they also tend to inhibit antiulcer activity *in vitro*, as well as urease activity. Their antiulcer potential can be further enhanced by lowering the pH of metabolites, reducing the Na+/K+ ATPase activity and transport of alanine in the gastrointestinal tract and regions of small intestine, respectively [89].

Antidiabetic Activity

Diabetes mellitus can be defined as a collection of metabolic disorders in which chronic hyperglycemia arises from an abnormality in both the production of insulin and its mode of action. The deleterious effect poses continuous damage, organ dysfunction, and malfunction of eyes, kidneys, lungs, nerves, heart, and blood vessels [90]. Plants containing phenolic acids, glycosides, saponins, stilbenes, vitamins, organic acids, and other beneficial nutrients have various therapeutic mechanisms, both in the management and prevention of diabetes mellitus [91].

Many antidiabetic pharmaceuticals frequently used are generally extracted from natural secondary metabolites, which can be traced back to the development of the popular antihyperglycemic drug metformin from *Galega officinalis*. Botanicals that can help to manage elevated glucose levels include bitter melon, nopal, fenugreek, ivy gourd, ginseng, cinnamon, psyllium, and garlic. Barberry (family Berberidaceae), rich in isoquinoline alkaloid berberine, has been effective for metabolic diseases. Zhang *et al.* proved that it has a positive effect on the gut microbiome, mediated through inhibition of DNA biotransformation by *Ruminococcusbromii* [92]. Curcumin, a valuable polyphenol from turmeric rhizome, is a biologically active molecule that can delay diabetes by improving beta cell function, preventing their death, and simultaneously reducing insulin resistance [93]. More recently, the antidiabetic activity of *M. Charantia L.* Fruits, pulp, and seeds focuses on improving pancreatic insulin secretion, glucose uptake, consumption by peripheral and skeletal muscle cells, and decreasing insulin resistance because of the presence of charantin and vicine. They also act as antidiabetics by inhibiting glucose absorption in the intestine along with suppression of key enzymes involved in gluconeogenic pathways [94]. Ginseng supplementation intake appreciably alters fasting glucose concentrations in serum, low-density lipoprotein cholesterol levels, insulin resistance index, and tumor necrosis factor levels [95]. A recent study by Jovanovski *et al.* shows that American ginseng and Korean red ginseng, both widely consumed species, can improve glycemic index significantly by lowering glucose levels. These are enriched with ginsenosides and malonylginsenosides, which are the main active compounds responsible for their hypoglycemic activity. *Rhodiolarosea L.* extracts are quite popular in the category of dietary supplements because of the presence of their active ingredient, the root p-hydroxyphenethyl-glucoside compound. In accordance with the latest studies rhodiola and salidroside possess strong AMP-

Activated Protein Kinase (AMPK) and signaling that can be attributed in the cure of diabetes [96]. Stevia, a popular natural calorie-free glycoside and sweetener obtained from the leaves of *Stevia rebaudiana* can be effectively used in replacement for artificial sweeteners in diabetic patients due to the inhibition of glycation end products [97]. The plant metabolites like cinnamaldehyde and polyphenols procured from cinnamon extracts are effective in the treatment of diabetes by significantly reducing the triglycerides and cholesterol levels. They have the ability to increase the high-density lipoproteins cholesterol level and can thereby be used as hypolipidemic agents.

Neuroprotective Activity

Pharmacologically active secondary metabolites derived from various plants exhibit significant neuroprotective activity, which can lead to the gradual and irreversible loss of neuronal cells indispensable for normal brain function. Their continuous loss eventually causes the death of brain cells and the most prevalent neurodegenerative illnesses include Alzheimer's, Parkinson's disease, amyotrophic lateral sclerosis, prion disorder, motor neuron, spinocerebellar ataxia, Huntington's disease, traumatic brain injury, chronic traumatic encephalopathy and spinal muscular atrophy [98]. The bioactive metabolites like physostigmine, galantamine, huperzine A, resveratrol, and curcumin play an imperative role in their prevention and short-term treatment.

Antioxidant Activity

Secondary metabolites depict antioxidant activity by neutralizing free radicals, stimulating defensive antioxidant mechanisms, binding metals, increasing the activity of antioxidant enzymes, thereby reducing oxidative damage and stimulating cytoprotective mechanisms. Phenolic compounds, comprised of an aromatic benzene ring with hydroxyl groups fused to a phenyl ring, constitute a huge range of phytochemicals with numerous health benefits [99]. Fruits are a potential source of phenolic functions and their regular intake prevents the hazard of ailments like cancer, lung disorders, heart failure, and stroke and promotes good health. Fruit is rich in phytocompounds such as vitamins, pyridoxine, minerals, niacin, folic acid, iron, fiber, magnesium, malic acid, tartaric acid, and citric acid. These high-antioxidant-rich nutrients can alter the rate of metabolism, neutralize free radicals, and flush out carcinogens. Thus, plant-based moieties are one of the best sources of polyphenols for disease prevention. Numerous herbal species contain different classes of secondary metabolites and commonly used antioxidants are aronia, bilberry fruits, the turmeric rhizome, purine alkaloids from the green tea leaf, coffee seed, cola seed, mate leaf, grape seed extract, and ginger rhizome.

Antifertility Activity

A range of phytoconstituents, such as alkaloids, resins, glycosides, saponins, flavonoids, tannins, and terpenoids, can interrupt normal ovarian functions along with the estrous cycle through the interchange of hormones and thus can induce infertility. They can significantly influence the production and functions of hormones in the ovary and uterus, and interfere with implantation and production of sperm. These natural drugs can act as anti-implantation or antiovulation agents by easily passing through the vagina and exhibit their effect by varying the vaginal pH. They can cause alterations in the cervix, inhibit sperm propulsion in the fallopian tubes, and affect decidual embedding. They tend to cause disturbance in the balance of estrogen and progesterone levels, and at the same time deprive the uterus and the embryo from nutrition. Plants with antiestrogenic activities can influence pituitary action by peripheral modulation and decrease the secretions of both important hormones *i.e,* Luteinizing Hormone (LH) and Follicle-Stimulating Hormone (FSH), block ovulation, and have abortifacient effects [100].

CONCLUSION

Secondary metabolites are diverse organic compounds produced by plants, fungi, and microorganisms and are used in medicine due to their potent bioactive properties. These include phenolics, alkaloids, flavonoids, and terpenoids, which have been integral to both traditional and alternative medicine for centuries. Their broad therapeutic potential encompasses antibacterial, anticancer, anti-inflammatory, and antidiabetic treatments. Many pharmaceutical drugs originate from these metabolites, and their role in complementary and preventive medicine is gaining increasing recognition. As ongoing research unveils new applications, the importance of secondary metabolites in developing innovative and effective therapeutic solutions continues to be highlighted.

REFERENCES

[1] Evans WC. Pharmacognosy. 16th ed., Edinburgh, London, New York, Philadelphia, St Louis, Sydney, Toronto: Elsevier 2009.

[2] Bourgaud F, Gravot A, Milesi S, Gontier E. Production of plant secondary metabolites: a historical perspective. Plant Sci 2001; 161(5): 839-51. [http://dx.doi.org/10.1016/S0168-9452(01)00490-3]

[3] Kaur R, Arora S. Alkaloids—important therapeutic secondary metabolites of plant origin. J Crit Rev 2015; 2: 1-8.

[4] Tadeusz A. Alkaloids: Chemistry, Biology, Ecology, and Applications. 2nd ed., Amsterdam: Elsevier 2015.

[5] Heinrich M, Mah J, Amirkia V. Alkaloids used as medicines: structural phytochemistry meets biodiversity—an update and forward look. Molecules 2021; 26(7): 1836. [http://dx.doi.org/10.3390/molecules26071836] [PMID: 33805869]

[6] Goławska S, Sprawka I, Łukasik I, Goławski A. Are naringenin and quercetin useful chemicals in pest-management strategies?. J Pest Sci 2014; 87(1): 173-80. [http://dx.doi.org/10.1007/s10340-013-0535-5] [PMID: 24563648]

[7] Zhang Y, Cai P, Cheng G, Zhang Y. A brief review of phenolic compounds identified from plants: their extraction, analysis, and biological activity. Nat Prod Commun 2022; 17(1): 1934578X211069721. [http://dx.doi.org/10.1177/1934578X211069721]

[8] Amann R, Peskar BA. Anti-inflammatory effects of aspirin and sodium salicylate. Eur J Pharmacol 2002; 447(1): 1-9. [http://dx.doi.org/10.1016/S0014-2999(02)01828-9] [PMID: 12106797]

[9] Hoffmann D. Medical Herbalism: The Science and Practice of Herbal Medicine. Rochester: Healing Arts Press 2003.

[10] Xu L, Wu Y, Zhao X, Zhang W. The study on biological and pharmacological activity of coumarins. Asia-Pacific Energy Equipment Engineering Research Conference (AP3ER). 2015; pp. 135-8. [http://dx.doi.org/10.2991/ap3er-15.2015.33]

[11] Goenka P, Sarawgi A, Karun V, Nigam A, Dutta S, Marwah N. Camellia sinensis (Tea): Implications and role in preventing dental decay. Pharmacogn Rev 2013; 7(14): 152-6. [http://dx.doi.org/10.4103/0973-7847.120515] [PMID: 24347923]

[12] Jepson RG, Craig JC. Cranberries for preventing urinary tract infections. Cochrane Database Syst Rev 2008; 1(1): CD001321. [http://dx.doi.org/10.1002/14651858.CD001321.pub4] [PMID: 18253990]

[13] Motsei ML, Lindsey KL, van Staden J, Jäger AK. Screening of traditionally used South African plants for antifungal activity against Candida albicans. J Ethnopharmacol 2003; 86(2-3): 235-41. [http://dx.doi.org/10.1016/S0378-8741(03)00082-5] [PMID: 12738093]

[14] Serafini M, Peluso I, Raguzzini A. Flavonoids as anti-inflammatory agents. Proc Nutr Soc 2010; 69(3): 273-8. [http://dx.doi.org/10.1017/S002966511000162X] [PMID: 20569521]

[15] Kumar S, Pandey AK. Chemistry and biological activities of flavonoids: an overview. ScientificWorldJournal 2013; 2013(1): 162750. [http://dx.doi.org/10.1155/2013/162750] [PMID: 24470791]

[16] Barker D. Lignans. Molecules 2019; 24(7): 1424. [http://dx.doi.org/10.3390/molecules24071424] [PMID: 30978936]

[17] Mbaze LM, Lado JA, Wansi JD, *et al.* Oxidative burst inhibitory and cytotoxic amides and lignans from the stem bark of *Fagara heitzii* (Rutaceae). Phytochemistry 2009; 70(11-12): 1442-7. [http://dx.doi.org/10.1016/j.phytochem.2009.08.007] [PMID: 19747699]

[18] Gehm BD, McAndrews JM, Chien PY, Jameson JL. Resveratrol, a polyphenolic compound found in grapes and wine, is an agonist for the estrogen receptor. Proc Natl Acad Sci USA 1997; 94(25): 14138-43. [http://dx.doi.org/10.1073/pnas.94.25.14138] [PMID: 9391166]

[19] Güçlü-Üstündağ Ö, Mazza G. Saponins: properties, applications and processing. Crit Rev Food Sci Nutr 2007; 47(3): 231-58. [http://dx.doi.org/10.1080/10408390600698197] [PMID: 17453922]

[20] Seigler DS. Plant Secondary Metabolism. New York: Springer Science: Business Media 1995.

[21] Ninkuu V, Zhang L, Yan J, Fu Z, Yang T, Zeng H. Biochemistry of terpenes and recent advances in plant protection. Int J Mol Sci 2021; 22(11): 5710. [http://dx.doi.org/10.3390/ijms22115710] [PMID: 34071919]

[22] Asif HM, Akram M, Saeed TM, Khan I, Akhtar N, Ur Rehman R, *et al.* Review paper carbohydrates. Int Res J BiochemBioinform 2011; 1(1): 1-5.

[23] Anbalahan N. Pharmacological activity of mucilage isolated from medicinal plants. Int J Appl Pure Sci Agric 2017; 3(1): 98-113.

[24] Fahy E, Subramaniam S, Murphy RC, *et al.* Update of the LIPID MAPS comprehensive classification system for lipids. J Lipid Res 2009; 50(Suppl) (Suppl.): S9-S14. [http://dx.doi.org/10.1194/jlr.R800095-JLR200] [PMID: 19098281]

[25] Ali S, Ekbbal R, Salar S, *et al.* Quality standards and pharmacological interventions of natural oils: current scenario and future perspectives. ACS Omega 2023; 8(43): 39945-63. [http://dx.doi.org/10.1021/acsomega.3c05241] [PMID: 37953833]

[26] de Sousa DP, Damasceno ROS, Amorati R, *et al.* Essential oils: chemistry and pharmacological activities. Biomolecules 2023; 13(7): 1144. [http://dx.doi.org/10.3390/biom13071144] [PMID: 37509180]

[27] Pagare S, Bhatia M, Tripathi N, Bansal YK. Secondary metabolites of plants and their role: overview. Curr Trends Biotechnol Pharm 2015; 9: 293-304.

[28] Erb M, Kliebenstein DJ. Plant secondary metabolites as defenses, regulators, and primary metabolites: the blurred functional trichotomy. Plant Physiol 2020; 184(1): 39-52. [http://dx.doi.org/10.1104/pp.20.00433] [PMID: 32636341]

[29] Savithramma N, Rao ML, Suhrulatha D. Screening of medicinal plants for secondary metabolites 2011; 2(4): 643-7.

[30] Behl T, Gupta A, Albratty M, *et al.* Alkaloidalphytoconstituents for diabetes management: Exploring the unrevealed potential. Molecules 2022; 27(18): 5851. [http://dx.doi.org/10.3390/molecules27185851] [PMID: 36144587]

[31] Marchiosi R, dos Santos WD, Constantin RP, *et al.* Biosynthesis and metabolic actions of simple phenolic acids in plants. Phytochem Rev 2020; 19(4): 865-906. [http://dx.doi.org/10.1007/s11101-020-09689-2]

[32] Al-Shawi AAA, Hameed MF, Ali NH, Hussein KA. Investigations of phytoconstituents, antioxidant and anti-liver cancer activities of sauedamonoicaforssk extracted by microwave-assisted extraction. Asian Pac J Cancer Prev 2020; 21(8): 2349. [http://dx.doi.org/10.31557/APJCP.2020.21.8.2349]

[33] Botha LE, Prinsloo G, Deutschländer MS. Variations in the accumulation of three secondary metabolites in Euclea undulata Thunb. var. myrtina as a function of seasonal changes. S Afr J Bot 2018; 117: 34-40. [http://dx.doi.org/10.1016/j.sajb.2018.04.016]

[34] Kaushik B, Sharma J, Yadav K, Kumar P, Shourie A. Phytochemical properties and pharmacological role of plants: Secondary metabolites. Biosci Biotechnol Res Asia 2021; 18(1): 23-35. [http://dx.doi.org/10.13005/bbra/2894]

[35] Good G. Angew Chem Int Ed. 2015; 6: pp. (11)951-2.

[36] Ayabe SI, Uchiyama H, Aoki T, Akashi T. Plant phenolics: Phenylpropanoids. Compr Nat Prod II Chem Biol 2010; 1: 929-76. [http://dx.doi.org/10.1016/B978-008045382-8.00023-X]

[37] Jepson W, Brown JC, Koeppe M. Agricultural intensification on Brazil's soybean frontier in southern

Rondônia. In: Millington A, Jepson W, Eds. Land Change Science in the Tropics. Springer Publications 2008.

[38] Xue , *et al.* TGG 2015 Suppl Fig1 [Internet]. [cited 2024 Jul 22].

[39] Li J, Saunders JC, Gilmour RS, Silver M, Fowden AL. Insulin-like growth factor-II messenger ribonucleic acid expression in fetal tissues of the sheep during late gestation: effects of cortisol. Endocrinology 1993; 132(5): 2083-9.https://pubmed.ncbi.nlm.nih.gov/8477658/ [http://dx.doi.org/10.1210/endo.132.5.8477658] [PMID: 8477658]

[40] De Klerk GJ, Guan H, Huisman P, Marinova S. Effects of phenolic compounds on adventitious root formation and oxidative decarboxylation of applied indoleacetic acid in Malus 'Jork 9'. Plant Growth Regul 2011; 63(2): 175-85. [http://dx.doi.org/10.1007/s10725-010-9555-9]

[41] Salvador JM, Brown-Clay JD, Fornace AJ Jr. Gadd45 in stress signaling, cell cycle control, and apoptosis. Adv Exp Med Biol 2013; 793: 1-19. [http://dx.doi.org/10.1007/978-1-4614-8289-5_1] [PMID: 24104470]

[42] Smith AR, Pryer KM, Schuettpelz E, Korall P, Schneider H, Wolf PG. A classification for extant ferns. Taxon 2006; 55(3): 705-31. [http://dx.doi.org/10.2307/25065646]

[43] Koyama H, Kawamura A, Kihara T, Hara T, Takita E, Shibata D. Overexpression of mitochondrial citrate synthase in Arabidopsis thaliana improved growth on a phosphorus-limited soil. Plant Cell Physiol 2000; 41(9): 1030-7. [http://dx.doi.org/10.1093/pcp/pcd029] [PMID: 11100775]

[44] Gao W, Zhang W, Meldrum DR. RT-qPCR based quantitative analysis of gene expression in single bacterial cells. J Microbiol Methods 2011; 85(3): 221-7. [http://dx.doi.org/10.1016/j.mimet.2011.03.008] [PMID: 21440012]

[45] Stratton K, Shetty P, Wallace R, Bondurant S. Nicotine pharmacology. Reducing Tobacco Harm: A Public Health Imperative 2001. Available from: https://www.ncbi.nlm.nih.gov/books/NBK222359/

[46] Zhang J, Davies WJ. Increased synthesis of ABA in partially dehydrated root tips and ABA transport from roots to leaves. J Exp Bot 1987; 38(12): 2015-23. [http://dx.doi.org/10.1093/jxb/38.12.2015]

[47] Chun KS, Kim DH, Raut PK, Surh YJ. Anticancer natural products targeting immune checkpoint protein network. Semin Cancer Biol 2022; 86(Pt 3): 1008-32. [http://dx.doi.org/10.1016/j.semcancer.2021.11.006] [PMID: 34838956]

[48] Jing S, Zou H, Wu Z, *et al.* Cucurbitacins: Bioactivities and synergistic effect with small-molecule drugs. J Funct Foods 2020; 72: 104042. [http://dx.doi.org/10.1016/j.jff.2020.104042]

[49] Szlasa W, Janicka N, Sauer N, *et al.* Chemotherapy and physical therapeutics modulate antigens on cancer cells. Front Immunol 2022; 13: 889950. [http://dx.doi.org/10.3389/fimmu.2022.889950] [PMID: 35874714]

[50] Thakur K, Partap M, Kumar P, Sharma R, Warghat AR. Understandings of bioactive composition, molecular regulation, and biotechnological interventions in the development and usage of specialized metabolites as health-promoting substances in Siraitia grosvenorii (Swingle) C. Jeffrey. J Food Compos Anal 2023; 116: 105070. [http://dx.doi.org/10.1016/j.jfca.2022.105070]

[51] Szakiel A, Pączkowski C, Henry M. Influence of environmental abiotic factors on the content of saponins in plants. Phytochem Rev 2011; 10(4): 471-91. [http://dx.doi.org/10.1007/s11101-010-9177-x]

[52] Thirumurugan D, Cholarajan A, Raja SS, Vijayakumar R. An introductory chapter: secondary metabolites. Secondary Metabolites-Sources and Applications 2018; 1: 13.

[53] Twaij BM, Hasan MN. Bioactive secondary metabolites from plant sources: types, synthesis, and their therapeutic uses. Int J Plant Biol 2022; 13(1): 4-14.
[http://dx.doi.org/10.3390/ijpb13010003]

[54] Reshi ZA, Ahmad W, Lukatkin AS, Javed SB. From nature to lab: A review of secondary metabolite biosynthetic pathways, environmental influences, and *in vitro* approaches. Metabolites 2023; 13(8): 895.
[http://dx.doi.org/10.3390/metabo13080895] [PMID: 37623839]

[55] Demain AL, Fang A. The natural functions of secondary metabolites. Adv Biochem Eng Biotechnol 2000; 69: 1-39.
[http://dx.doi.org/10.1007/3-540-44964-7_1] [PMID: 11036689]

[56] Wink M. Modes of action of herbal medicines and plant secondary metabolites. Medicines (Basel) 2015; 2(3): 251-86.
[http://dx.doi.org/10.3390/medicines2030251] [PMID: 28930211]

[57] Mikail HG, Mohammed M, Umar HD, Suleiman MM. Secondary metabolites: The natural remedies

[58] Divekar PA, Narayana S, Divekar BA, *et al.* Plant secondary metabolites as defense tools against herbivores for sustainable crop protection. Int J Mol Sci 2022; 23(5): 2690.
[http://dx.doi.org/10.3390/ijms23052690] [PMID: 35269836]

[59] Claros Cuadrado JL, Pinillos EO, Tito R, Mirones CS, Gamarra Mendoza NN. Insecticidal properties of capsaicinoids and glucosinolates extracted from *Capsicum chinense* and *Tropaeolumtuberosum*. Insects 2019; 10(5): 132.
[http://dx.doi.org/10.3390/insects10050132] [PMID: 31064092]

[60] Demain AL. Pharmaceutically active secondary metabolites of microorganisms. Appl Microbiol Biotechnol 1999; 52(4): 455-63.
[http://dx.doi.org/10.1007/s002530051546] [PMID: 10570792]

[61] Caputi L, Aprea E. Use of terpenoids as natural flavouring compounds in food industry. Recent Pat Food Nutr Agric 2011; 3(1): 9-16.
[http://dx.doi.org/10.2174/2212798411103010009] [PMID: 21114471]

[62] Sarkic A, Stappen I. Essential oils and their single compounds in cosmetics—A critical review. Cosmetics 2018; 5(1): 11.
[http://dx.doi.org/10.3390/cosmetics5010011]

[63] Stępniowska A, Cieplińska P, Fac W, Górska J. Selected alkaloids used in the cosmetics industry. J Cosmet Sci 2021; 72(2): 229-45.
[PMID: 35361327]

[64] Sadegh N, Haddadi H, Sadegh F, Asfaram A. Recent advances and perspectives of tannin-based adsorbents for wastewater pollutants elimination: A review. Environ Nanotechnol Monit Manag 2023; 19: 100763.
[http://dx.doi.org/10.1016/j.enmm.2022.100763]

[65] Nirmala L. PadminiAmma ZD, Jalaj AV Plant secondary metabolites as nutraceuticals Plant Metabolites: Methods. Applications and Prospects 2020; pp. 239-53.

[66] Huang X, Gull N, Hussain L, Bazmi RR, Jamshed A, Siddique R, *et al.* The emerging trend of phytochemicals and nutraceuticals-based traditional medicines and their role in chronic disease management. J Biol Regul Homeost Agents 2024; 38(1): 31-45.
[http://dx.doi.org/10.23812/j.biol.regul.homeost.agents.20243801.3]

[67] Kopple JD, Massry SG, Kalantar-Zadeh K, Fouque D, Eds. Nutritional management of renal disease. 4th ed. United States: Academic Press 2022; pp. 907-19.

[68] Wang Z, Zu X, Xiong S, *et al.* The role of colchicine in different clinical phenotypes of Behcet disease. Clin Ther 2023; 45(2): 162-76.

[http://dx.doi.org/10.1016/j.clinthera.2023.01.004] [PMID: 36732153]

[69] Bu N, Liaqat H, Anam Y, Syed Haroon K, Yun W, Imran I, *et al.* Management of polycystic ovarian syndrome; a metabolic morbidity of reproductive age, special focus on the role of natural and alternative medicine. J Biol Regul Homeost Agents 2023; 37(9): 4531-46. [http://dx.doi.org/10.23812/j.biol.regul.homeost.agents.20233709.443]

[70] Bérdy J. Bioactive microbial metabolites. J Antibiot (Tokyo) 2005; 58(1): 1-26. [http://dx.doi.org/10.1038/ja.2005.1] [PMID: 15813176]

[71] Rajeev L. Antibiotic Discovery. Materials and Methods 2018; 8: 2671. [http://dx.doi.org/10.13070/mm.en.8.2671]

[72] Shamsudin, N. F., Ahmed, Q. U., Mahmood, S., *et al.* (2022). Antibacterial effects of flavonoids and their structure-activity relationship study: A comparative interpretation. Molecules, 27(4), 1149. [http://dx.doi.org/10.3390/molecules27041149] [PMID: 24470791]

[73] Newman DJ, Cragg GM. Natural products as sources of new drugs over the nearly four decades from 01/1981 to 09/2019. J Nat Prod 2020; 83(3): 770-803. [http://dx.doi.org/10.1021/acs.jnatprod.9b01285] [PMID: 32162523]

[74] Gorlenko CL, Kiselev HY, Budanova EV, Zamyatnin AA Jr, Ikryannikova LN. ZamyatninJr AA, Ikryannikova LN. Plant secondary metabolites in the battle of drugs and drug-resistant bacteria: new heroes or worse clones of antibiotics?. Antibiotics (Basel) 2020; 9(4): 170. [http://dx.doi.org/10.3390/antibiotics9040170] [PMID: 32290036]

[75] Valeeva LR, Dague AL, Hall MH, *et al.* Antimicrobial activities of secondary metabolites from model mosses. Antibiotics (Basel) 2022; 11(8): 1004. [http://dx.doi.org/10.3390/antibiotics11081004] [PMID: 35892395]

[76] Ghasemian M, Owlia S, Owlia MB. Review of anti-inflammatory herbal medicines. Adv Pharmacol Sci 2016; 2016: 1-11. [http://dx.doi.org/10.1155/2016/9130979] [PMID: 27247570]

[77] Jakhetia V, Patel R, Khatri P, Pahuja N, Garg S, Pandey A, *et al.* Cinnamon: a pharmacological review. Int J Adv Sci Res 2010; 1(2): 19-23.

[78] Block KI, Gyllenhaal C, Lowe L, *et al.* Designing a broad-spectrum integrative approach for cancer prevention and treatment. Semin Cancer Biol 2015; 35(Suppl) (Suppl.): S276-304. [http://dx.doi.org/10.1016/j.semcancer.2015.09.007] [PMID: 26590477]

[79] Huang M, Lu JJ, Ding J. Natural products in cancer therapy: past, present and future. Nat Prod Bioprospect 2021; 11(1): 5-13. [http://dx.doi.org/10.1007/s13659-020-00293-7] [PMID: 33389713]

[80] Theofylaktou D, Takan I, Karakülah G, *et al.* Mining natural products with anticancer biological activity through a systems biology approach. Oxid Med Cell Longev 2021; 2021(1): 9993518. [http://dx.doi.org/10.1155/2021/9993518] [PMID: 34422220]

[81] Sammar M, Abu-Farich B, Rayan I, Falah M, Rayan A. Correlation between cytotoxicity in cancer cells and free radical-scavenging activity: *In-vitro* evaluation of 57 medicinal and edible plant extracts. Oncol Lett 2019; 18(6): 6563-71. [http://dx.doi.org/10.3892/ol.2019.11054] [PMID: 31819777]

[82] Moore A, Pinkerton R. Vincristine: Can its therapeutic index be enhanced?. Pediatr Blood Cancer 2009; 53(7): 1180-7. [http://dx.doi.org/10.1002/pbc.22161] [PMID: 19588521]

[83] Almagro L, Fernández-Pérez F, Pedreño M. Indole alkaloids from Catharanthus roseus: bioproduction and their effect on human health. Molecules 2015; 20(2): 2973-3000. [http://dx.doi.org/10.3390/molecules20022973] [PMID: 25685907]

[84] Bernabeu E, Cagel M, Lagomarsino E, Moretton M, Chiappetta DA. Paclitaxel: What has been done

and the challenges remain ahead. Int J Pharm 2017; 526(1-2): 474-95.
[http://dx.doi.org/10.1016/j.ijpharm.2017.05.016] [PMID: 28501439]

[85] Kantarjian HM, O'Brien S, Cortes J. Homoharringtonine/omacetaxine mepesuccinate: the long and winding road to food and drug administration approval. Clin Lymphoma Myeloma Leuk 2013; 13(5): 530-3.
[http://dx.doi.org/10.1016/j.clml.2013.03.017] [PMID: 23790799]

[86] Ali M, Khan T, Fatima K, *et al.* Selected hepatoprotective herbal medicines: Evidence from ethnomedicinal applications, animal models, and possible mechanism of actions. Phytother Res 2018; 32(2): 199-215.
[http://dx.doi.org/10.1002/ptr.5957] [PMID: 29047177]

[87] Meng X, Li Y, Li S, Gan RY, Li HB. Natural products for prevention and treatment of chemical-induced liver injuries. Compr Rev Food Sci Food Saf 2018; 17(2): 472-95.
[http://dx.doi.org/10.1111/1541-4337.12335] [PMID: 33350084]

[88] Mirza Alizadeh A, Golzan SA, Mahdavi A, Dakhili S, Torki Z, Hosseini H. Recent advances on the efficacy of essential oils on mycotoxin secretion and their mode of action. Crit Rev Food Sci Nutr 2022; 62(17): 4726-51.
[http://dx.doi.org/10.1080/10408398.2021.1878102] [PMID: 33523705]

[89] Velu G, Palanichamy V, Rajan AP. Phytochemical and pharmacological importance of plant secondary metabolites in modern medicine. Bioorg Phase Nat Food 2018; 135-56.
[http://dx.doi.org/10.1007/978-3-319-74210-6_8]

[90] Report of the expert committee on the diagnosis and classification of diabetes mellitus. Diabetes Care 2003; 26 (Suppl. 1): s5-s20.
[http://dx.doi.org/10.2337/diacare.26.2007.S5] [PMID: 12502614]

[91] Sukhikh S, Babich O, Prosekov A, *et al.* Antidiabetic properties of plant secondary metabolites. Metabolites 2023; 13(4): 513.
[http://dx.doi.org/10.3390/metabo13040513] [PMID: 37110171]

[92] Zhang Y, Gu Y, Ren H, *et al.* Gut microbiome-related effects of berberine and probiotics on type 2 diabetes (the PREMOTE study). Nat Commun 2020; 11(1): 5015.
[http://dx.doi.org/10.1038/s41467-020-18414-8] [PMID: 33024120]

[93] Mi J, He W, Lv J, Zhuang K, Huang H, Quan S. Effect of berberine on the HPA-axis pathway and skeletal muscle GLUT4 in type 2 diabetes mellitus rats. Diabetes Metab Syndr Obes 2019; 12: 1717-25.
[http://dx.doi.org/10.2147/DMSO.S211188] [PMID: 31564939]

[94] Mahwish , Saeed F, Sultan MT, *et al.* Bitter melon (*Momordicacharantia L.*) fruit bioactivescharantin and vicine potential for diabetes prophylaxis and treatment. Plants 2021; 10(4): 730.
[http://dx.doi.org/10.3390/plants10040730] [PMID: 33918062]

[95] Naseri K, Saadati S, Sadeghi A, *et al.* The efficacy of ginseng (Panax) on human prediabetes and type 2 diabetes mellitus: A systematic review and meta-analysis. Nutrients 2022; 14(12): 2401.
[http://dx.doi.org/10.3390/nu14122401] [PMID: 35745129]

[96] Zheng T, Bian F, Chen L, Wang Q, Jin S. Beneficial effects of Rhodiola and salidroside in diabetes: potential role of AMP-activated protein kinase. Mol Diagn Ther 2019; 23(4): 489-98.
[http://dx.doi.org/10.1007/s40291-019-00402-4] [PMID: 31069710]

[97] Aswar U, Gogawale V, Miniyar P, Patil Y. Beneficial effects of Stevioside on AGEs, blood glucose, lipid profile and renal status in streptozotocin-induced diabetic rats. J Appl Biomed 2019; 17(3): 190-7.
[http://dx.doi.org/10.32725/jab.2019.013] [PMID: 34907701]

[98] Iriti M, Vitalini S, Fico G, Faoro F. Neuroprotective herbs and foods from different traditional medicines and diets. Molecules 2010; 15(5): 3517-55.

[http://dx.doi.org/10.3390/molecules15053517] [PMID: 20657497]

[99] Ghasemzadeh A, Jaafar HZE. Optimization of reflux conditions for total flavonoid and total phenolic extraction and enhanced antioxidant capacity in Pandan (*Pandanus amaryllifolius Roxb.*) using response surface methodology. ScientificWorldJournal 2014; 2014: 1-10. [http://dx.doi.org/10.1155/2014/523120] [PMID: 25147852]

[100] Bhatt N, Deshpande M. A critical review and scientific prospective on contraceptive therapeutics from Ayurveda and allied ancient knowledge. Front Pharmacol 2021; 12: 629591. [http://dx.doi.org/10.3389/fphar.2021.629591] [PMID: 34149405]

CHAPTER 4

Harnessing The Role of Terpenoids in Type 1 Diabetes Mellitus

Vishakha Saini[1,*], **Jasmeen Kaur**[1], **Rashmi Bhamra**[2], **Kulvinder Kaur**[2], **Varinder Kaur**[2], **Rupa Devi**[1] and **Ashwani K. Dhingra**[3]

[1] *Department of Pharmaceutics, Global Research Institute of Pharmacy, Radaur, Yamuna Nagar 135133, Haryana, India*

[2] *Department of Pharmacy, Global Research Institute of Pharmacy, Radaur, Yamuna Nagar 135133, Haryana, India*

[3] *Department of Pharmaceutical Chemistry, Global Research Institute of Pharmacy, Radaur, Yamuna Nagar 135133, Haryana, India*

Abstract: Type-1 Diabetes Mellitus (T1DM) poses major complications due to its autoimmune nature, which is characterized by pancreatic β-cell breakdown, resulting in a lack of insulin as well as dysregulated glucose metabolism. While insulin therapy remains the cornerstone of T1DM management, emerging research investigating adjunctive therapies includes natural compounds, such as terpenoids derived from plants. Regenerative medicine aims to generate new insulin-producing cells derived from various cell kinds to treat T1DM, which is caused by the loss of pancreatic β cells. Terpenoids, also known as isoprenoids, are natural chemicals derived from isoprene that play important functions in all species' metabolisms. Natural terpenoid compounds have been classified into five different categories based on their structure: monoterpenoids (Paeoniflorin, Catalpol, Geniposide), sesquiterpenoids (Curcumol, β-Patchoulene), diterpenoids (Carnosic Acid, Ginkgolide), triterpenoids (Ginsenoside, Ursolic Acid), and tetraterpenoids (Lycopene, Astaxanthin). Terpenoids appear to have a therapeutic impact on non-alcoholic fatty liver disease, largely *via* insulin resistance, regulating lipid metabolism, inflammation, and oxidative stress. Terpenoids can help diagnose diabetic nephropathy by decreasing the production of pro-inflammatory cytokines (α-amylase and α-glucosidase), controlling glycolipid metabolism, and lowering renal inflammation. We look at some of the most beneficial and promising terpenoids that are now being employed in medicine and research, as well as the most recent information on their natural occurrence, biosynthesis, and mechanism of action in the body. Terpenoids promote the proliferation and development of osteoblast cells in high-glucose circumstances. These findings demonstrated that terpenoids stimulated glycogenesis *via* the PI3K/AKT pathway while inhibiting glucosamine-induced gluconeogenesis by downregulating gluconeogenesis enzymes. Despite these encouraging findings, the therapeutic potential of terpenoids in T1DM has to be further investigated through rigorous preclinical and clinical trials.

* **Corresponding author Vishakha Saini:** Global research institute of pharmacy, Radaur, Yamuna Nagar 135133, Haryana, India; E-mail: vishakhabanwait@gmail.com

M.S. Ashawat, Aditi Kaushik, Akash Jain, Jasmine Chaudhary & Manish Kaushik (Eds.)
All rights reserved-© 2025 Bentham Science Publishers

Keywords: Diabetes, Gluconeogenesis, Insulin, Pro-inflammatory cytokines, Terpenoids.

INTRODUCTION

Hyperglycemia, the hallmark of diabetes mellitus, is a chronic metabolic state that has spread like an epidemic over the globe. Diabetes mellitus can lead to limb blindness, kidney amputation, cardiovascular disease, failure, and other problems. Diabetes mellitus patients' lives are affected as a result of these consequences [1]. Diabetes is a vast public health concern around the world. Currently, one in every eleven adults has the illness, and some forecasts suggest that by 2050, more than one-third of humans will have the disorder. Diabetes-related problems claim the lives of over 4 million individuals globally each year. Diabetes healthcare spending was expected to reach $727 billion globally per year in 2017, with medication therapy accounting for 40% of total diabetes spending [2]. Diabetes can be triggered by a lack of insulin production, damage to pancreatic β cells, or insulin resistance from non-use. Sedentary lifestyles may contribute to the increasing proportion of diabetic patients worldwide, projected to spread to 366 million in 2030 among the elderly. Diabetes may lead to consequences such as kidney disease, neuropathy, cardiac and renal problems, retinopathy, and food-related illnesses [3].

T1DM is triggered by the autoimmune destruction of endocrine pancreas cells. TIDM pathophysiology is distinct from that of type 2 diabetes mellitus, where reduced cell production of insulin and insulin resistance coexist [4]. T1DM is a fatal disease that results in insulin insufficiency and diabetes due to the autoimmune destruction of β cells. Ten million individuals worldwide suffer from the illness, and many of its side effects, such as nephropathy, retinopathy, neuropathy, and cardiovascular problems, are fatal [5, 6]. Because T1DM includes several pathways and is controlled by both the immune and endocrine systems, its pathophysiology is complex. Genetic, immunological, or environmental factors are the leading causes of T1DM development [4, 6, 7]. The development and consequences of type 1 diabetes are attributed to immune system dysregulation and β-cell homeostasis. Dendritic cells, macrophages, β cells, and antigen-presenting cells convey auto-antigens, including insulin and glutamic acid decarboxylase, to T-cells during the development of T1DM. Following activation, T-cells divide into several subsets of T cells. Local inflammatory cytokines, such as TNF-α, perforin, and IFN-γ, are generated when cells invade the pancreas, causing insulitis. Furthermore, misdirected autoimmunity Myeloid-Derived Suppressor Cells (MDSC) and other immune cells are influenced by regulatory T cells and natural killer cells [5, 8 - 10]. As a result, β cells undergo apoptosis, leading to dysfunction. The pathogenic situation of diabetes is associated with β-cell bulk and function decline [11]. The most common endocrine and metabolic disorder affecting children is T1DM. For those with T1DM, insulin treatment may be both life-saving and permanent. A person with T1DM has to follow a thorough self-management plan like blood glucose monitoring, insulin use, exercise, and a balanced diet [12]. Three interconnected processes—genetic susceptibility, autoimmunity, and environmental factors—contribute to the pathophysiology of T1DM. The two main insulin formulations utilized in the pharmacological treatment of T1DM are insulin lispro and insulin aspart, both of which are rapid-acting insulin. Insulin that acts quickly includes regular Humulin, Velosulin BR, and long-acting or intermediate-acting insulin, such as insulin glargine (Lantus), Lente Humulin, and NPH (Neutral Protamine Hagedorn).

The most important and most varied class of complexes derived from plants is called terpenoids, as shown in Table **1**. Food and pharmaceutical companies, among others, have made substantial use of these plant-derived terpenoids [13]. Terpenoids, alkaloids, and phenylpropane chemicals make up the majority of the biologically active components found in therapeutic plants [14]. Terpenoids are one of the most abundant and structurally varied classes of naturally occurring chemicals [15]. There are about 80,000 different types of terpenoids found in almost all living things. Because of their structural variety, terpenoids may be used in flavors, biofuels, and pharmaceutical applications. The Methylerythritol-Phosphate (MEP) pathway in prokaryotes and plant plastids, as well as the Mevalonate (MVA) route in eukaryotes, naturally produce isopentenyl diphosphate and its isomer, dimethylallyl diphosphate. The skeletons of terpenoids are made up of these parts [16]. One of the most structurally diverse classes of natural materials is composed of tens of thousands of naturally occurring hydrocarbons [17]. Terpenoids, of which there have been over 25,000 identified chemical species, are the most prevalent class of secondary metabolites in plants. Based on the quantity of five-carbon units in their structure, terpenes are classified as monoterpenes, sesquiterpenes, diterpenes, triterpenes, tetraterpenes, and high polyterpenes. Terpenes are structurally constituted of one or more five-carbon units. Important volatile plant compounds called monoterpenes and sesquiterpenes support interactions between plants, microorganisms, and animals as well as defensive reactions [18]. These include pain-relieving anti-malarial artemisinins, cannabinoids, anti-cardiovascular tanshinones, anti-tumor paclitaxel, and ginkgolides [13].

Table 1. Source of Terpenoids

Plant Species	Terpenes	References
Nicotiana attenuata	Sesquiterpenes: (E)-α-Bergamotene, (E)-β-Farnesene	[19, 20]
Oryza sativa	Monoterpenes:α-terpinolene, sabinene, limonene; myrcene; β-ocimene; α-terpinene; γ-terpinene	[21]
Vitis vinifera cv. Chardonay	monoterpenes	[22]
Pseudotsuga menziesii (douglas fir)	Monoterpenes: 3-carene; β-pinene; β-citronellol; α-pinene; camphene	[23]
Zea mays	Sesquiterpenoid: diterpenoid: zealexin, kaulalexins, together with ABA	[24]
Salvia fruticose, Salvia officinalis, Rosmarinus officinalis	Diterpene: carnosic acid	[25]
Cinnomon and clove	Eugenol, α-pinene, caryophyllene oxide, α-phellandrene and α-humulene	[25]
Panax notoginseng	P.notoginseng saponins	[13]
Ginko biloba	Ginkgolide	[13]
Cannabis sativa	Tetrahydrocannabinol	[13]
Taxus media	Paclitaxel	[13]
Panax ginseng	Ginsenoside	[13]

Terpenoid Pathways

The carbon backbone of highly modified terpenoids is designed by the combination of two key terpenoid metabolic intermediates, isopentenyl and dimethylallyl diphosphate, as shown in Fig. (**1**). Two insufficient metabolic pathways-the 2C-Methyl-D-Erythritol-4-Phosphate (MEP) route and the Mevalonic Acid (MVA) mechanism-are used by nature to produce them [26 - 28]. The MEP pathway is active in eubacteria, as well as the plastids of higher plants, protists, and algae, whereas the cytosolic MVA system supplies IDP as well as DMADP to nearly all archaea and eukaryotes [29]. Both precursor pathways are used by photosynthetic species; however, they are divided into different subcellular compartments. There is not much information on plants about the exchange of DMADP/IDP pools between the cytosol and plastid, which usually takes place during secondary metabolism [30 - 34]. For the synthesis of C40 tetraterpenes, C20 diterpenes, C10 monoterpenes, and the MEP route typically produces C5 prenyl diphosphates, but the MVA pathway does not. Terpenoids and their derivatives have been proven in numerous biological studies to possess a diverse range of pharmacological and physiological characteristics [35]. Terpenoids, which originate in therapeutic plants, are diverse and have a wide variety of medical applications. With many terpenoid chemicals being secondary metabolites, terpenoid chemical diversity is very beneficial in plants.

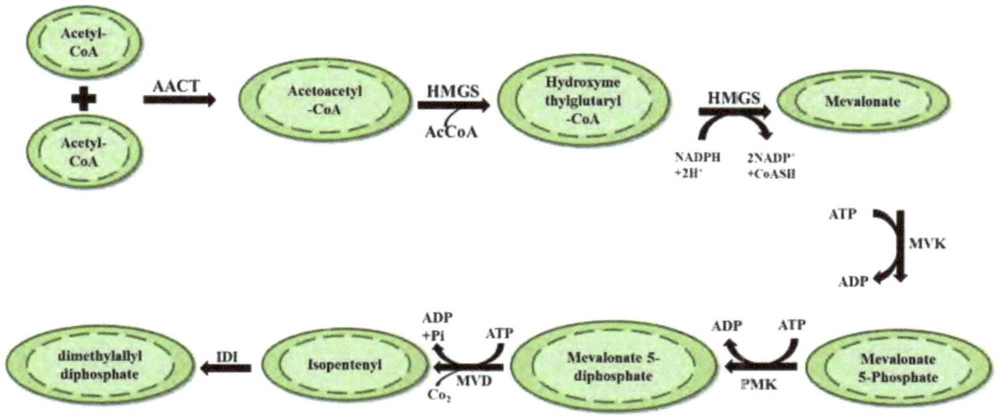

Fig. (1). Biosynthesis of isopentenyl & dimethylallyl diphosphate *via* MVA.

Classification of Terpenoids

The typical formula for most naturally occurring terpenoid hydrocarbons is $(C_5H_8)_n$. They can be divided into groups based on the value of n or the number of carbon atoms in the structure, as shown in Table **2** [36 - 38].

Table 2. Classification of terpenoids according to the number of carbon atoms present in the ring.

Sr. No.	No. of Carbon(C) atoms present	Value of n	Classifications of terpenoids	Formula
1	10	2	Monoterpenoids	$(C_{10}H_{16})$
2	15	3	Sesquiterpenoinds	$(C_{15}H_{24})$
3	20	4	Diterpenoids	$(C_{20}H_{32})$
4	25	5	Sesterpenoids	$(C_{25}H_{40})$
5	30	6	Triterpenoids	$(C_{30}H_{48})$
6	40	8	Tetraterpenoids	$(C_{40}H_{64})$
7	More than 40	More than 8	Polyterpenoids	$(C_5H_8)n$

Subclasses of Terpenoids

Depending on how many rings are in the structure, each class can be further divided into subclasses as shown in Table **3** [39 - 41].

Table 3. Classification of terpenoids according to the number of rings present in the structure.

Sr. No.	No. of the ring in the structure	Sub-Class	Examples	Structure
1	Open Ring	Acyclic Terpenoids	Linalool	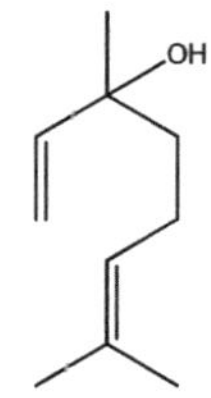
2	1	Monocyclic Terpenoids:	Citral,	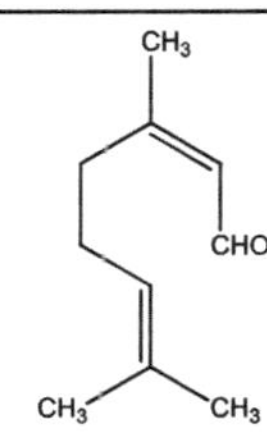
			Graniol	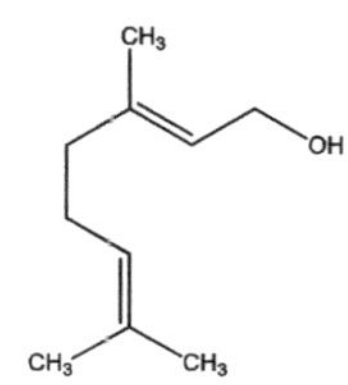
3	2	Bicyclic Terpenoids	Thujane	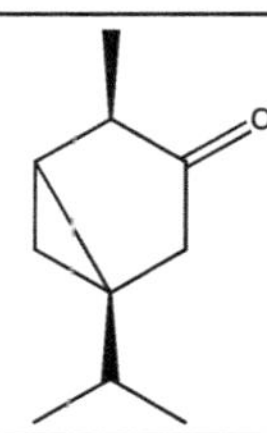
			Carane	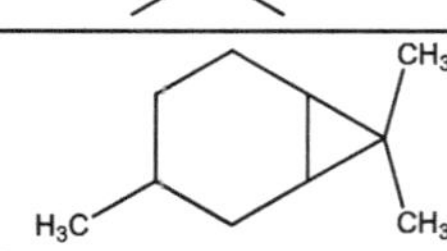
4	3	Tricyclic Terpenoids	Abietane,	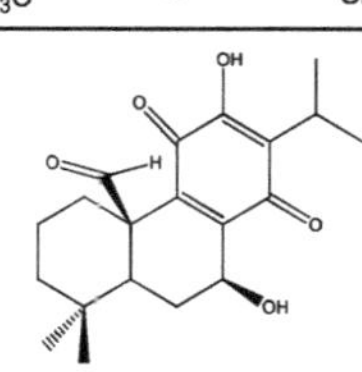
			Pimarane	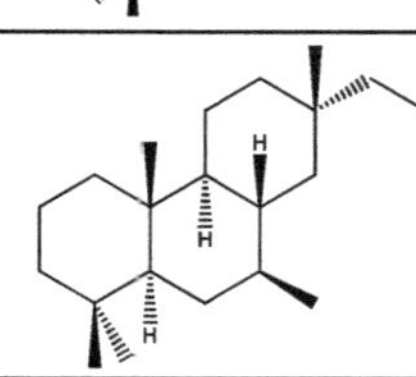

(Table 3) cont.....

Sr. No.	No. of the ring in the structure	Sub-Class	Examples	Structure
5	4	Tetracyclic Terpenoids	Lanosterol	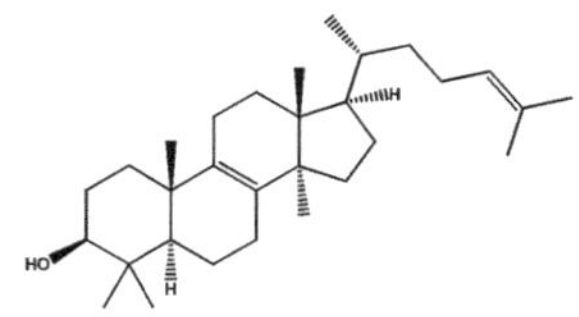
			Parkeol	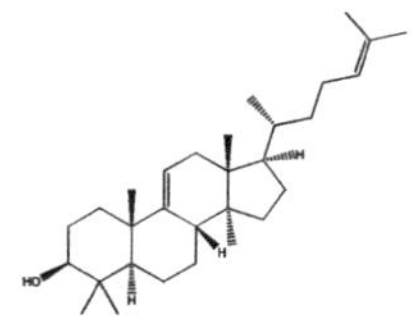

Terpenoids Antidiabetic Properties

There are several compounds that are used for the treatment or diagnosis of T1DM and some of them are shown in Table **4** [42 - 44].

Mechanism of Type 1 Diabetes Mellitus

Terpenoids treatment significantly reduces the level of blood glucose (by 23%) in STZ-induced diabetic rats [45, 46]. Furthermore, terpenoids were shown by Wang *et al.* to reduce FBG concentrations in STZ diabetic rats by 59% and 72%, respectively, during four weeks [47]. In High-Fat Diet (HFD)/Streptozotocin (STZ)-induced diabetic mice, it suggestively reduced serum insulin, Fasting Blood Glucose (FBG), triglycerides, total cholesterol, low-density lipoprotein and enhanced the insulin tolerance test and oral glucose tolerance test [48 - 52].

Activity of Terpenoids on Diabetes Mellitus

Monoterpenes are a type of secondary metabolite found in plants that are classified as terpenoids. In recent years, several drugs have been discovered to have antidiabetic characteristics. Terpenoids are secondary metabolites that originate in several types of plants. They are produced through the mevalonic acid pathway and have a role in the plant's defense mechanism and flavor profile [53].

Paeoniflorin effectively reduced the detrimental effects of STZ-induced mitochondrial dysfunction and enhanced the defective insulin signaling by promoting the expression of p-PI3K and pAkt proteins, while inhibiting the expression of p-IRS-1 protein.

The naturally occurring substance catalpol is derived from the roots of *Rehmannia glutinosa*. It has been discovered to have activity against diabetes. By modifying the expression of several genes, including Irs1, SOCS3, Idh2, and catalpol, G6pd2 produces a hypoglycemic effect [54].

Table 4. Terpenoids that have antidiabetic properties along with the structure.

Sr. No.	Class of Terpenoids	Antidiabetic Agents	Structure
1	Monoterpenoids	D-limonene	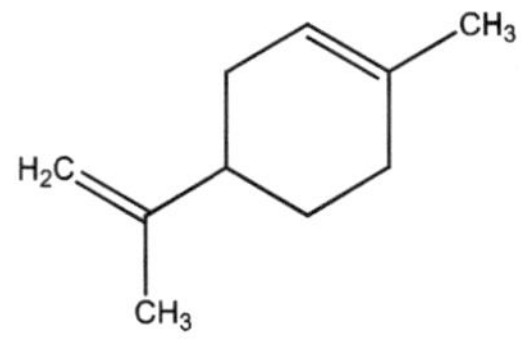
		Citronellol	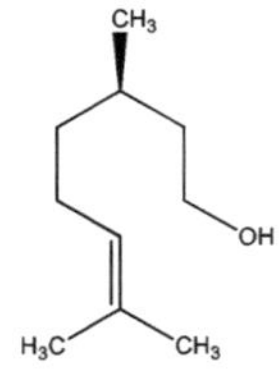
		Catalpol	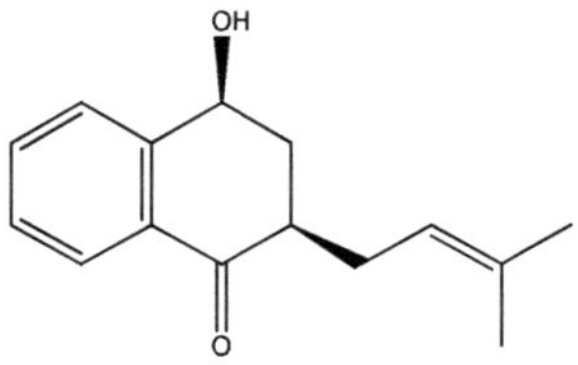
2	Sesquiterpenoinds	Caryophyllene	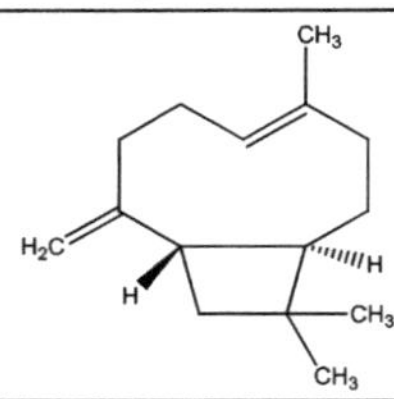
		Dysidine	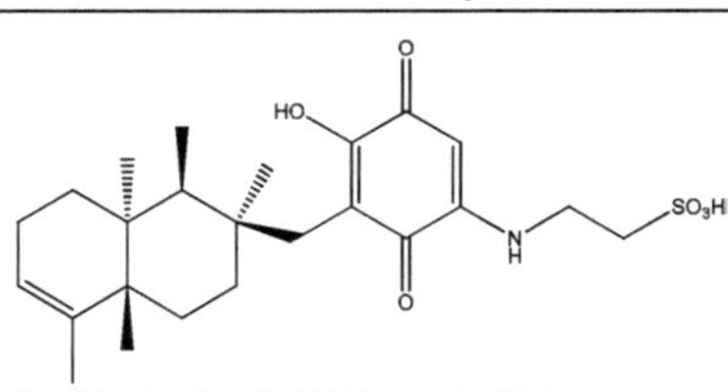
		Farnesol	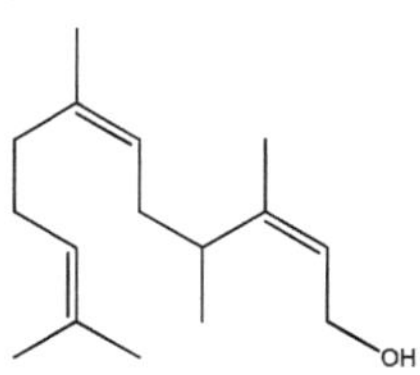

(Table 4) cont.....

Sr. No.	Class of Terpenoids	Antidiabetic Agents	Structure
3	Diterpenoids	Labdane	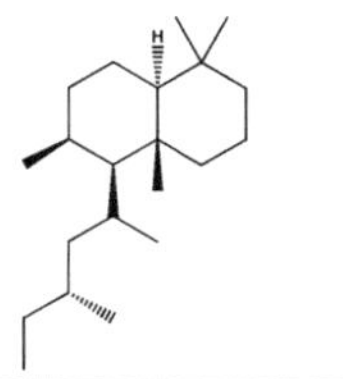
		Kaurane	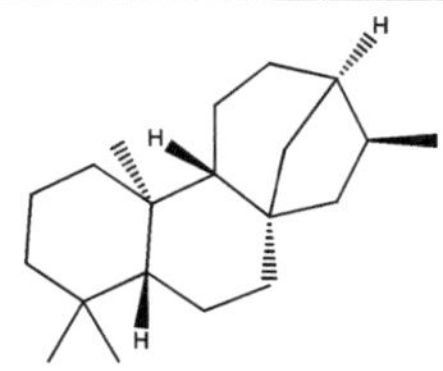
		Pimarane,	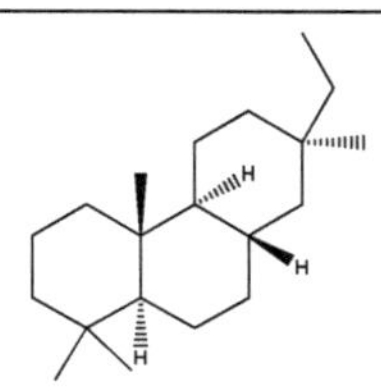
4	Triterpenoids	Limonoids	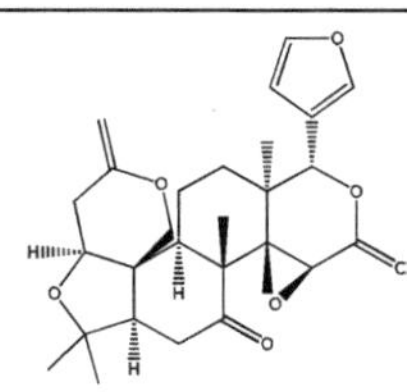
		Quassinoids	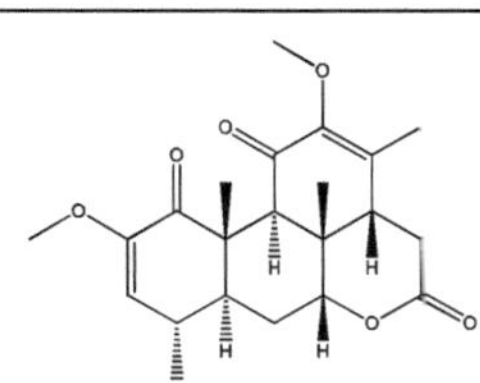
5	Tetraterpenoids	Betacarotene	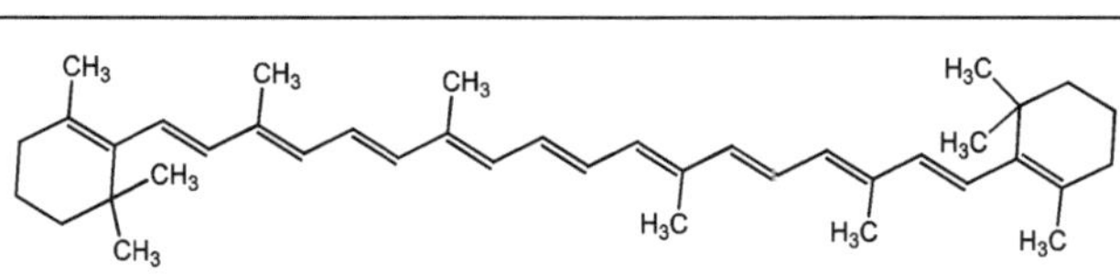

The lower blood glucose levels and enhanced insulin sensitivity can be activated through the Phosphatidylinositol-3-Kinase (PI3K)/protein kinase B (AKT) pathway. This showed increased amounts of myogenic differentiation markers, including MyoD, MyoG, and MHC, and enhanced muscle development [55].

In diabetic mice, the administration of carvacrol intraperitoneally at a dose of 20 mg/kg dramatically decreases the levels of plasma LDH and triglycerides.

However, there was no change in the levels of AST, ALT, or ALP. Carvacrol also increased the activities of Citrate Synthase (CS), 6-Phosphofructokinase (PFK), and Hexokinase (HK) [56].

One type of phenolic chemical that belongs to the monoterpene class is thymol. It possesses a diverse array of pharmacological properties. Thymol treatment decreased levels of adiponectin, HbA1c, insulin resistance, insulin, plasma glucose, and leptin. Plasma levels of HDL increased, while those of free fatty acids, triglycerides, low-density lipoprotein, and total cholesterol were considerably reduced when thymol was administered [57].

Genipin, the primary active compound found in Gardeniae fructus, has been shown to enhance diabetes management and reduce insulin resistance in rat models. The intervention increased dyslipidemia, insulin intolerance, hepatic steatosis, glucose intolerance, and adipocyte hypertrophy in diet-induced obese mice, while lowering blood levels of tumor necrosis factor α. The text is referenced by the number [58].

It has been demonstrated that giving diabetic rats geraniol supplements preserves their pancreatic beta cells and liver cells in normal histological structure [59]. Myrtenal decreases plasma glucose levels while increasing insulin levels. It also increases the levels of GLUT2, Akt, as well as IRS2 in the liver, and GLUT 4, Akt, or IRS2 in the skeletal muscle [60]. Skeletal muscle absorbs more glucose when glucose transporters are well-regulated. Myrtenal is a promising phytochemical option for developing a novel antidiabetic medication due to its antihyperglycemic and β-cell protection capabilities [61].

Cymene, a monoterpene often present in Cuminum cyminum, enhanced the levels of HbA1c and serum fructosamine, resulting in their normalization. P-cymene was used to raise blood glucose levels and improve triglycerides, VLDL cholesterol, lipid profiles, and LDL cholesterol in mice with STZ-induced diabetes. Citrus fruit peels contain large amounts of the monoterpene Limonene (LM), which may be produced quite cheaply [62]. To demonstrate the effect of monoterpenes, several studies have been conducted. D-limonene administration led to significant decreases in MDA levels, GR enzyme activity, and DNA damage. It also showed a significant increase in GSH levels and the activity of the enzymes SOD, GSH-Px and CAT. Additionally, it altered liver and lipid markers in rats with diabetes [63].

Citronellol is a naturally occurring monoterpene alcohol found in citrus oils, which has health benefits. Significant reductions in glucose and HbA1C were seen as a result of citronellol's enhancement of insulin, hemoglobin, and liver glycogen levels. Administration of citronellol reduces hyperglycemia in diabetic rats produced by STZ by enhancing crucial carbohydrate metabolic enzymes, suggesting its potential efficacy in treating diabetes mellitus [64, 65].

Menthol exerted a notable effect on diabetic rats by considerably decreasing glycosylated hemoglobin levels and blood glucose while significantly increasing plasma insulin, total hemoglobin, and liver glycogen levels. The rarity and lack of any apparent adverse effects suggest the potential to utilize this monoterpene as a beneficial supplement in the management of diabetic complications [66].

Sesquiterpenes can be found in the human diet and are commonly consumed as constituents of several traditional remedies and dietary supplements. Sesquiterpenes have diverse biological actions, including anticancer, antiinflammatory, immunomodulatory, antidiabetic, and antibacterial effects. These attributes render them auspicious contenders for the creation of innovative therapies and their utilization in the medical field. The world has taken notice of natural goods because of their extensive range of biological activity, exceptional safety, and few side effects. Sesquiterpenes, including βcaryophyllene, dysidine, farnesol, and eremanthin, are bioactive compounds that belong to a class of terpenoids. Because these substances can reduce blood glucose levels, they may be utilized in the diagnosis or retardation of diabetes. The specific mechanisms by which they have this effect are still being studied [67].

Diterpenes are secondary metabolites that play a crucial role in controlling various disorders. Numerous interesting biological actions, including the control of diabetes, have been demonstrated for polyphenols, flavonoids, terpenoids, alkaloids, and other components [68]. Many diterpenes have been studied for their antidiabetic properties during the past 25 years; some have even advanced to the point of clinical testing. Preclinical assessments against diabetes consistently show good activity from all tested primaries. The most widely utilized models to investigate the antidiabetic effect of diterpenes include the inhibition of α-glucosidase and Protein Tyrosine Phosphatase 1B (PTP 1B) actions, as well as the agonistic characteristics of receptors activated by Peroxisome Proliferator (PPAR-γ). Increased GLUT4 translocation and the activation of signaling pathways involving Phosphoinositide 3-Kinase (PI3K) and AMP-activated protein kinase (AMPK) are two of the biological mechanisms that govern the action of diterpenes [69, 70].

Triterpenes have the potential to be effective in treating diabetic neuropathy, retinopathy, nephropathy, and impaired wound healing. They achieve this by blocking many pathways that are implicated in diabetes and its related problems. However, research is scarce on the molecular mechanisms and clinical trials exploring the use of triterpenes for diabetes treatment. Therefore, it is crucial to give particular focus to investigating the therapeutic capabilities of these substances and offering novel insights to the scientific community [71].

Advancement of Treatment of Type 1 Diabetes

The field of T1DM patient treatment has seen a boom in the use of artificial intelligence-driven developments in recent years. Insulin pumps and closed-loop devices, or "artificial pancreas," for example, have been shown to significantly enhance T1DM management and patient outcomes to give a summary of the most current studies on TIDM therapy using AI [72, 73]. The randomized clinical trial, conducted in a well-designed multicenter setting with a six-month follow-up, provided the most recent data [74]. A cost-effectiveness evaluation contrasting a hybrid closed-loop system with ongoing subcutaneous insulin administration and a comparison of real-time and intermittently scanning continuous glucose monitoring (CGM) [75]. Interestingly, it has been shown that the use of algorithms for machine learning in CGMs can lead to a considerable decrease in postprandial hypoglycemia, a decrease in the frequency of closed-loop exits and alarms, and an improvement in glycaemic management, all without causing appreciable modifications to psychological results. In terms of *in vivo* studies, the non-obese diabetic mouse model is a well-researched method that is widely utilized to assess therapeutic drugs and investigate various facets of the molecular and cellular pathways underlying T1DM [76]. Antigen-loaded or -unloaded lDCs can be used in immunotherapies, and both approaches have demonstrated efficacy in preventing T1DM [77]. But the antigen-loaded approaches appear more practical, and as a result, they ought to precisely prevent autoreactive T cell activity. Currently underway is a phase 1 trial assessing the use of lDC as an immunotherapy vaccine for the treatment of T1DM patients who use insulin and do not have any other health issues connected to diabetes. Vaccination seeks to prevent the autoimmune process and safeguard βcells, which in turn leads to effective insulin production, blood glucose management, and a decrease in problems associated with T1DM [78]. Nephrin protein levels decrease in diabetic nephropathy, presumably due to the synthesis and subsequent loss of isoforms of the splice variant nephrin that lack a transmembrane domain, resulting in their excretion into the urine. Numerous investigations have been conducted about the role of angiotensin II activity in podocyte damage in individuals with diabetes [79]. In diabetics, angiotensin II activity contributes to nephrin suppression and podocyte damage. T1DM can be reversed with βcell replacement through islet transplantation or allogenic solid organ pancreas, although graft rejection prevention needs lifelong immunosuppression [80].

FUTURE PERSPECTIVE

The fact that medicine is still developing is encouraging for future type 1 diabetes mellitus treatment options. Here are some potential development directions: Insulin pumps and closed-loop devices, or artificial pancreas, have been shown to significantly enhance T1DM management and patient outcomes. Research has developed novel techniques that are less invasive, more effective, and less likely to have negative side effects than present practices. These could be cutting-edge methods like insulin therapy. Pharmacological advancements, including new medications or other treatments, may be developed to target specific T1DM symptoms or treat their underlying causes.

Medical technology advancements may lead to the development of enhanced minimally invasive therapies for T1DM. The most important thing to keep in mind is that these possibilities are just that—possibilities. Additional clinical evidence and research would be required to validate their efficacy and safety. It is always preferable to seek medical advice or any other treatment if you have T1DM symptoms or any other concerns. They can point you in the direction of the most recent knowledge and the best treatments.

CONCLUSION

The significance of terpenoids is systematically illustrated in this review, aiming to advance our understanding of and research into their therapeutic activity. The objective of this book is to convey the prevailing understanding of the treatment of T1DM, highlighting its significant impact on pancreatic β cell destruction, reducing insulin deficiency and dysregulated glucose metabolism, as well as advancing the disease. We elaborate on the mechanism by which terpenoids exhibit a significant effect on type 1 diabetes mellitus. This book chapter intends to present the latest developments in the field of terpenoid chemistry, including their derivatives, biological interventions, and therapeutic applications. The focus is particularly on their role in diabetes and related illnesses.

REFERENCES

[1] Li Y, Zhang W, Zhao R, Zhang X. Advances in oral peptide drug nanoparticles for diabetes mellitus treatment. Bioact Mater 2022; 15: 392-408.
[http://dx.doi.org/10.1016/j.bioactmat.2022.02.025] [PMID: 35386357]

[2] Hussain S, Chowdhury TA. The impact of comorbidities on the pharmacological management of type 2 diabetes mellitus. Drugs 2019; 79(3): 231-42.
[http://dx.doi.org/10.1007/s40265-019-1061-4] [PMID: 30742277]

[3] Padhi S, Nayak AK, Behera A. Type II diabetes mellitus: a review on recent drug based therapeutics. Biomed Pharmacother 2020; 131: 110708.
[http://dx.doi.org/10.1016/j.biopha.2020.110708] [PMID: 32927252]

[4] Paschou SA, Papadopoulou-Marketou N, Chrousos GP, Kanaka-Gantenbein C. On type 1 diabetes mellitus pathogenesis. Endocr Connect 2018; 7(1): R38-46. [http://dx.doi.org/10.1530/EC-17-0347] [PMID: 29191919]

[5] Bluestone JA, Herold K, Eisenbarth G. Genetics, pathogenesis and clinical interventions in type 1 diabetes. Nature 2010; 464(7293): 1293-300. [http://dx.doi.org/10.1038/nature08933] [PMID: 20432533]

[6] Atkinson MA, Eisenbarth GS, Michels AW. Type 1 diabetes. Lancet 2014; 383(9911): 69-82. [http://dx.doi.org/10.1016/S0140-6736(13)60591-7] [PMID: 23890997]

[7] Chen W, Xie A, Chan L. Mechanistic basis of immunotherapies for type 1 diabetes mellitus. Transl Res 2013; 161(4): 217-29. [http://dx.doi.org/10.1016/j.trsl.2012.12.017] [PMID: 23348026]

[8] Lodoen M, Ogasawara K, Hamerman JA, *et al.* NKG2D-mediated natural killer cell protection against cytomegalovirus is impaired by viral gp40 modulation of retinoic acid early inducible 1 gene molecules. J Exp Med 2003; 197(10): 1245-53. [http://dx.doi.org/10.1084/jem.20021973] [PMID: 12756263]

[9] Yin B, Ma G, Yen CY, *et al.* Myeloid-derived suppressor cells prevent type 1 diabetes in murine models. J Immunol 2010; 185(10): 5828-34. [http://dx.doi.org/10.4049/jimmunol.0903636] [PMID: 20956337]

[10] O'reilly LA, Hutchings PR, Crocker PR, *et al.* Characterization of pancreatic islet cell infiltrates in NOD mice: effect of cell transfer and transgene expression. Eur J Immunol 1991; 21(5): 1171-80. [http://dx.doi.org/10.1002/eji.1830210512] [PMID: 1674689]

[11] Chang CL, Chen YC, Chen HM, Yang NS, Yang WC. Natural cures for type 1 diabetes: a review of phytochemicals, biological actions, and clinical potential. Curr Med Chem 2013; 20(7): 899-907. [PMID: 23210779]

[12] Patterson CC, Karuranga S, Salpea P, *et al.* Worldwide estimates of incidence, prevalence and mortality of type 1 diabetes in children and adolescents: Results from the International Diabetes Federation Diabetes Atlas, 9th edition. Diabetes Res Clin Pract 2019; 157: 107842. [http://dx.doi.org/10.1016/j.diabres.2019.107842] [PMID: 31518658]

[13] Wang Q, Zhao X, Jiang Y, Jin B, Wang L. Functions of representative terpenoids and their biosynthesis mechanisms in medicinal plants. Biomolecules 2023; 13(12): 1725. [http://dx.doi.org/10.3390/biom13121725] [PMID: 38136596]

[14] Li J, Li B, Luo L, *et al.* Increased phenolic acid and tanshinone production and transcriptional responses of biosynthetic genes in hairy root cultures of Salvia przewalskii Maxim. treated with methyl jasmonate and salicylic acid. Mol Biol Rep 2020; 47(11): 8565-78. [http://dx.doi.org/10.1007/s11033-020-05899-1] [PMID: 33048323]

[15] Yang W, Chen X, Li Y, Guo S, Wang Z, Yu X. Advances in pharmacological activities of terpenoids. Nat Prod Commun 2020; 15(3) [http://dx.doi.org/10.1177/1934578X20903555]

[16] Zhang C, Hong K. Production of terpenoids by synthetic biology approaches. Front Bioeng Biotechnol 2020; 8: 347. [http://dx.doi.org/10.3389/fbioe.2020.00347] [PMID: 32391346]

[17] Proshkina E, Plyusnin S, Babak T, *et al.* Terpenoids as potential geroprotectors. Antioxidants 2020; 9(6): 529. [http://dx.doi.org/10.3390/antiox9060529] [PMID: 32560451]

[18] Li C, Zha W, Li W, Wang J, You A. Advances in the biosynthesis of terpenoids and their ecological functions in plant resistance. Int J Mol Sci 2023; 24(14): 11561. [http://dx.doi.org/10.3390/ijms241411561] [PMID: 37511319]

[19] Palmer-Young EC, Veit D, Gershenzon J, Schuman MC. The sesquiterpenes (E)-ß-farnesene and (E)-α-bergamotene quench ozone but fail to protect the wild tobacco Nicotiana attenuata from ozone, UVB, and drought stresses. PLoS One 2015; 10(6): e0127296.
[http://dx.doi.org/10.1371/journal.pone.0127296] [PMID: 26030663]

[20] Loreto F, Mannozzi M, Maris C, Nascetti P, Ferranti F, Pasqualini S. Ozone quenching properties of isoprene and its antioxidant role in leaves. Plant Physiol 2001; 126(3): 993-1000.
[http://dx.doi.org/10.1104/pp.126.3.993] [PMID: 11457950]

[21] Lee GW, Lee S, Chung MS, Jeong YS, Chung BY. Rice terpene synthase 20 (OsTPS20) plays an important role in producing terpene volatiles in response to abiotic stresses. Protoplasma 2015; 252(4): 997-1007.
[http://dx.doi.org/10.1007/s00709-014-0735-8] [PMID: 25430981]

[22] Bertamini M, Grando MS, Zocca P, Pedrotti M, Lorenzi S, Cappellin L. Linking monoterpenes and abiotic stress resistance in grapevines. BIO Web Conf. 13: 01003.
[http://dx.doi.org/10.1051/bioconf/20191301003]

[23] Kleiber A, Duan Q, Jansen K, *et al.* Drought effects on root and needle terpenoid content of a coastal and an interior Douglas fir provenance. Tree Physiol 2017; 37(12): 1648-58.
[http://dx.doi.org/10.1093/treephys/tpx113] [PMID: 29036462]

[24] Vaughan MM, Christensen S, Schmelz EA, *et al.* Accumulation of terpenoid phytoalexins in maize roots is associated with drought tolerance. Plant Cell Environ 2015; 38(11): 2195-207.
[http://dx.doi.org/10.1111/pce.12482] [PMID: 25392907]

[25] Boncan DAT, Tsang SSK, Li C, *et al.* Terpenes and terpenoids in plants: Interactions with environment and insects. Int J Mol Sci 2020; 21(19): 7382.
[http://dx.doi.org/10.3390/ijms21197382] [PMID: 33036280]

[26] Banerjee A, Sharkey TD. Methylerythritol 4-phosphate (MEP) pathway metabolic regulation. Nat Prod Rep 2014; 31(8): 1043-55.
[http://dx.doi.org/10.1039/C3NP70124G] [PMID: 24921065]

[27] Frank A, Groll M. The methylerythritol phosphate pathway to isoprenoids. Chem Rev 2017; 117(8): 5675-703.
[http://dx.doi.org/10.1021/acs.chemrev.6b00537] [PMID: 27995802]

[28] Phillips M, León P, Boronat A, Rodríguezconcepción M. The plastidial MEP pathway: unified nomenclature and resources. Trends Plant Sci 2008; 13(12): 619-23.
[http://dx.doi.org/10.1016/j.tplants.2008.09.003] [PMID: 18948055]

[29] Lombard J, Moreira D. Origins and early evolution of the mevalonate pathway of isoprenoid biosynthesis in the three domains of life. Mol Biol Evol 2011; 28(1): 87-99.
[http://dx.doi.org/10.1093/molbev/msq177] [PMID: 20651049]

[30] Dudareva N, Andersson S, Orlova I, *et al.* The nonmevalonate pathway supports both monoterpene and sesquiterpene formation in snapdragon flowers. Proc Natl Acad Sci USA 2005; 102(3): 933-8.
[http://dx.doi.org/10.1073/pnas.0407360102] [PMID: 15630092]

[31] Hemmerlin A, Hoeffler JF, Meyer O, *et al.* Cross-talk between the cytosolic mevalonate and the plastidial methylerythritol phosphate pathways in tobacco bright yellow-2 cells. J Biol Chem 2003; 278(29): 26666-76.
[http://dx.doi.org/10.1074/jbc.M302526200] [PMID: 12736259]

[32] Opitz S, Nes WD, Gershenzon J. Both methylerythritol phosphate and mevalonate pathways contribute to biosynthesis of each of the major isoprenoid classes in young cotton seedlings. Phytochemistry 2014; 98: 110-9.
[http://dx.doi.org/10.1016/j.phytochem.2013.11.010] [PMID: 24359633]

[33] Adam KP, Thiel R, Zapp J. Incorporation of 1-[1-13C] deoxy-D-xylulose in chamomile sesquiterpenes. Arch Biochem Biophys 1999; 369(1): 127-32.

[http://dx.doi.org/10.1006/abbi.1999.1346] [PMID: 10462448]

[34] Laule O, Fürholz A, Chang HS, *et al.* Crosstalk between cytosolic and plastidial pathways of isoprenoid biosynthesis in Arabidopsis thaliana. Proc Natl Acad Sci USA 2003; 100(11): 6866-71. [http://dx.doi.org/10.1073/pnas.1031755100] [PMID: 12748386]

[35] El-Baba C, Baassiri A, Kiriako G, *et al.* Terpenoids' anti-cancer effects: focus on autophagy. Apoptosis 2021; 26(9-10): 491-511. [http://dx.doi.org/10.1007/s10495-021-01684-y] [PMID: 34269920]

[36] Ludwiczuk A, Skalicka-Woźniak K, Georgiev MI. Terpenoids. Pharmacognosy 2017; 233-66.

[37] Mabou FD, Yossa IB. TERPENES: Structural classification and biological activities. IOSR J Pharm Biol Sci 2021; 16: 25-40.

[38] Jiang H, Wang X. Biosynthesis of monoterpenoid and sesquiterpenoid as natural flavors and fragrances. Biotechnol Adv 2023; 65: 108151. [http://dx.doi.org/10.1016/j.biotechadv.2023.108151] [PMID: 37037288]

[39] Li SW, Xue BX, Yang TT, *et al.* Sesquiterpenoids and monoterpenoids from the water decoction of Valeriana officinalis L. Phytochemistry 2023; 205: 113474. [http://dx.doi.org/10.1016/j.phytochem.2022.113474] [PMID: 36273590]

[40] Zhao JX, Ge ZP, Yue JM. Cephalotane diterpenoids: structural diversity, biological activity, biosynthetic proposal, and chemical synthesis. Nat Prod Rep 2024; 41(7): 1152-79. [http://dx.doi.org/10.1039/D3NP00067B] [PMID: 38482919]

[41] Semmar N. Secondary metabolites in plant stress adaptation: Analytic space of secondary metabolites. Springer Nature 2024. [http://dx.doi.org/10.1007/978-3-031-52595-7]

[42] Aly SH, Elbadry AMM, Doghish AS, El-Nashar HAS. Unveiling the pharmacological potential of plant triterpenoids in breast cancer management: an updated review. Naunyn Schmiedebergs Arch Pharmacol 2024; 397(8): 5571-96. [http://dx.doi.org/10.1007/s00210-024-03054-2] [PMID: 38563878]

[43] Shao YM, Li TT, Wu CE, *et al.* A review on extraction and biological activities of triterpenoid from *Cyclocarya paliurus*. Food Rev Int 2024; 40(5): 1374-94. [http://dx.doi.org/10.1080/87559129.2023.2213307]

[44] Barras BJ, Ling T, Rivas F. Recent advances in chemistry and antioxidant/anticancer biology of monoterpene and meroterpenoid natural product. Molecules 2024; 29(1): 279. [http://dx.doi.org/10.3390/molecules29010279] [PMID: 38202861]

[45] Chen D, Zhang X, Vorobieva AA, *et al.* An evolved artificial radical cyclase enables the construction of bicyclic terpenoid scaffolds *via* an H-atom transfer pathway. Nat Chem 2024; 16(10): 1656-64. [http://dx.doi.org/10.1038/s41557-024-01562-5] [PMID: 39030420]

[46] Shieh JP, Cheng KC, Chung HH, Kerh YF, Yeh CH, Cheng JT. Plasma glucose lowering mechanisms of catalpol, an active principle from roots of Rehmannia glutinosa, in streptozotocin-induced diabetic rats. J Agric Food Chem 2011; 59(8): 3747-53. [http://dx.doi.org/10.1021/jf200069t] [PMID: 21391677]

[47] Wang CF, Li DQ, Xue HY, Hu B. Oral supplementation of catalpol ameliorates diabetic encephalopathy in rats. Brain Res 2010; 1307: 158-65. [http://dx.doi.org/10.1016/j.brainres.2009.10.034] [PMID: 19852947]

[48] Yan J, Wang C, Jin Y, *et al.* Catalpol ameliorates hepatic insulin resistance in type 2 diabetes through acting on AMPK/NOX4/PI3K/AKT pathway. Pharmacol Res 2018; 130: 466-80. [http://dx.doi.org/10.1016/j.phrs.2017.12.026] [PMID: 29284152]

[49] Xu Z, Zhang L, Li X, *et al.* Mitochondrial fusion/fission process involved in the improvement of catalpol on high glucose-induced hepatic mitochondrial dysfunction. Acta Biochim Biophys Sin

(Shanghai) 2015; 47(9): 730-40.
[http://dx.doi.org/10.1093/abbs/gmv061] [PMID: 26140925]

[50] Xu D, Huang X, Hassan HM, *et al.* Hypoglycaemic effect of catalpol in a mouse model of high-fat diet-induced prediabetes. Appl Physiol Nutr Metab 2020; 45(10): 1127-37.
[http://dx.doi.org/10.1139/apnm-2020-0075] [PMID: 32294390]

[51] Li X, Xu Z, Jiang Z, *et al.* Hypoglycemic effect of catalpol on high-fat diet/streptozotocin-induced diabetic mice by increasing skeletal muscle mitochondrial biogenesis. Acta Biochim Biophys Sin (Shanghai) 2014; 46(9): 738-48.
[http://dx.doi.org/10.1093/abbs/gmu065] [PMID: 25178463]

[52] Zhou J, Xu G, Ma S, *et al.* Catalpol ameliorates high-fat diet-induced insulin resistance and adipose tissue inflammation by suppressing the JNK and NF-κB pathways. Biochem Biophys Res Commun 2015; 467(4): 853-8.
[http://dx.doi.org/10.1016/j.bbrc.2015.10.054] [PMID: 26474703]

[53] Sarkar T, Bharadwaj KK, Salauddin M, Pati S, Chakraborty R. Phytochemical characterization, antioxidant, antiinflammatory, antidiabetic properties, molecular docking, pharmacokinetic profiling, and network pharmacology analysis of the major phytoconstituents of raw and differently dried mangifera indica (himsagar cultivar): an *in vitro* and *in silico* investigations. Appl Biochem Biotechnol 2022; 194(2): 950-87.
[http://dx.doi.org/10.1007/s12010-021-03669-8] [PMID: 34591254]

[54] Liu J, Zhang HR, Hou YB, Jing XL, Song XY, Shen XP. Global gene expression analysis in liver of db/db mice treated with catalpol. Chin J Nat Med 2018; 16(8): 590-8.
[http://dx.doi.org/10.1016/S1875-5364(18)30096-7] [PMID: 30197124]

[55] Xu D, Wang L, Jiang Z, *et al.* A new hypoglycemic mechanism of catalpol revealed by enhancing MyoD/MyoG-mediated myogenesis. Life Sci 2018; 209: 313-23.
[http://dx.doi.org/10.1016/j.lfs.2018.08.028] [PMID: 30118770]

[56] Li Y, Mai Y, Qiu X, *et al.* Effect of long-term treatment of carvacrol on glucose metabolism in streptozotocin-induced diabetic mice. BMC Complement Med Ther 2020; 20: 1-8.
[http://dx.doi.org/10.1186/s12906-020-02937-0]

[57] Saravanan S, Pari L. Role of thymol on hyperglycemia and hyperlipidemia in high fat diet-induced type 2 diabetic C57BL/6J mice. Eur J Pharmacol 2015; 761: 279-87.
[http://dx.doi.org/10.1016/j.ejphar.2015.05.034] [PMID: 26007642]

[58] Guan L, Gong D, Yang S, *et al.* Genipin ameliorates diet-induced obesity *via* promoting lipid mobilization and browning of white adipose tissue in rats. Phytother Res 2018; 32(4): 723-32.
[http://dx.doi.org/10.1002/ptr.6022] [PMID: 29377296]

[59] Babukumar S, Vinothkumar V, Sankaranarayanan C, Srinivasan S. Geraniol, a natural monoterpene, ameliorates hyperglycemia by attenuating the key enzymes of carbohydrate metabolism in streptozotocin-induced diabetic rats. Pharm Biol 2017; 55(1): 1442-9.
[http://dx.doi.org/10.1080/13880209.2017.1301494] [PMID: 28330423]

[60] Rathinam A, Pari L. Myrtenal ameliorates hyperglycemia by enhancing GLUT2 through Akt in the skeletal muscle and liver of diabetic rats. Chem Biol Interact 2016; 256: 161-6.
[http://dx.doi.org/10.1016/j.cbi.2016.07.009] [PMID: 27417257]

[61] Rathinam A, Pari L, Chandramohan R, Sheikh BA. Histopathological findings of the pancreas, liver, and carbohydrate metabolizing enzymes in STZ-induced diabetic rats improved by administration of myrtenal. J Physiol Biochem 2014; 70(4): 935-46.
[http://dx.doi.org/10.1007/s13105-014-0362-z] [PMID: 25292424]

[62] Vigushin DM, Poon GK, Boddy A, *et al.* Phase I and pharmacokinetic study of d -limonene in patients with advanced cancer. Cancer Chemother Pharmacol 1998; 42(2): 111-7.
[http://dx.doi.org/10.1007/s002800050793] [PMID: 9654110]

[63] Bacanlı M, Anlar HG, Aydın S, *et al.* d-limonene ameliorates diabetes and its complications in streptozotocin-induced diabetic rats. Food Chem Toxicol 2017; 110: 434-42. [http://dx.doi.org/10.1016/j.fct.2017.09.020] [PMID: 28923438]

[64] Srinivasan S, Muruganathan U. Antidiabetic efficacy of citronellol, a citrus monoterpene by ameliorating the hepatic key enzymes of carbohydrate metabolism in streptozotocin-induced diabetic rats. Chem Biol Interact 2016; 250: 38-46. [http://dx.doi.org/10.1016/j.cbi.2016.02.020] [PMID: 26944432]

[65] Karthikeyan R, Kanimozhi G, Prasad NR, Agilan B, Ganesan M, Srithar G. Alpha pinene modulates UVA-induced oxidative stress, DNA damage and apoptosis in human skin epidermal keratinocytes. Life Sci 2018; 212: 150-8. [http://dx.doi.org/10.1016/j.lfs.2018.10.004] [PMID: 30292828]

[66] Muruganathan U, Srinivasan S, Vinothkumar V. Antidiabetogenic efficiency of menthol, improves glucose homeostasis and attenuates pancreatic β-cell apoptosis in streptozotocin–nicotinamide induced experimental rats through ameliorating glucose metabolic enzymes. Biomed Pharmacother 2017; 92: 229-39. [http://dx.doi.org/10.1016/j.biopha.2017.05.068] [PMID: 28549291]

[67] Maurya A, Mohan S, Verma SC. Antidiabetic potential of naturally occurring sesquiterpenes: A review. Curr Top Med Chem 2021; 21(10): 851-62. [http://dx.doi.org/10.2174/1568026621666210305102500] [PMID: 33676391]

[68] Etsassala NGER, Cupido CN, Iwuoha EI, Hussein AA. Abietane diterpenes as potential candidates for the management of type 2 diabetes. Curr Pharm Des 2020; 26(24): 2885-91. [http://dx.doi.org/10.2174/1381612826666200331082917] [PMID: 32228419]

[69] Kusumah J, Gonzalez de Mejia E. Coffee constituents with antiadipogenic and antidiabetic potentials: A narrative review. Food Chem Toxicol 2022; 161: 112821. [http://dx.doi.org/10.1016/j.fct.2022.112821] [PMID: 35032569]

[70] de Oliveira A, Tirapelli C, Ambrosio S, da Costa F. Diterpenes: a therapeutic promise for cardiovascular diseases. Recent Adv Cardiovasc Drug Discov 2008; 3(1): 1-8. [http://dx.doi.org/10.2174/157489008783331689] [PMID: 18221123]

[71] Putta S, Sastry Yarla N, Kumar Kilari E, *et al.* Therapeutic potentials of triterpenes in diabetes and its associated complications. Curr Top Med Chem 2016; 16(23): 2532-42. [http://dx.doi.org/10.2174/1568026616666160414123343] [PMID: 27086788]

[72] Mackenzie SC, Sainsbury CAR, Wake DJ. Diabetes and artificial intelligence beyond the closed loop: a review of the landscape, promise and challenges. Diabetologia 2024; 67(2): 223-35. [http://dx.doi.org/10.1007/s00125-023-06038-8] [PMID: 37979006]

[73] Fuchs J, Hovorka R. Closed-loop control in insulin pumps for type-1 diabetes mellitus: safety and efficacy. Expert Rev Med Devices 2020; 17(7): 707-20. [http://dx.doi.org/10.1080/17434440.2020.1784724] [PMID: 32569476]

[74] Nimri R, Phillip M, Kovatchev B. Closed-loop and artificial intelligence–based decision support systems. Diabetes Technol Ther 2023; 25(S1): S-70-89. [http://dx.doi.org/10.1089/dia.2023.2505] [PMID: 36802182]

[75] O'Meara M, Mateus Acuña JC, Uribe A. Long-term benefits of an integrated continuous glucose monitoring and insulin pump system for emergency admissions, hospitalization, and metabolic control in a cohort of people with diabetes: Retrospective Cohort Study. JMIR Diabetes 2023; 8(1): e46880. [http://dx.doi.org/10.2196/46880] [PMID: 37610810]

[76] Chatterjee A, Tumarin J, Prabhakar S. Role of inflammation in the progression of diabetic kidney disease. Vessel Plus 2024; 8. [N-A.]. [http://dx.doi.org/10.20517/2574-1209.2024.21]

[77] Theaker SM. Developing peptide vaccines for breast cancer (Doctoral dissertation, Cardiff University)

[78] Roep BO, Thomaidou S, van Tienhoven R, Zaldumbide A. Type 1 diabetes mellitus as a disease of the β-cell (do not blame the immune system?). Nat Rev Endocrinol 2021; 17(3): 150-61. [http://dx.doi.org/10.1038/s41574-020-00443-4] [PMID: 33293704]

[79] Barutta F, Bellini S, Gruden G. Mechanisms of podocyte injury and implications for diabetic nephropathy. Clin Sci (Lond) 2022; 136(7): 493-520. [http://dx.doi.org/10.1042/CS20210625] [PMID: 35415751]

[80] Aggarwal S. Targeting apoptosis and necroptosis inhibition to improve islet graft function

CHAPTER 5

Advances in Therapeutic Modulation of Cannabinoids for Effective Treatment and Research in Multiple Sclerosis

Balaji Govindaswamy[1,*], Sarath Perumal[2], Chandrasekar Ponnusamy[3] and **Murugappan Kumarappan[4]**

[1] *Department of Biotechnology, Bhupat and Jyoti Mehta School of Biosciences, Indian Institute of Technology Madras, Chennai 600042 ,Tamil Nadu, India*

[2] *Department of Biotechnology, School of Bio-science and Technology, Vellore Institute of Technology, Vellore 632014, Tamil Nadu, India*

[3] *Department of Biotechnology, Rathinam College of Arts and Science, Coimbatore 641021, Tamil Nadu, India*

[4] *Department of Biotechnology, School of Biotechnology and Genetic Engineering, Bharathidasan University, Tiruchirappalli 620024, Tamil Nadu, India*

Abstract: A complicated and long-lasting neurodegenerative illness, Multiple Sclerosis (MS) is characterized by lesions in the Central Nervous System (CNS). Although the exact etiology of MS and the processes behind this rise are yet unknown, complex gene-environment interactions most likely have a significant impact. Growing research indicates that certain symptoms of multiple sclerosis and spinal cord damage, such as pain and spasticity, are effectively suppressed by Cannabinoids. Natural cannabis products and single Cannabinoids are often smoked or taken orally, with different administration routes. Transdermal, sublingual, ocular, and aerosols have only been employed in a few studies and are not highly relevant in modern practice. This chapter focuses on novel approaches of Cannabinoids drugs with synthetic material, co-drug development, mechanism of action, and demonstrating the use of Cannabinoids receptor agonists in the treatment of multiple sclerosis. Furthermore, the chapter explains the preclinical and clinical approaches, suggesting that Cannabinoids CB1 and/or CB2 receptors may decrease some of the pathological alterations that lead to the signs and symptoms of multiple sclerosis in addition to alleviating them and using synthetically derived Cannabinoids, also explains how it reduces the effects of MS and prolongs 'patient's lifespan. Thus, the chapter delivers the potentiality of using Cannabinoids with advances to overcome the Pharmacokinetic and Pharmacodynamic pathways.

[*] **Corresponding author Balaji Govindaswamy:** Department of Biotechnology, Bhupat and Jyoti Mehta School of Biosciences, Indian Institute of Technology Madras, Chennai 600042, Tamil Nadu, India; E-mail: balajishilou.08@gmail.com

M.S. Ashawat, Aditi Kaushik, Akash Jain, Jasmine Chaudhary & Manish Kaushik (Eds.)
All rights reserved-© 2025 Bentham Science Publishers

Keywords: Aetiology of MS, Blood Brain Barrier, Cannabinoids, Cannabis, Cellular pathway, Central Nervous System, Endocannabinoid, Genes, Immune cells, Lesions, Lifespan, Multiple Sclerosis, Muscle atrophy, Myelin sheath, Neurodegenerative, Pathology, Receptors, Sativex, Spasticity, Spinal cord.

INTRODUCTION

A common and crippling autoimmune illness, Multiple Sclerosis (MS) primarily affects the Central Nervous System (CNS), which includes the brain and spinal cord. The immune ' 'system's breakdown of myelin, the coating that protects nerve fibres, is a defining feature of multiple sclerosis [1]. The effective conduction of electrical impulses along the nerves is disrupted by this demyelination process, which results in a variety of neurological symptoms and gradual impairment [2]. The abnormal activation of CD4+ T lymphocytes, which identify myelin antigens presented by Major Histocompatibility Complex (MHC) class II molecules, is central to the pathophysiology of multiple sclerosis [3, 4]. These auto-reactive T cells multiply and release pro-inflammatory cytokines, such as aggravating inflammation and drawing more immune cells to the central nervous system [5]. Through the generation of myelin-specific antibodies and the development of ectopic lymphoid follicles inside the meninges [6], B cells also contribute to the pathology associated with multiple sclerosis. Microglia and astrocytes are activated in MS due to the inflammatory milieu, which results in the production of neurotoxic chemicals such as nitric oxide and reactive oxygen species [7]. Demyelination, axonal damage, and the death of oligodendrocytes are the outcomes of this inflammatory cascade [8]. Sclerotic plaques are a hallmark of MS lesions seen on MRI and are linked to chronic demyelination and axonal degeneration [9]. Myelin sheaths are necessary for the quick and accurate transfer of electrical impulses between neurons in a healthy central nervous system [2, 10]. In the CNS, oligodendrocytes create myelin, which insulates nerve fibres and helps action potentials spread by saltatory conduction [11]. Auto-reactive lymphocytes in MS cause demyelination and damage to neuro-axons by piercing the blood-brain barrier and starting anti-inflammatory responses against myelin and oligodendrocytes [12]. Genetic predisposition and environmental stimuli interact intricately during the pathophysiology of multiple sclerosis [13]. Numerous genetic loci, many of which are involved in immune modulation, have been discovered by genome-wide association studies as being related to an elevated risk for multiple sclerosis [14]. The genesis of MS has also been linked to environmental variables, including smoking, vitamin D insufficiency, and viral infections (Epstein-Barr virus) [15].

The development of synthetic Disease-Modifying Therapies (DMTs) such as fingolimod, alemtuzumab, and ocrelizumab has completely changed the way that

MS is managed [16]. Through their targeting of different components of the immune response, these drugs have been shown to be effective in decreasing the number of relapses, slowing the course of the illness, and enhancing the quality of life for patients [17 - 19]. However, a variety of adverse effects are associated with its usage, including flu-like symptoms, bradycardia, gastrointestinal issues, and increased risk of infections and secondary cancers [20]. Beyond immunomodulation, these synthetic drugs can also negatively impact normal inflammations, elevated oxidative stress, impaired cell division, and increased susceptibility to CNS [21, 22]. Additional difficulties with long-term treatment include cumulative toxicity, the possibility of developing secondary autoimmune illness, and the requirement for therapeutic medication because neutralizing antibodies or tolerance develop [23, 24]. These treatments have long-lasting impacts, so ' 'it's critical to have tailored treatment plans and routine monitoring to optimize positive results and reduce negative ones [25]. In order to maximize the therapeutic use of these medications and enhance the quality of life and prognosis for MS patients, ongoing research into the mechanism and long-term effects of these treatments is necessary [26, 27].

Natural drugs may be less likely to cause adverse effects than synthetic medicines and have the potential for neuro-protection, immunomodulation and symptomatic alleviation. Moreover, natural medications are gaining attention in the therapy of multiple sclerosis [28 - 31]. These natural substances, which come from a variety of plants and food sources, have demonstrated potential in MS ' 'patient's treatment of chronic pain, reduction of neuroinflammation, and alleviation of spasticity [32 - 34] using their interaction with the ' 'body's own regulatory systems which are vital to the preservation of Central Nervous System (CNS) homeostasis [35]. They have antioxidant and anti-inflammatory qualities that might prevent neurodegeneration and encourage remyelination [36]. Some are renowned for their neuroprotective and cognitive-enhancing qualities, which may improve cognitive function and tiredness in MS patients [32, 37]. Others have shown promise in lowering the severity of relapses and inflammation in MS due to their immunomodulatory actions [38]. These organic substances provide an alternative method of treating multiple sclerosis, intending to optimize the effectiveness of current treatments while reducing side effects [39, 40]. But in the case of MS, thorough clinical trials are necessary to confirm their safety, effectiveness, and long-term advantages. Natural-based medications are relevant for MS because of their many modes of action that match the ' 'illness's intricate pathophysiology [27, 41]. This allows for a comprehensive approach to disease treatment and enhances ' 'patient's quality of life in general.

Research into cannabis as a potential treatment for multiple sclerosis is a promising and developing area. The key ingredients for *Cannabis sativa* known as

Cannabinoids, have attracted a lot of attention because of their possible anti-inflammatory, neuro-protective, and symptom-relieving effects [42, 43]. The endocannabinoid system, which is made up of endogenous ligands, metabolic enzymes, and Cannabinoid receptors (CB1 and CB2) [44 - 46], is essential for preserving CNS homeostasis and regulating immunological responses [47]. Cannabinoids can lessen neuroinflammation, encourage remyelination, and guard against neurodegeneration, according to preclinical research [48, 49]. Evidence from clinical trials suggests that Cannabinoids based medicines, including nabiximols (a THC and CBD combination) [50], help reduce bladder dysfunction, stiffness, and other symptoms associated with multiple sclerosis [51]. Notwithstanding these encouraging results, a more thorough study is still required to determine whether or not cannabis has a clinically meaningful effect on how quickly a disease progresses [52]. Challenges include individual heterogeneity in response, possible side effects, and the requirement for standardized formulations and dosage schedules that limit the therapeutic potential for cannabis in MS [53, 54]. Future studies should concentrate on clarifying the specific mechanism of action, improving treatment regimens, and creating long-term safety profiles as the field of cannabis research continues to grow [55]. In this chapter, cannabis provides a potentially beneficial supplement to the arsenal for treating multiple sclerosis. To completely grasp their therapeutic potential and incorporate Cannabinoids-based therapies into evidence-based clinical practice for MS patients, ongoing research and clinical evaluations are needed.

CANNABINOIDS AND ENDOCANNABINOIDS FOR MULTIPLE SCLEROSIS

MS is an inflammatory demyelinating condition; the idea that neurodegenerative processes are also significant events in this disorder has lately received more attention due to the advent of neuroimaging and histology tools [56]. As a result, MS frequently and extensively exhibits neuronal degeneration and axonal loss, as well as inflammatory lesions and typically looking white matter [57]. Moreover, even in the early stages of MS, brain shrinkage is primarily caused by neuronal death in the gray matter. Even so, it remains a reasonable theory that the inflammatory demyelinating aspect of multiple sclerosis dominates in the initial stages of the illness, whereas neuronal and axonal damage, although precocious, reaches critical levels, leading to prolonged impairment, which can result in permanent impairment [58, 59]. There is growing evidence that the ECS has a role in both neurodegeneration associated with multiple sclerosis and the inflammatory process that characterizes the illness. Since elevated amounts of AEA have been discovered in this tissue from inflammatory lesions of individuals with active or silent MS, it follows that MS profoundly modifies the ECS [27, 60, 61]. While AEA and 2-AG are either normal or down-regulated in the brains of other MS models, endocannabinoid also is elevated in the spinal cord of a mouse model of the disease [44, 62, 63].

Strong experimental evidence from several studies suggests that endocannabinoids may also affect the expression of the 'diseases' crippling clinical symptoms [64]. These findings lend credence to earlier reports that found marijuana to be beneficial for MS patients self-medicating because it reduces pain, spasticity, dystonia, and bladder control [65]. Testing the effects of oral Cannabinoids agonists in MS spastic patients was made possible by the discovery that central endocannabinoid levels rise in spastic with experimental MS and that pharmacological activation of CB receptors decreases spasticity in these animals [66, 67]. However, longer-term experiments are required to corroborate the optimistic outcomes that have been produced thus far.

ECS plays a part in the inflammatory process in experimental MS. For instance, the administration of cannabis agonists considerably reduces and delays the inflammatory infiltrates in the spinal cord and the clinical manifestations of experimentally produced MS in rats [68]. According to MS models, the anti-inflammatory qualities of cannabis against the pathophysiology of the disease appear to be linked to a decrease in the quantity of CD4T cells, MHC II molecules expression, and activated microglia in the spinal cord [60, 69]. Other significant effects of these substances in mice with experimental multiple sclerosis include decreased generation of pro-inflammatory cytokines such as TNF-, interleukin IL-1 and IL-6 [70, 71]. Since they downregulate macrophage function and inhibit microglial activation, thereby reducing nitric oxide production and significant histocompatibility complex class II antigen expression in the CNS, both exogenous and endogenous Cannabinoids offer an effective therapy for experimental multiple sclerosis [72, 73].

Higher amounts of functional CB2 receptors than CB1 receptors are expressed by immune cells implicated in the pathogenesis of multiple sclerosis. The protective effects of Cannabinoids in MS are explained by the complex inhibitory activities that are mediated in these cells by CB2 receptor stimulation [74]. Accordingly, CB2 receptor activation restricts the release of NO, prevents the synthesis of many inflammatory cytokines, and stops cell division and chemotaxis [75]. Each of these elements is crucial for the anti-inflammatory effects of Cannabinoids in MS. The inhibitory effect of Cannabinoids on astrocytes activation was also extended to non-CB1 and non-CB2 receptors, indicating a potential function for these receptors in the anti-inflammatory effects of exogenous and endogenous Cannabinoids in MS [76]. When activated, microglia or other immune cells invade the CNS, they release harmful cytokines and free radicals, which contribute to some of the neurodegenerative damage observed in MS [77].

Therefore, endocannabinoids have an indirect neuroprotective effect in MS by reducing inflammation. However, by acting through CB1 receptors, Cannabinoids directly inhibit glutamate release and toxic damage in several neurodegenerative diseases [78]. This involvement of excitotoxicity in MS-related to neuronal damage is significant, indicating that pharmacological CB1 activation may mitigate neurodegenerative damage in this condition as well [79, 80].

THERAPEUTIC POTENTIAL OF CANNABINOID IN MULTIPLE SCLEROSIS

Cannabinoids and Neuroinflammation

One of the hallmarks of MS is chronic neuroinflammation, which results from an abnormal immune response targeting the myelin sheath—a protective covering around nerve fibres. This immune-mediated attack leads to demyelination, axonal injury, and ultimately, neuronal death. Cannabinoids, particularly through the activation of CB2 receptors on immune cells, can exert potent anti-inflammatory effects, which are crucial in managing MS. Activation of CB2 receptors by cannabinoids such as CBD leads to the inhibition of pro-inflammatory cytokines like Tumor Necrosis Factor-alpha (TNF-α), Interleukin-1 Beta (IL-1β), and Interleukin-6 (IL-6). These cytokines play a critical role in perpetuating the inflammatory response in MS [81]. By reducing their production and release, cannabinoids can decrease the infiltration of immune cells into the CNS, thereby reducing the extent of demyelination and neuronal damage. Additionally, cannabinoids can modulate the activity of microglia, the resident immune cells of the CNS. In MS, microglia become overactivated and contribute to the chronic inflammatory environment. Cannabinoids, particularly THC, can induce a shift in microglial activity from a pro-inflammatory M1 phenotype to an anti-inflammatory M2 phenotype. This shift not only reduces the production of harmful cytokines but also promotes the release of neurotrophic factors that support neuronal survival and repair [82].

Cannabinoids and Neuroprotection

Beyond their anti-inflammatory effects, cannabinoids also offer neuroprotection in MS, which is essential for preserving neuronal function and preventing long-term disability. Neuroprotection involves safeguarding neurons from oxidative stress, excitotoxicity, and apoptosis—all of which are significant contributors to neurodegeneration in MS. Cannabinoids can reduce oxidative stress by scavenging free radicals and enhancing the activity of antioxidant enzymes. This is particularly important in MS, where excessive production of Reactive Oxygen Species (ROS) occurs due to chronic inflammation and mitochondrial dysfunction. By mitigating oxidative stress, cannabinoids can protect neurons from damage and preserve their function [83]. Excitotoxicity, another major factor in MS, results from excessive glutamate release and impaired glutamate reuptake in the CNS. High levels of glutamate can overstimulate glutamate receptors, leading to calcium overload, mitochondrial dysfunction, and ultimately, neuronal death. Cannabinoids, particularly through CB1 receptor activation, can inhibit glutamate release and modulate calcium influx, thereby reducing excitotoxic damage to neurons. Furthermore, cannabinoids have been shown to upregulate the expression of neurotrophic factors, such as Brain-Derived Neurotrophic Factor (BDNF) and Glial Cell Line-Derived Neurotrophic Factor (GDNF). These factors support neuronal survival, promote axonal growth, and enhance remyelination—processes that are crucial for recovery and functional improvement in patients with MS [84]. The neuroprotective effects against neuroinflammation are shown in Fig. (**1**).

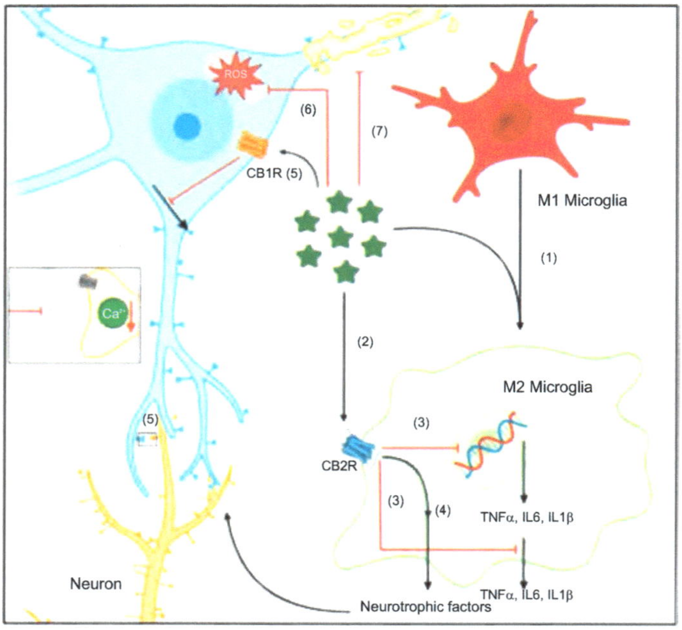

Fig. (1). Cannabinoids in neuroprotection (Cannabinoids reduce the degeneration of neurons in multiple sclerosis. The green star is labeled as a cannabinoid compound. (1) They induce a phenotype switch in microglia from the pro-inflammatory M1 phenotype to the M2 phenotype. (2) In microglia, cannabinoids act on the CB2 cannabinoid receptor and (3) inhibit the expression and release of pro-inflammatory cytokines such as TNF-α, IL-6, and IL-1β. (4) They also stimulate the release of neurotrophic factors. (5) Cannabinoids interact with neurons through the CB1 cannabinoid receptor and inhibit glutamate release. The reduced glutamate availability lowers calcium levels in the postsynaptic neuron, preventing excessive excitation. (6) Cannabinoids also inhibit reactive oxygen species (ROS) generation and (7) reduce demyelination caused by pro-inflammatory cytokines.

CANNABINOIDS IN SYMPTOM MANAGEMENT OF MULTIPLE SCLEROSIS

Pain Management

Chronic pain is a common and often debilitating symptom of MS. Conventional analgesics may provide limited relief, and many patients experience adverse effects. Cannabinoids have demonstrated potential in managing various pain types, including neuropathic pain, which is prevalent in MS. The Endocannabinoid System (ECS) is involved in pain modulation through multiple mechanisms. Cannabinoids can interact with the ECS to reduce pain perception. By activating cannabinoid receptors, particularly CB1, cannabinoids can inhibit the release of pain-inducing neurotransmitters, such as substance P and glutamate. Additionally, cannabinoids can modulate the activity of microglia as well as immune cells involved in pain processing, potentially reducing inflammation and pain. Clinical studies have shown that cannabinoids, such as Sativex, a combination of THC and CBD, can effectively reduce pain intensity and improve pain-related quality of life in MS patients. However, individual responses to cannabinoids vary, and further research is needed to optimize their use for pain management in MS [85].

Spasticity Management

Spasticity, characterized by muscle stiffness and involuntary contractions, is a common and disabling symptom of MS. It can significantly impair mobility and activities of daily living. Traditional treatments, such as muscle relaxants and botulinum toxin injections, often provide limited relief and have associated side effects. Cannabinoids have shown promise in managing spasticity. By interacting with the ECS, cannabinoids can modulate spinal cord excitability and reduce muscle tone. Studies have demonstrated that cannabinoids can alleviate spasticity-related symptoms, including muscle stiffness, pain, and impaired mobility. Sativex, a combination of THC and CBD, has been approved for the treatment of spasticity in several countries. It has shown efficacy in reducing spasticity scores and improving patient-reported outcomes. However, the optimal dosage and duration of treatment for spasticity management with cannabinoids require further investigation [86].

Fatigue Management

Fatigue is a pervasive symptom in MS, significantly impacting daily functioning and quality of life. While the exact mechanisms underlying MS-related fatigue are complex, the ECS is believed to play a role in energy regulation and sleep-wake cycles. Cannabinoids have shown potential in addressing fatigue in other conditions, such as cancer-related fatigue. While there is limited research specifically on cannabinoids for MS-related fatigue, some patients report improvements in energy levels and reduced fatigue after using cannabinoids. It is important to note that fatigue is a complex symptom with multiple contributing factors. A comprehensive approach to fatigue management should include lifestyle modifications, sleep hygiene, and other therapeutic interventions in addition to cannabinoids [87].

Bladder Dysfunction

Bladder dysfunction, including urinary incontinence and retention, is a common and distressing symptom of MS. It can significantly impact the quality of life and lead to social isolation. While the role of the ECS in bladder function is not fully understood, there is some evidence suggesting its involvement in bladder control. Cannabinoids have been investigated for the treatment of bladder dysfunction in other conditions, such as overactive bladder. Limited research is available on the use of cannabinoids for bladder dysfunction in MS. However, some patients report improvements in bladder symptoms after using cannabinoids. Further studies are needed to evaluate the efficacy and safety of cannabinoids for this condition [88].

Other Symptoms

In addition to the core symptoms discussed above, MS patients may experience a range of other symptoms, including tremors, dizziness, and cognitive impairment. While research on the use of cannabinoids for these symptoms is limited, some patients report improvements. For example, some studies suggest that cannabinoids may have anti-tremor effects. However, more research is needed to confirm these findings and to determine the optimal dosage and treatment duration [89]. While cannabinoids offer potential benefits for symptom management in MS, it is important to note that responses to cannabinoids vary significantly among individuals. Finding the optimal dosage and formulation may require trial and error. Cannabinoids can also cause side effects, such as dry mouth, dizziness, and fatigue. It is essential to weigh the potential benefits against the risks since the lack of standardized dosing guidelines for cannabinoids in MS is still under discussion. Moreover, the legal status of medical cannabis varies across countries and regions, limiting access to patients [90]. The cannabinoid's potential effects on the multiple sclerosis symptoms are shown in Fig. (**2**).

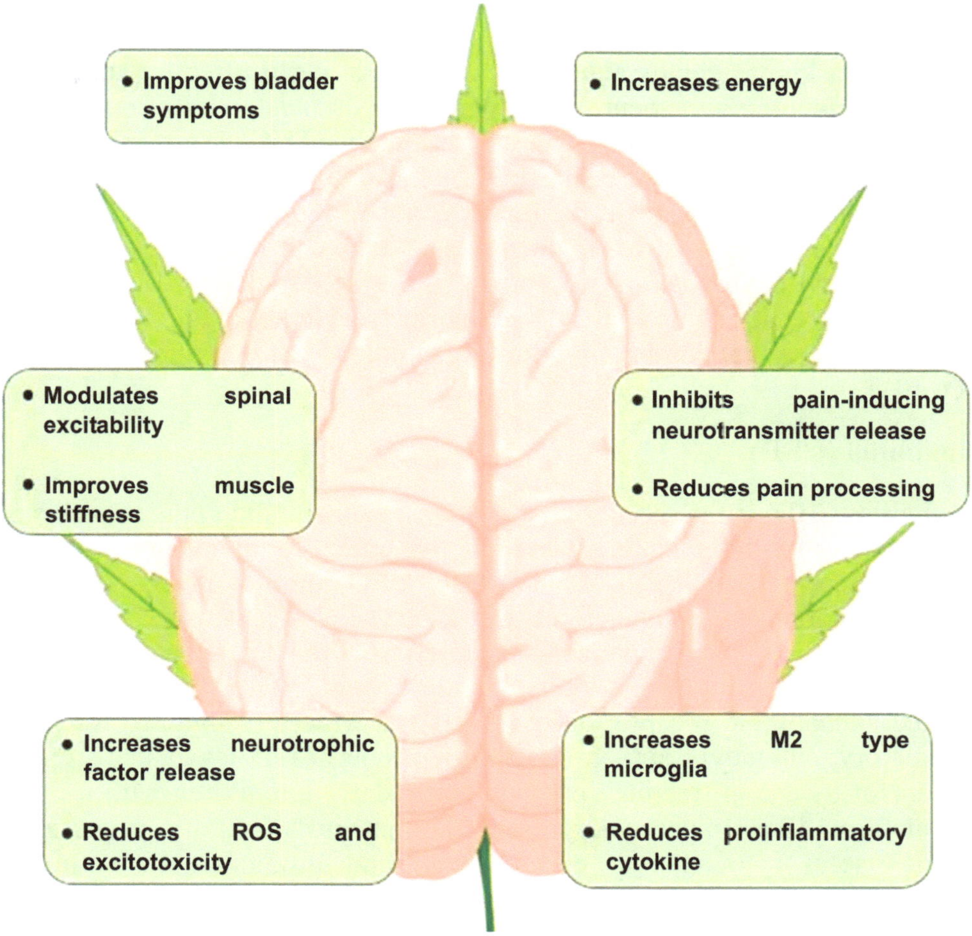

Fig. (2). Cannabinoids on Multiple Sclerosis symptoms (Cannabinoid products have the potential to reduce the symptoms of multiple sclerosis by managing pain, spasticity, and fatigue. They help improve energy levels by decreasing fatigue and bladder symptoms. Pain management occurs through the suppression of pain neurotransmitters and a reduction in immune cell activity related to pain perception. Motor symptoms, including spasticity, are improved by muscle relaxation and reduced spinal excitability. Additionally, cannabinoids provide neuronal protection by reducing inflammatory responses).

KEY CANNABINOIDS IN MEDICAL USE

Tetrahydrocannabinol (THC)

Tetrahydrocannabinol (THC) is the most well-known and psychoactive compound in the cannabis plant. It exerts its effects primarily through partial agonism at the CB1 receptors located in the brain and central nervous system. THC's psychoactive effects are due to its ability to activate CB1 receptors, leading to alterations in neurotransmitter release and affecting mood, memory, and perception. Beyond its psychoactive properties, THC has significant therapeutic potential. It is known for its analgesic effects, making it effective in managing chronic pain, including the neuropathic pain often associated with conditions like multiple sclerosis and fibromyalgia. Additionally, THC has muscle relaxant properties, which can alleviate spasticity, a common symptom in MS patients. The compound also has anti-inflammatory and neuroprotective effects, which contribute to its potential in treating neurodegenerative diseases. However, the use of THC is limited by its psychoactive side effects, which include anxiety, paranoia, and cognitive impairment. These effects have led to the development of THC formulations that combine it with Cannabidiol (CBD) to mitigate these side effects [91].

Cannabidiol (CBD)

Cannabidiol (CBD) is the second most abundant cannabinoid in the cannabis plant and is non-psychoactive, making it an attractive option for therapeutic use without the "high" associated with THC. Unlike THC, CBD does not directly bind to CB1 or CB2 receptors but exerts its effects through several mechanisms, including the modulation of the ECS. It enhances the signaling of the endogenous cannabinoid anandamide by inhibiting its reuptake and breakdown, which can lead to increased cannabinoid receptor activity. CBD is widely recognized for its anti-inflammatory, anticonvulsant, and anxiolytic properties. It has gained significant attention for its use in treating epilepsy, particularly in children with treatment-resistant forms like Dravet syndrome. CBD's anti-inflammatory properties also make it useful in managing chronic pain and inflammation, without the psychoactive side effects associated with THC. Moreover, CBD has been shown to have neuroprotective effects, potentially offering benefits in neurodegenerative diseases like Alzheimer's and Parkinson's disease. Its ability to modulate immune responses also suggests potential use in autoimmune conditions such as MS [92].

Cannabinol (CBN)

Cannabinol (CBN) is a mildly psychoactive cannabinoid that is primarily a product of THC degradation. As cannabis ages, THC is slowly converted to CBN, which has a much lower affinity for CB1 receptors than THC, resulting in milder psychoactive effects. CBN is gaining attention for its potential sedative effects, making it a possible treatment for insomnia. Some studies suggest that CBN might be more effective as a sleep aid when combined with other cannabinoids like THC and CBD, leveraging the "entourage effect," where multiple cannabinoids work together to enhance therapeutic outcomes. Additionally, CBN has shown potential as an anti-inflammatory agent and may have applications in pain management, particularly when inflammation is a contributing factor. Its antibacterial properties have also been noted, although this aspect of CBN is less explored. While research on CBN is still in its early stages, its mild psychoactive profile and potential therapeutic benefits make it an interesting candidate for further study, particularly in formulations designed for sleep disorders and chronic pain [93].

Cannabigerol (CBG)

Cannabigerol (CBG) is often referred to as the "mother cannabinoid" because it is the precursor from which other cannabinoids, including THC and CBD, are synthesized. CBG itself is non-psychoactive and interacts with both CB1 and CB2 receptors. However, it has a higher affinity for CB2 receptors, which are primarily involved in immune response regulation. CBG has been shown to possess a variety of therapeutic properties, including anti-inflammatory, antibacterial, and neuroprotective effects. It is particularly noted for its potential in treating conditions like Inflammatory Bowel Disease (IBD) due to its ability to reduce inflammation in the gut. CBG also shows promise in neuroprotective applications, potentially offering benefits for neurodegenerative diseases such as Huntington's disease, where it has been shown to protect neurons in preclinical models. Additionally, CBG's antibacterial properties have sparked interest in its use against resistant bacterial strains, such as MRSA (methicillin-resistant Staphylococcus aureus). Although less researched than THC or CBD, CBG's broad therapeutic potential and non-psychoactive nature make it a valuable candidate for further investigation [94].

Cannabichromene (CBC)

Cannabichromene (CBC) is one of the lesser-known cannabinoids, but it plays a significant role in the plant's pharmacological profile. Like CBD and CBG, CBC is non-psychoactive and does not bind strongly to CB1 or CB2 receptors. Instead, CBC interacts with other receptor systems in the body, such as the Transient Receptor Potential (TRP) channels, which are involved in the perception of pain and inflammation. CBC is particularly noted for its anti-inflammatory, analgesic, and antidepressant properties. It has been shown to inhibit the uptake of anandamide, an endocannabinoid that plays a role in pain and mood regulation, thereby enhancing anandamide's effects. This makes CBC a potential candidate for managing chronic pain and depression. Additionally, CBC has demonstrated potential in promoting neurogenesis, particularly in the hippocampus, an area of the brain crucial for memory and learning. This property suggests that CBC might have applications in treating neurodegenerative diseases and cognitive disorders.

While CBC is not as well-studied as THC or CBD, its unique interactions with the body's endocannabinoid and other receptor systems make it a promising area for future research [95].

NOVEL SYNTHETIC CANNABINOID ANALOGUES

HU-210

HU-210 is a synthetic cannabinoid that is a potent agonist of both CB1 and CB2 receptors. It was developed in the 1980s and is significantly more potent than THC, up to 100 times more so. HU-210 has been used extensively in research to understand the effects of cannabinoid receptor activation. Due to its high potency and affinity for cannabinoid receptors, HU-210 is a valuable tool for studying the endocannabinoid system and its role in various physiological and pathological processes. In preclinical studies, HU-210 has demonstrated strong anti-inflammatory and neuroprotective effects, suggesting potential applications in neurodegenerative diseases like Alzheimer's and Parkinson's disease. However, its potent psychoactive effects limit its use as a therapeutic agent in humans. The extreme potency of HU-210 can lead to significant side effects, including anxiety, paranoia, and cognitive impairment, similar to or more severe than those seen with high doses of THC. Despite these limitations, HU-210 continues to be an important compound in cannabinoid research, particularly in the development of new therapies that aim to maximize the therapeutic benefits of cannabinoid receptor activation while minimizing adverse effects [96].

JWH-133

JWH-133 is a synthetic cannabinoid with a high affinity for CB2 receptors and negligible activity at CB1 receptors, making it non-psychoactive. It was developed by Dr. John W. Huffman, who synthesized numerous cannabinoid analogues for research purposes. JWH-133's selectivity for CB2 receptors makes it particularly interesting for its potential therapeutic applications, especially in the context of inflammation and immune-related conditions. CB2 receptor activation is known to modulate immune cell function and reduce the release of pro-inflammatory cytokines, which are implicated in various autoimmune diseases and chronic inflammatory conditions. In preclinical studies, JWH-133 has shown promise in reducing inflammation in models of MS and rheumatoid arthritis. Additionally, it has demonstrated potential neuroprotective effects, particularly in reducing the progression of neuroinflammation and neuronal damage in models of neurodegenerative diseases. The lack of psychoactive effects makes JWH-133 an attractive candidate for therapeutic use, as it can potentially offer the benefits of cannabinoid therapy without the cognitive and psychological side effects associated with CB1 receptor activation. Ongoing research is focused on understanding the full therapeutic potential of JWH-133, particularly in chronic inflammatory and neurodegenerative conditions [97].

CP 55,940

CP 55,940 is another synthetic cannabinoid that was developed in the late 1970s as part of efforts to understand the ECS better. It is a potent agonist at both CB1 and CB2 receptors, with an affinity that is higher than that of THC. CP 55,940 is widely used in research as a reference compound to study the binding and activity of cannabinoid receptors. In preclinical studies, CP 55,940 has shown significant analgesic, anti-inflammatory, and neuroprotective effects. Its ability to activate both CB1 and CB2 receptors makes it a powerful tool for investigating the therapeutic potential of cannabinoids in various conditions, including pain, inflammation, and neurodegeneration. However, like HU-210, CP 55,940's potent activation of CB1 receptors also leads to strong psychoactive effects, which limit its therapeutic use in humans. The compound's high potency can result in pronounced side effects, including alterations in mood, cognition, and motor function. Despite these limitations, CP 55,940 remains an important compound in cannabinoid research, particularly for its role in elucidating the functions of the ECS and guiding the development of new therapeutic agents that target cannabinoid receptors [98].

WIN 55,212-2

WIN 55,212-2 is a synthetic cannabinoid that acts as a potent agonist at both CB1 and CB2 receptors. It was developed as part of research into the ECS and has been extensively used in studies exploring the physiological effects of cannabinoid receptor activation. WIN 55,212-2 has demonstrated a range of pharmacological effects, including analgesia, anti-inflammatory activity, and neuroprotection. In preclinical models, WIN 55,212-2 has been shown to reduce pain and inflammation, making it a valuable compound for studying [99]. The cannabinoid compounds and their various effects are shown in Fig. (**3**).

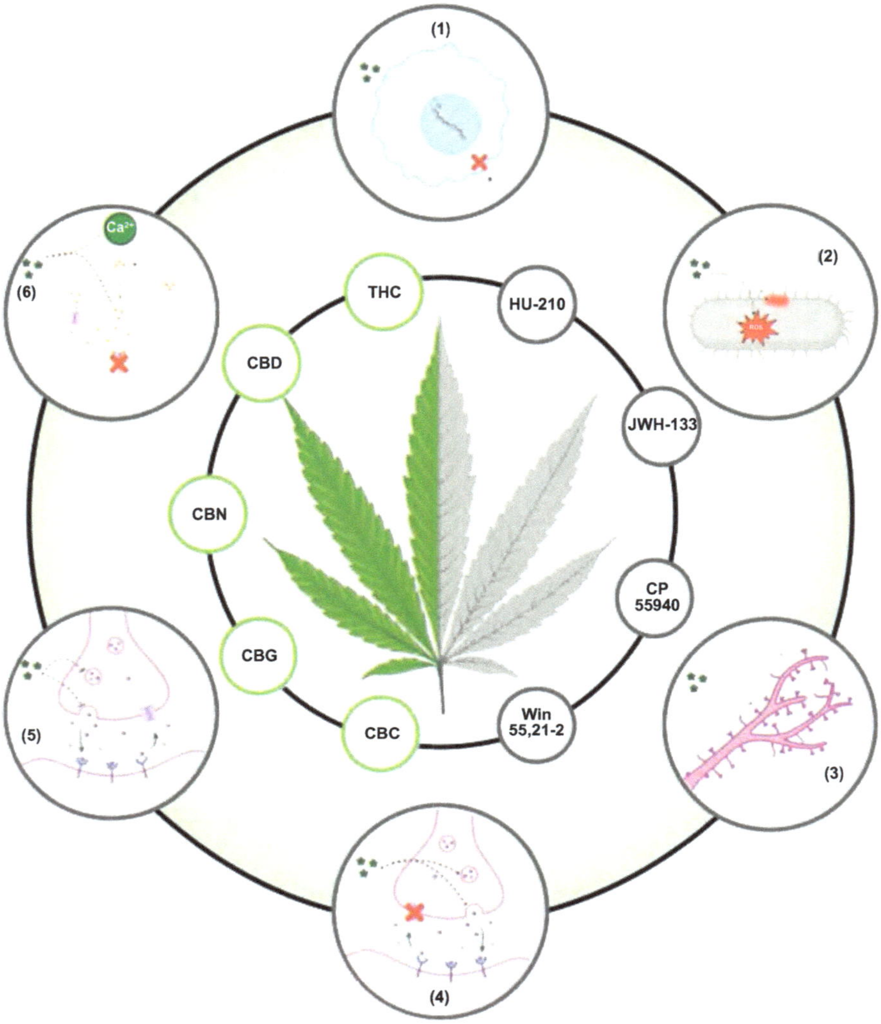

Fig. (3). Effects of Cannabinoids (The neuroprotective effects of cannabinoids are important in the treatment of multiple sclerosis. Various cannabinoid compounds are used in cannabinoid-based therapies. These compounds are shown with green and grey markers, representing naturally derived and synthetically produced compounds, respectively. The naturally derived compounds include Tetrahydrocannabinol (THC), cannabidiol (CBD), cannabinol (CBN), cannabigerol (CBG), and cannabichromene (CBC). The synthetic compounds include HU-210, JWH-133, CP 55940, and WIN 55,212-2. These compounds exhibit various activities, collectively categorized under neuroprotective effects as follows: (1) Anti-inflammatory activity by reducing the expression and release of pro-inflammatory cytokines; (2) Antibacterial activity by generating reactive oxygen species (ROS) and causing cell wall damage; (3) Neuroprotection through the promotion of synaptogenesis; (4) Antidepressant effects by increasing serotonin availability at 5HT/α receptors; (5) Anxiolytic effects through increased serotonin uptake and inhibition of serotonin release; (6) Anticonvulsant activity by reducing glutamate availability through increased calcium influx.).

NANOTECHNOLOGY IN CANNABINOID DELIVERY

Nanotechnology has emerged as a promising approach to enhancing Cannabinoid delivery in medical applications. By creating nano-formulations, it is possible to improve bioavailability and optimize the therapeutic potential of cannabinoids, overcoming challenges associated with their administration [100]. When combined with other therapeutic agents, cannabinoids can be more effective in treating conditions like pain, anxiety, and inflammatory disorders. This multi-modal approach leverages the complementary actions of different compounds, potentially leading to better patient outcomes. Nano-encapsulated cannabinoids are particularly promising for treating Inflammatory Bowel Diseases (IBD), as these formulations can target specific areas in the gastrointestinal tract, reducing inflammation and alleviating symptoms more effectively than traditional therapies.

Enhancement of Neuro-regulatory Mechanisms

The integration of nanotechnology into Cannabinoid therapies may also extend the regulatory action of neurotrophic factors like nerve growth factors. Carbon nanotubes have shown potential in promoting neuronal growth, suggesting a pathway through which cannabinoids could provide prolonged therapeutic effects in neurological conditions [101]. One of the main challenges in administering cannabinoids is their poor bioavailability, which refers to the proportion of a drug that reaches systemic circulation. Cannabinoids often have low water solubility and variable absorption rates, complicating their effective medicinal use [102]. Nanotechnology offers innovative strategies to address these issues by encapsulating cannabinoids in nanocarriers, which enhances their solubility, stability, and targeted distribution. These carriers also enable controlled release, maximizing therapeutic effects while minimizing side effects. Studies have shown that nano-formulations can significantly improve the solubility and stability of cannabinoids, allowing for more effective delivery and consistent therapeutic outcomes.

Enhanced Bioavailability of Cannabinoids

Research indicates that nanocarriers can significantly improve the bioavailability of cannabinoids, with some studies reporting enhanced absorption rates and sustained release profiles. This improvement is crucial for maintaining therapeutic levels in the bloodstream, thereby maximizing the pharmacological effects of cannabinoids in various clinical conditions, such as pain, anxiety, and inflammation. Cannabidiol (CBD), a non-psychoactive component of cannabis, has shown positive effects on specific body systems and has been effective in reducing seizures in some individuals with epilepsy.

Epilepsy

Clinical trials have demonstrated the effectiveness of cannabinoids, particularly CBD, in treating epilepsy, especially in patients with treatment-resistant forms like Dravet syndrome and Lennox-Gastaut syndrome [103]. Epidiolex, a CBD oral solution, has received FDA approval for these conditions, making it the first cannabis-derived medication authorized for treating seizures related to these syndromes [104]. Additionally, studies have shown that CBD can reduce seizure frequency by 37-42% in treated groups compared to lower rates in placebo groups.

Multiple Sclerosis

Numerous clinical trials have explored the benefits of cannabinoids in managing Multiple Sclerosis (MS) symptoms, particularly spasticity, neuropathic pain, and sleep disturbances. Evidence suggests that cannabinoids can alleviate spasticity and improve the quality of life for MS patients, with systematic reviews offering moderate-quality evidence for these effects. Nabiximols, an oromucosal spray containing THC and CBD, has been used effectively to treat MS-related spasticity [105].

Parkinson's disease

Research on the effects of cannabinoids on Parkinson's disease has yielded mixed results, particularly concerning motor symptoms. Some clinical trials suggest potential benefits for non-motor symptoms, such as anxiety and pain relief, indicating that cannabinoids may improve overall well-being in patients [106]. However, more comprehensive and controlled studies are needed to fully assess the effectiveness and optimal administration methods for cannabinoids in treating Parkinson's disease [107].

EVIDENCE-BASED STUDIES AND SAFETY CONCERNS

While the therapeutic potential of cannabinoids for neurological disorders is clear, safety and side effect profiles must be carefully considered. Clinical trials report various adverse events associated with cannabinoid use, including dizziness, dry mouth, fatigue, and sedation. Although there may be an increased risk of short-term adverse events, many side effects are generally mild to moderate and often dose-related. This underscores the importance of balancing benefits and potential risks when using cannabinoids in clinical practice for neurological disorders. Moreover, MS patients strive to obtain easy medications for their symptoms according to the stage of MS, as shown in Table **1**. It describes modern products that are FDA standard approved drug molecules which can be used for multi-neuro-disorder treatment, these products are combined with cannabinoids and their derivatives.

Table 1. Modern products of Cannabinoids for neuro-disease management.

S. No	Product name	Treated disorder	Mechanism of action	References
1	Charlotte's Web	Epilepsy	CBD acts as an agonist at cannabinoid receptors in the brain, leading to neuromodulatory effects that can reduce symptoms like pain, spasticity, and seizures.	[108]
2	Koi CBD	Anxiety	Modulates endocannabinoid receptors.	[109]
3	PlusCBD Oil	Sleep disorders	Enhances endocannabinoid system functioning.	[110]
4	Epidiolex	Seizures	Cannabidiol (CBD) modulates intracellular calcium levels, which can stabilize neuronal activity and reduce the likelihood of seizures.	[111]
5	NuLeaf Naturals	Anxiety, depression	CBD interacts with cannabinoid receptors (CB1 and CB2) distributed throughout the body, influencing various physiological processes like pain perception, mood, and immune response.	[112]
6	PureKana	Anxiety, depression	CBD interacts with cannabinoid receptors (CB1 and CB2) distributed throughout the body, influencing various physiological processes like pain perception, mood, and immune response.	[113]
7	CBD American Shaman	Stress and anxiety	CBD acts as an agonist at cannabinoid receptors in the brain, leading to neuromodulatory effects that can reduce symptoms like pain, spasticity, and seizures.	[114]
8	CBDfx	Stress and anxiety	CBD acts as an agonist at cannabinoid receptors in the brain, leading to neuromodulatory effects that can reduce symptoms like pain, spasticity, and seizures.	[115]
9	Veritas Farms	Depression	CBD acts as an agonist at cannabinoid receptors in the brain, leading to neuromodulatory effects that can reduce symptoms like pain, spasticity, and seizures.	[116]
10	Sativex	Multiple sclerosis	CBD acts as an agonist at cannabinoid receptors in the brain, leading to neuromodulatory effects that can reduce symptoms like pain, spasticity, and seizures.	[117]
11	CBD oral solution	Seizures	CBD modulates the activity of the endocannabinoid system by interacting with cannabinoid receptors, leading to a range of therapeutic effects, including seizure reduction and anxiety relief.	[118]
12	Medterra CBD	Anxiety	CBD interacts with cannabinoid receptors (CB1 and CB2) distributed throughout the body, influencing various physiological processes like pain perception, mood, and immune response.	[119]

(Table 1) cont.....

S. No	Product name	Treated disorder	Mechanism of action	References
13	Hemp Bombs	Anxiety, epilepsy	Enhances endocannabinoid system functioning.	[120]
14	Green Roads CBD	Stress	CBD interacts with cannabinoid receptors (CB1 and CB2) distributed throughout the body, influencing various physiological processes like pain perception, mood, and immune response.	[121]
15	Nabiximols	Multiple sclerosis	CBD enhances the signaling of the endocannabinoid system by inhibiting the breakdown of endocannabinoids, which can alleviate symptoms like pain, anxiety, and inflammation.	[117]
16	Royal CBD	Anxiety, depression, ' 'Alzheimer's disease	Modulates endocannabinoid receptors.	[122]
17	Funky Farms	Stress and anxiety	Enhances endocannabinoid system functioning.	[123]
18	Bluebird Botanicals	Stress and anxiety	Enhances endocannabinoid system functioning.	[124]
19	Joy Organics	Stress and anxiety	Modulates endocannabinoid receptors.	[125]

CONCLUSION

The administration of cannabinoids has significant impacts on several organ systems, including the Central Nervous System (CNS), some of which are medicinal. The complicated side effect profile of various cannabinoids, especially THC and other CB1 agonists, is their main disadvantage. THC and synthetics that resemble it have some potential for treating pain and anxiety, but they can seriously impair cognitive function. However, by changing how pain and anxiety are perceived, THC and related synthetics may have some therapeutic benefits due to their psychotropic effects. Creating synthetic cannabinoids that positively activate CB1 receptors in specific brain areas and peripheral neurons without noticeable cognitive impact is one of the main research problems going forward. There may be greater potential for CBD, a non-psychotropic cannabis compound, to treat some neurodegenerative illnesses. The regulated administration of CBD therapies to the correct location of action can provide a hurdle. Research has unequivocally demonstrated the safety of CBD, which suggests that the development of more potent and stable CBD analogs is likely underway.

REFERENCES

[1] Prineas JW, Parratt JDE. Oligodendrocytes and the early multiple sclerosis lesion. Ann Neurol 2012; 72(1): 18-31. [http://dx.doi.org/10.1002/ana.23634] [PMID: 22829266]

[2] Stadelmann C, Timmler S, Barrantes-Freer A, Simons M. Myelin in the central nervous system: Structure, function, and pathology. Physiol Rev 2019; 99(3): 1381-431. [http://dx.doi.org/10.1152/physrev.00031.2018] [PMID: 31066630]

[3] Fakhoury M. Role of immunity and inflammation in the pathophysiology of neurodegenerative diseases. Neurodegener Dis 2015; 15(2): 63-9. [http://dx.doi.org/10.1159/000369933] [PMID: 25591815]

[4] Safaralizadeh R, Eslahi M, Nematbakhsh N, Dastmalchi N, Teimourian S. An updated review of epigenetic-related mechanisms and their contribution to multiple sclerosis disease. CNS Neurol Disord Drug Targets 2023; 22(3): 381-93. [http://dx.doi.org/10.2174/1871527321666220119104649] [PMID: 35043771]

[5] Thompson K, Tsirka S. The diverse roles of microglia in the neurodegenerative aspects of central nervous system (CNS) autoimmunity. Int J Mol Sci 2017; 18(3): 504. [http://dx.doi.org/10.3390/ijms18030504] [PMID: 28245617]

[6] Pachner AR, Li L, Lagunoff D. Plasma cells in the central nervous system in the Theiler's virus model of multiple sclerosis. J Neuroimmunol 2011; 232(1-2): 35-40. [http://dx.doi.org/10.1016/j.jneuroim.2010.09.026] [PMID: 20961623]

[7] Simpson DSA, Oliver PL. ROS generation in microglia: Understanding oxidative stress and inflammation in neurodegenerative disease. Antioxidants 2020; 9(8): 743. [http://dx.doi.org/10.3390/antiox9080743] [PMID: 32823544]

[8] Brück W. The pathology of multiple sclerosis is the result of focal inflammatory demyelination with axonal damage. J Neurol 2005; 252(S5) (Suppl. 5): v3-9. [http://dx.doi.org/10.1007/s00415-005-5002-7] [PMID: 16254699]

[9] Kutzelnigg A, Lassmann H. Pathology of multiple sclerosis and related inflammatory demyelinating diseases Handbook of Clinical Neurology. Elsevier 2014; Vol. 122: pp. 15-58. [http://dx.doi.org/10.1016/B978-0-444-52001-2.00002-9]

[10] Klingseisen A, Lyons DA. Axonal regulation of central nervous system myelination: Structure and function. Neuroscientist 2018; 24(1): 7-21. [http://dx.doi.org/10.1177/1073858417703030] [PMID: 28397586]

[11] Caon M. Nervous system examination questions and answers in basic anatomy and physiology. Cham: Springer International Publishing 2020; pp. 503-84. [http://dx.doi.org/10.1007/978-3-030-47314-3_14]

[12] Niu J, Tsai HH, Hoi KK, *et al.* Aberrant oligodendroglial–vascular interactions disrupt the blood–brain barrier, triggering CNS inflammation. Nat Neurosci 2019; 22(5): 709-18. [http://dx.doi.org/10.1038/s41593-019-0369-4] [PMID: 30988524]

[13] Grigorian A, Mkhikian H, Li CF, Newton BL, Zhou RW, Demetriou M. Pathogenesis of multiple sclerosis *via* environmental and genetic dysregulation of N-glycosylation. Semin Immunopathol 2012; 34(3): 415-24. [http://dx.doi.org/10.1007/s00281-012-0307-y] [PMID: 22488447]

[14] Kemppinen A, Sawcer S, Compston A. Genome-wide association studies in multiple sclerosis: lessons and future prospects. Brief Funct Genomics 2011; 10(2): 61-70. [http://dx.doi.org/10.1093/bfgp/elr004] [PMID: 21310812]

[15] Wingerchuk DM. Environmental factors in multiple sclerosis: Epstein-Barr virus, vitamin D, and cigarette smoking. Mt Sinai J Med 2011; 78(2): 221-30. [http://dx.doi.org/10.1002/msj.20240] [PMID: 21425266]

[16] Bross M, Hackett M, Bernitsas E. Approved and emerging disease modifying therapies on neurodegeneration in multiple sclerosis. Int J Mol Sci 2020; 21(12): 4312. [http://dx.doi.org/10.3390/ijms21124312] [PMID: 32560364]

[17] Mancuso S, Mattana M, Carlisi M, Santoro M, Siragusa S. Effects of B-cell lymphoma on the immune system and immune recovery after treatment: The paradigm of targeted therapy. Int J Mol Sci 2022; 23(6): 3368. [http://dx.doi.org/10.3390/ijms23063368] [PMID: 35328789]

[18] Steinman L. Immunology of relapse and remission in multiple sclerosis. Annu Rev Immunol 2014; 32(1): 257-81. [http://dx.doi.org/10.1146/annurev-immunol-032713-120227] [PMID: 24438352]

[19] Piehl F. Current and emerging disease-modulatory therapies and treatment targets for multiple sclerosis. J Intern Med 2021; 289(6): 771-91. [http://dx.doi.org/10.1111/joim.13215] [PMID: 33258193]

[20] Gharwan H, Groninger H. Kinase inhibitors and monoclonal antibodies in oncology: clinical implications. Nat Rev Clin Oncol 2016; 13(4): 209-27. [http://dx.doi.org/10.1038/nrclinonc.2015.213] [PMID: 26718105]

[21] Berríos-Cárcamo P, Quezada M, Quintanilla ME, *et al.* Oxidative stress and neuroinflammation as a pivot in drug abuse. A focus on the therapeutic potential of antioxidant and anti-inflammatory agents and biomolecules. Antioxidants 2020; 9(9): 830. [http://dx.doi.org/10.3390/antiox9090830] [PMID: 32899889]

[22] Maurya SK, Bhattacharya N, Mishra S, *et al.* Microglia specific drug targeting using natural products for the regulation of redox imbalance in neurodegeneration. Front Pharmacol 2021; 12: 654489. [http://dx.doi.org/10.3389/fphar.2021.654489] [PMID: 33927630]

[23] Klotz L, Havla J, Schwab N, *et al.* Risks and risk management in modern multiple sclerosis immunotherapeutic treatment. Ther Adv Neurol Disord 2019; 12: 1756286419836571. [http://dx.doi.org/10.1177/1756286419836571] [PMID: 30967901]

[24] Boyman O, Comte D, Spertini F. Adverse reactions to biologic agents and their medical management. Nat Rev Rheumatol 2014; 10(10): 612-27. [http://dx.doi.org/10.1038/nrrheum.2014.123] [PMID: 25112605]

[25] Hamine S, Gerth-Guyette E, Faulx D, Green BB, Ginsburg AS. Impact of mHealth chronic disease management on treatment adherence and patient outcomes: a systematic review. J Med Internet Res 2015; 17(2): e52. [http://dx.doi.org/10.2196/jmir.3951] [PMID: 25803266]

[26] Montalban X, Gold R, Thompson AJ, *et al.* ECTRIMS/EAN Guideline on the pharmacological treatment of people with multiple sclerosis. Mult Scler 2018; 24(2): 96-120. [http://dx.doi.org/10.1177/1352458517751049] [PMID: 29353550]

[27] Correale J, Gaitán MI, Ysrraelit MC, Fiol MP. Progressive multiple sclerosis: from pathogenic mechanisms to treatment. Brain 2016; aww258. [http://dx.doi.org/10.1093/brain/aww258] [PMID: 27794524]

[28] Yadav DK. Potential therapeutic strategies of phytochemicals in neurodegenerative disorders. Curr Top Med Chem 2021; 21(31): 2814-38. [http://dx.doi.org/10.2174/1568026621666211201150217] [PMID: 34852737]

[29] Fong J, Rae-Grant A, Huang D. Neurodegeneration and neuroprotective agents in multiple sclerosis. Recent Patents CNS Drug Discov 2008; 3(3): 153-65. [http://dx.doi.org/10.2174/157488908786242498] [PMID: 18991805]

[30] Hussain MS, Chaturvedi V, Goyal S, Singh S, Mir RH. An update on the application of nano phytomedicine as an emerging therapeutic tool for neurodegenerative diseases. Curr Bioact Compd 2024; 20(5): e251023222648.

[http://dx.doi.org/10.2174/011573407225865623101308531 8]

[31] Miljković D, Spasojević I. Multiple sclerosis: molecular mechanisms and therapeutic opportunities. Antioxid Redox Signal 2013; 19(18): 2286-334.
[http://dx.doi.org/10.1089/ars.2012.5068] [PMID: 23473637]

[32] Farzaei MH, Shahpiri Z, Bahramsoltani R, nia MM, Najafi F, Rahimi R. Efficacy and tolerability of phytomedicines in multiple sclerosis patients: A Review. CNS Drugs 2017; 31(10): 867-89.
[http://dx.doi.org/10.1007/s40263-017-0466-4] [PMID: 28948486]

[33] Bhatti GK, Singh HV, Sharma E, Sehrawat A, Mishra J, Navik U, *et al.* Protective role of natural products and bioactive compounds in multiple sclerosis. Treatments, Nutraceuticals, Supplements, and Herbal Medicine in Neurological Disorders 2023; 453-82.
[http://dx.doi.org/10.1016/B978-0-323-90052-2.00026-3]

[34] Rehman MU, Wali AF, Ahmad A, Shakeel S, Rasool S, Ali R, *et al.* Neuroprotective strategies for neurological disorders by natural products: an update. CN 2019; 17: 247-67.
[http://dx.doi.org/10.2174/1570159X16666180911124605]

[35] De Luca C, Colangelo AM, Alberghina L, Papa M. Neuro-immune hemostasis: Homeostasis and diseases in the central nervous system. Front Cell Neurosci 2018; 12: 459.
[http://dx.doi.org/10.3389/fncel.2018.00459] [PMID: 30534057]

[36] Stangel M. Remyelinating and neuroprotective treatments in multiple sclerosis. Expert Opin Investig Drugs 2004; 13(4): 331-47.
[http://dx.doi.org/10.1517/13543784.13.4.331] [PMID: 15102584]

[37] Miller E, Morel A, Redlicka J, Miller I, Saluk J. Pharmacological and non-pharmacological therapies of cognitive impairment in multiple sclerosis. CN 2018; 16: 475-83.
[http://dx.doi.org/10.2174/1570159X15666171109132650]

[38] Yong H, Chartier G, Quandt J. Modulating inflammation and neuroprotection in multiple sclerosis. J Neurosci Res 2018; 96(6): 927-50.
[http://dx.doi.org/10.1002/jnr.24090] [PMID: 28580582]

[39] Zeng Y, Li Z, Zhu H, Gu Z, Zhang H, Luo K. Recent advances in nanomedicines for multiple sclerosis therapy. ACS Appl Bio Mater 2020; 3(10): 6571-97.
[http://dx.doi.org/10.1021/acsabm.0c00953] [PMID: 35019387]

[40] Allanach JR, Farrell JW III, Mésidor M, Karimi-Abdolrezaee S. Current status of neuroprotective and neuroregenerative strategies in multiple sclerosis: A systematic review. Mult Scler 2022; 28(1): 29-48.
[http://dx.doi.org/10.1177/13524585211008760] [PMID: 33870797]

[41] Faissner S, Plemel JR, Gold R, Yong VW. Progressive multiple sclerosis: from pathophysiology to therapeutic strategies. Nat Rev Drug Discov 2019; 18(12): 905-22.
[http://dx.doi.org/10.1038/s41573-019-0035-2] [PMID: 31399729]

[42] Hourfane S, Mechqoq H, Bekkali AY, Rocha JM, El Aouad N. A comprehensive review on *Cannabis sativa* ethnobotany, phytochemistry, molecular docking and biological activities. Plants 2023; 12(6): 1245.
[http://dx.doi.org/10.3390/plants12061245] [PMID: 36986932]

[43] Gupta P, Singh A, Shafi S, *et al.* Cannabis sativa in phytotherapy: Reappraisal of therapeutic potential and regulatory aspects. Curr Pharm Biotechnol 2024; 25(1): 58-76.
[http://dx.doi.org/10.2174/1389201024666230508142114] [PMID: 37157219]

[44] Lu HC, Mackie K. Review of the endocannabinoid system. Biol Psychiatry Cogn Neurosci Neuroimaging 2021; 6(6): 607-15.
[http://dx.doi.org/10.1016/j.bpsc.2020.07.016] [PMID: 32980261]

[45] Wu J. Cannabis, cannabinoid receptors, and endocannabinoid system: yesterday, today, and tomorrow. Acta Pharmacol Sin 2019; 40(3): 297-9.
[http://dx.doi.org/10.1038/s41401-019-0210-3] [PMID: 30670816]

[46] Chanda D, Neumann D, Glatz JFC. The endocannabinoid system: Overview of an emerging multi-faceted therapeutic target. Prostaglandins Leukot Essent Fatty Acids 2019; 140: 51-6. [http://dx.doi.org/10.1016/j.plefa.2018.11.016] [PMID: 30553404]

[47] Tian L, Rauvala H, Gahmberg CG. Neuronal regulation of immune responses in the central nervous system. Trends Immunol 2009; 30(2): 91-9. [http://dx.doi.org/10.1016/j.it.2008.11.002] [PMID: 19144568]

[48] Maurya N, Velmurugan BK. Therapeutic applications of cannabinoids. Chem Biol Interact 2018; 293: 77-88. [http://dx.doi.org/10.1016/j.cbi.2018.07.018] [PMID: 30040916]

[49] Seghetti F, Gobbi S, Belluti F, Rampa A, Bisi A. Interplay between endocannabinoid system and neurodegeneration: Focus on Polypharmacology. Curr Med Chem 2022; 29(28): 4796-830. [http://dx.doi.org/10.2174/0929867328666211115124639] [PMID: 34781863]

[50] Russo E, Guy GW. A tale of two cannabinoids: The therapeutic rationale for combining tetrahydrocannabinol and cannabidiol. Med Hypotheses 2006; 66(2): 234-46. [http://dx.doi.org/10.1016/j.mehy.2005.08.026] [PMID: 16209908]

[51] Ben-Zacharia AB. Therapeutics for multiple sclerosis symptoms. Mt Sinai J Med 2011; 78(2): 176-91. [http://dx.doi.org/10.1002/msj.20245] [PMID: 21425263]

[52] MacCallum CA, Russo EB. Practical considerations in medical cannabis administration and dosing. Eur J Intern Med 2018; 49: 12-9. [http://dx.doi.org/10.1016/j.ejim.2018.01.004] [PMID: 29307505]

[53] Schlag AK, Hindocha C, Zafar R, Nutt DJ, Curran HV. Cannabis based medicines and cannabis dependence: A critical review of issues and evidence. J Psychopharmacol 2021; 35(7): 773-85. [http://dx.doi.org/10.1177/0269881120986393] [PMID: 33593117]

[54] Legare CA, Raup-Konsavage WM, Vrana KE. Therapeutic potential of cannabis, cannabidiol, and cannabinoid-based pharmaceuticals. Pharmacology 2022; 107(3-4): 131-49. [http://dx.doi.org/10.1159/000521683] [PMID: 35093949]

[55] Russo EB. Current therapeutic cannabis controversies and clinical trial design issues. Front Pharmacol 2016; 7: 309. [http://dx.doi.org/10.3389/fphar.2016.00309] [PMID: 27683558]

[56] Kuchling J, Paul F. Visualizing the central nervous system: Imaging tools for multiple sclerosis and neuromyelitis optica spectrum disorders. Front Neurol 2020; 11: 450. [http://dx.doi.org/10.3389/fneur.2020.00450] [PMID: 32625158]

[57] Haider L, Zrzavy T, Hametner S, *et al.* The topograpy of demyelination and neurodegeneration in the multiple sclerosis brain. Brain 2016; 139(3): 807-15. [http://dx.doi.org/10.1093/brain/awv398] [PMID: 26912645]

[58] Höftberger R, Lassmann H. Inflammatory demyelinating diseases of the central nervous system Handbook of Clinical Neurology. Elsevier 2018; Vol. 145: pp. 263-83. [http://dx.doi.org/10.1016/B978-0-12-802395-2.00019-5]

[59] Williams A. Remyelination in multiple sclerosis: What do we know and where are we going?. Neurodegener Dis Manag 2015; 5(1): 49-59. [http://dx.doi.org/10.2217/nmt.14.40] [PMID: 25711454]

[60] Rossi S, Bernardi G, Centonze D. The endocannabinoid system in the inflammatory and neurodegenerative processes of multiple sclerosis and of amyotrophic lateral sclerosis. Exp Neurol 2010; 224(1): 92-102. [http://dx.doi.org/10.1016/j.expneurol.2010.03.030] [PMID: 20353778]

[61] Derada Troletti C, Fontijn RD, Gowing E, *et al.* Inflammation-induced endothelial to mesenchymal transition promotes brain endothelial cell dysfunction and occurs during multiple sclerosis

pathophysiology. Cell Death Dis 2019; 10(2): 45.
[http://dx.doi.org/10.1038/s41419-018-1294-2] [PMID: 30718504]

[62] Bisogno T, Di Marzo V. Cannabinoid receptors and endocannabinoids: role in neuroinflammatory and neurodegenerative disorders. CNS Neurol Disord Drug Targets 2010; 9(5): 564-73.
[http://dx.doi.org/10.2174/187152710793361568] [PMID: 20632970]

[63] Di Marzo V. The endocannabinoid system for the development of new drugs for spasticity. Drugs Future 2007; 32: 341.
[http://dx.doi.org/10.1358/dof.2007.032.04.1083482]

[64] Bourke SL, Schlag AK, O'Sullivan SE, Nutt DJ, Finn DP. Cannabinoids and the endocannabinoid system in fibromyalgia: A review of preclinical and clinical research. Pharmacol Ther 2022; 240: 108216.
[http://dx.doi.org/10.1016/j.pharmthera.2022.108216] [PMID: 35609718]

[65] Ware MA, Adams H, Guy GW. The medicinal use of cannabis in the UK: results of a nationwide survey. Int J Clin Pract 2005; 59(3): 291-5.
[http://dx.doi.org/10.1111/j.1742-1241.2004.00271.x] [PMID: 15857325]

[66] Giacoppo S, Mandolino G, Galuppo M, Bramanti P, Mazzon E. Cannabinoids: new promising agents in the treatment of neurological diseases. Molecules 2014; 19(11): 18781-816.
[http://dx.doi.org/10.3390/molecules191118781] [PMID: 25407719]

[67] Baker D, Pryce G. The endocannabinoid system and multiple sclerosis. Curr Pharm Des 2008; 14(23): 2326-36.
[http://dx.doi.org/10.2174/138161208785740036] [PMID: 18781983]

[68] Rodríguez Mesa XM, Moreno Vergara AF, Contreras Bolaños LA, Guevara Moriones N, Mejía Piñeros AL, Santander González SP. Therapeutic prospects of cannabinoids in the immunomodulation of prevalent autoimmune diseases. Cannabis Cannabinoid Res 2021; 6(3): 196-210.
[http://dx.doi.org/10.1089/can.2020.0183] [PMID: 34030476]

[69] Mecha M, Feliú A, Iñigo PM, Mestre L, Carrillo-Salinas FJ, Guaza C. Cannabidiol provides long-lasting protection against the deleterious effects of inflammation in a viral model of multiple sclerosis: A role for A2A receptors. Neurobiol Dis 2013; 59: 141-50.
[http://dx.doi.org/10.1016/j.nbd.2013.06.016] [PMID: 23851307]

[70] Jahan-Abad AJ, Karima S, Shateri S, *et al.* Serum pro-inflammatory and anti-inflammatory cytokines and the pathogenesis of experimental autoimmune encephalomyelitis. Neuropathology 2020; 40(1): 84-92.
[http://dx.doi.org/10.1111/neup.12612] [PMID: 31709666]

[71] Musella A, Fresegna D, Rizzo FR, *et al.* 'Prototypical' proinflammatory cytokine (IL-1) in multiple sclerosis: role in pathogenesis and therapeutic targeting. Expert Opin Ther Targets 2020; 24(1): 37-46.
[http://dx.doi.org/10.1080/14728222.2020.1709823] [PMID: 31899994]

[72] Minghetti L, Carnevale D, Simone R. Microglia-neuron interaction in inflammatory and degenerative diseases: role of cholinergic and noradrenergic systems. CNS Neurol Disord Drug Targets 2007; 6(6): 388-97.
[http://dx.doi.org/10.2174/187152707783399193] [PMID: 18220778]

[73] Jeffrey J. Bajramovic. Regulation of innate immune responses in the central nervous system, CNS & neurological disorders. Drug Targets 2011; 10(1).
[http://dx.doi.org/10.2174/187152711794488610]

[74] Lago E, Fernández-Ruiz J. Cannabinoids and neuroprotection in motor-related disorders. CNS Neurol Disord Drug Targets 2007; 6(6): 377-87.
[http://dx.doi.org/10.2174/187152707783399210] [PMID: 18220777]

[75] Pisanti S, Malfitano AM, Ciaglia E, *et al.* Cannabidiol: State of the art and new challenges for therapeutic applications. Pharmacol Ther 2017; 175: 133-50.

[http://dx.doi.org/10.1016/j.pharmthera.2017.02.041] [PMID: 28232276]

[76] Ashton J, Glass M. The cannabinoid CB2 receptor as a target for inflammation-dependent neurodegeneration. CN 2007; 5: 73-80. [http://dx.doi.org/10.2174/157015907780866884]

[77] Yıldızhan K, Nazıroğlu M. Microglia and its role in neurodegenerative diseases. Journal of Cellular Neuroscience and Oxidative Stress 2019; 11(2): 861-73. [http://dx.doi.org/10.37212/jcnos.683407]

[78] Micale V, Mazzola C, Drago F. Endocannabinoids and neurodegenerative diseases. Pharmacol Res 2007; 56(5): 382-92. [http://dx.doi.org/10.1016/j.phrs.2007.09.008] [PMID: 17950616]

[79] Docagne F, Muñetón V, Clemente D, *et al.* Excitotoxicity in a chronic model of multiple sclerosis: Neuroprotective effects of cannabinoids through CB1 and CB2 receptor activation. Mol Cell Neurosci 2007; 34(4): 551-61. [http://dx.doi.org/10.1016/j.mcn.2006.12.005] [PMID: 17229577]

[80] Paloczi J, Varga ZV, Hasko G, Pacher P. Neuroprotection in oxidative stress-related neurodegenerative diseases: Role of endocannabinoid system modulation. Antioxid Redox Signal 2018; 29(1): 75-108. [http://dx.doi.org/10.1089/ars.2017.7144] [PMID: 28497982]

[81] Pertwee RG. The diverse CB_1 and CB_2 receptor pharmacology of three plant cannabinoids: Δ^9-tetrahydrocannabinol, cannabidiol and Δ^9-tetrahydrocannabivarin. Br J Pharmacol 2008; 153(2): 199-215. [http://dx.doi.org/10.1038/sj.bjp.0707442] [PMID: 17828291]

[82] Bhunia S, Kolishetti N, Arias AY, Vashist A, Nair M. Cannabidiol for neurodegenerative disorders: A comprehensive review. Front Pharmacol 2022; 13: 989717. [http://dx.doi.org/10.3389/fphar.2022.989717] [PMID: 36386183]

[83] Al-Khazaleh AK, Zhou X, Bhuyan DJ, *et al.* The neurotherapeutic arsenal in *cannabis sativa*: Insights into anti-neuroinflammatory and neuroprotective activity and potential entourage effects. Molecules 2024; 29(2): 410. [http://dx.doi.org/10.3390/molecules29020410] [PMID: 38257323]

[84] Neri S, Mastroianni G, Gardella E, Aguglia U, Rubboli G. Epilepsy in neurodegenerative diseases. Epileptic Disord 2022; 24(2): 249-73. [http://dx.doi.org/10.1684/epd.2021.1406] [PMID: 35596580]

[85] Shkodina AD, Bardhan M, Chopra H, *et al.* Pharmacological and non-pharmacological approaches for the management of neuropathic pain in multiple sclerosis. CNS Drugs 2024; 38(3): 205-24. [http://dx.doi.org/10.1007/s40263-024-01072-5] [PMID: 38421578]

[86] Amatya B, Khan F. Are cannabis and cannabinoids effective for symptomatic treatment in people with multiple sclerosis?. Am J Phys Med Rehabil 2023; 102(1): 83-4. [http://dx.doi.org/10.1097/PHM.0000000000002106] [PMID: 36099645]

[87] Campos MG, China M, Cláudio M, *et al.* Drug–cannabinoid interactions in selected therapeutics for symptoms associated with epilepsy, autism spectrum disorder, cancer, multiple sclerosis, and pain. Pharmaceuticals (Basel) 2024; 17(5): 613. [http://dx.doi.org/10.3390/ph17050613] [PMID: 38794183]

[88] Stasiłowicz-Krzemień A, Nogalska W, Maszewska Z, *et al.* The use of compounds derived from *Cannabis sativa* in the treatment of epilepsy, painful conditions, and neuropsychiatric and neurodegenerative disorders. Int J Mol Sci 2024; 25(11): 5749. [http://dx.doi.org/10.3390/ijms25115749] [PMID: 38891938]

[89] Marini P, Maccarrone M, Saso L, Tucci P. The effect of phytocannabinoids and endocannabinoids on Nrf2 activity in the central nervous system and periphery. Neurol Int 2024; 16(4): 776-89.

[http://dx.doi.org/10.3390/neurolint16040057] [PMID: 39051218]

[90] Khaspekov LG, Illarioshkin SN. Therapeutic application of modulators of endogenous cannabinoid system in Parkinson's disease. Int J Mol Sci 2024; 25(15): 8520. [http://dx.doi.org/10.3390/ijms25158520] [PMID: 39126088]

[91] Choi S, Joseph E. A Novel tetrahydrocannabinol (THC) analog, 3,10,10-Trimethy--1,2,3,4,4a,6,7,8,10,10a-decahydro-9-oxa-5-phenanthrenone (TDP), mitigates the decrease in cell viability in oxidatively-stressed osteosarcoma bone-like cell cultures, UMR 106-01 BSP (UMR cells). Physiology (Bethesda) 2024; 39(S1): 1406. [http://dx.doi.org/10.1152/physiol.2024.39.S1.1406]

[92] Raïch I, Lillo J, Rivas-Santisteban R, *et al.* Potential of CBD acting on cannabinoid receptors CB_1 and CB_2 in ischemic stroke. Int J Mol Sci 2024; 25(12): 6708. [http://dx.doi.org/10.3390/ijms25126708] [PMID: 38928415]

[93] Khouchlaa A, Khouri S, Hajib A, *et al.* Health benefits, pharmacological properties, and metabolism of cannabinol: A comprehensive review. Ind Crops Prod 2024; 213: 118359. [http://dx.doi.org/10.1016/j.indcrop.2024.118359]

[94] Pires HFO, da Silva PR, Dias AL, *et al.* Mechanisms involved in the therapeutic effect of cannabinoid compounds on gliomas: A review with experimental approach. Curr Protein Pept Sci 2024; 25(1): 27-43. [http://dx.doi.org/10.2174/1389203724666230830125423] [PMID: 37649287]

[95] Anand R, Painuli R, Kumar V, Singh PP. Chemistry and pharmacological aspects of furanoid cannabinoids and related compounds: Is furanoid cannabinoids open a new dimension towards the non-psychoactive cannabinoids?. Eur J Med Chem 2024; 268: 116164. [http://dx.doi.org/10.1016/j.ejmech.2024.116164] [PMID: 38417219]

[96] Li G, Choi J, Stephens KL, DeGeorge BR Jr. Vasoactive and antifibrotic properties of cannabinoids and applications to vasospastic/vaso-occlusive disorders. Ann Plast Surg 2024; 92(6S) (Suppl. 4): S445-52. [http://dx.doi.org/10.1097/SAP.0000000000003985] [PMID: 38857012]

[97] Das S, Ghosh A, Karmakar V, *et al.* Cannabis effectiveness on immunologic potency of pulmonary contagion. J Basic Clin Physiol Pharmacol 2024; 35(3): 129-42. [http://dx.doi.org/10.1515/jbcpp-2023-0030] [PMID: 38635412]

[98] Heal DJ, Gosden J, Smith SL. A critical assessment of the abuse, dependence and associated safety risks of naturally occurring and synthetic cannabinoids. Front Psychiatry 2024; 15: 1322434. [http://dx.doi.org/10.3389/fpsyt.2024.1322434] [PMID: 38915848]

[99] Barker H, Ferraro MJ. Exploring the versatile roles of the endocannabinoid system and phytocannabinoids in modulating bacterial infections. Infect Immun 2024; 92(6): e00020-24. [http://dx.doi.org/10.1128/iai.00020-24] [PMID: 38775488]

[100] Reddy TS, Zomer R, Mantri N. Nanoformulations as a strategy to overcome the delivery limitations of cannabinoids. Phytother Res 2023; 37(4): 1526-38. [http://dx.doi.org/10.1002/ptr.7742] [PMID: 36748949]

[101] Hassanzadeh P, Arbabi E, Atyabi F, Dinarvand R. Nerve growth factor-carbon nanotube complex exerts prolonged protective effects in an *in vitro* model of ischemic stroke. Life Sci 2017; 179: 15-22. [http://dx.doi.org/10.1016/j.lfs.2016.11.029] [PMID: 27919823]

[102] Bruni N, Della Pepa C, Oliaro-Bosso S, Pessione E, Gastaldi D, Dosio F. Cannabinoid delivery systems for pain and inflammation treatment. Molecules 2018; 23(10): 2478. [http://dx.doi.org/10.3390/molecules23102478] [PMID: 30262735]

[103] Espinosa-Jovel C. Cannabinoids in epilepsy: clinical efficacy and pharmacological considerations. Neurología (English Edition) 2023; 38(1): 47-53. [http://dx.doi.org/10.1016/j.nrleng.2020.02.012] [PMID: 34824031]

[104] Abu-Sawwa R, Scutt B, Park Y. Emerging use of epidiolex (Cannabidiol) in epilepsy. J Pediatr Pharmacol Ther 2020; 25(6): 485-99.
[http://dx.doi.org/10.5863/1551-6776-25.6.485] [PMID: 32839652]

[105] Flachenecker P, Henze T, Zettl UK. Nabiximols (THC/CBD oromucosal spray, Sativex®) in clinical practice--results of a multicenter, non-interventional study (MOVE 2) in patients with multiple sclerosis spasticity. Eur Neurol 2014; 71(5-6): 271-9.
[http://dx.doi.org/10.1159/000357427] [PMID: 24525548]

[106] Pagano C, Navarra G, Coppola L, Avilia G, Bifulco M, Laezza C. Cannabinoids: Therapeutic use in clinical practice. Int J Mol Sci 2022; 23(6): 3344.
[http://dx.doi.org/10.3390/ijms23063344] [PMID: 35328765]

[107] Patel RS, Kamil S, Shah MR, Bhimanadham NN, Imran S. Pros and cons of marijuana in treatment of Parkinson's disease. Cureus 2019; 11(6): e4813.
[http://dx.doi.org/10.7759/cureus.4813] [PMID: 31403009]

[108] Lowe H, Toyang N, Steele B, Bryant J, Ngwa W. The endocannabinoid system: A potential target for the treatment of various diseases. Int J Mol Sci 2021; 22(17): 9472.
[http://dx.doi.org/10.3390/ijms22179472] [PMID: 34502379]

[109] De Gregorio D, McLaughlin RJ, Posa L, *et al.* Cannabidiol modulates serotonergic transmission and reverses both allodynia and anxiety-like behavior in a model of neuropathic pain. Pain 2019; 160(1): 136-50.
[http://dx.doi.org/10.1097/j.pain.0000000000001386] [PMID: 30157131]

[110] Gajender MA, Mazumder A, Sharma A, Azad MAK. A comprehensive review of the pharmacological importance of dietary flavonoids as hepatoprotective agents. Evid Based Complement Alternat Med 2023; 2023(1): 4139117.
[http://dx.doi.org/10.1155/2023/4139117] [PMID: 37123086]

[111] Raucci U, Pietrafusa N, Paolino MC, *et al.* Cannabidiol treatment for refractory epilepsies in pediatrics. Front Pharmacol 2020; 11: 586110.
[http://dx.doi.org/10.3389/fphar.2020.586110] [PMID: 33117180]

[112] Maggirwar SB, Khalsa JH. The link between cannabis use, immune system, and viral infections. Viruses 2021; 13(6): 1099.
[http://dx.doi.org/10.3390/v13061099] [PMID: 34207524]

[113] Ho C, Martinusen D, Lo C. A review of cannabis in chronic kidney disease symptom management. Can J Kidney Health Dis 2019; 6: 2054358119828391.
[http://dx.doi.org/10.1177/2054358119828391] [PMID: 30828459]

[114] Henson J, Vitetta L, Quezada M, Hall S. Enhancing endocannabinoid control of stress with cannabidiol. J Clin Med 2021; 10(24): 5852.
[http://dx.doi.org/10.3390/jcm10245852] [PMID: 34945148]

[115] Melas PA, Scherma M, Fratta W, Cifani C, Fadda P. Cannabidiol as a potential treatment for anxiety and mood disorders: Molecular targets and epigenetic insights from preclinical research. Int J Mol Sci 2021; 22(4): 1863.
[http://dx.doi.org/10.3390/ijms22041863] [PMID: 33668469]

[116] Wiese BM, Liktor-Busa E, Couture SA, *et al.* Brain penetrant, but not peripherally restricted, synthetic cannabinoid 1 receptor agonists promote morphine-mediated respiratory depression. Cannabis Cannabinoid Res 2022; 7(5): 621-7.
[http://dx.doi.org/10.1089/can.2021.0090] [PMID: 34935460]

[117] Dykukha I, Essner U, Schreiber H, Raithel LM, Penner IK. Effects of Sativex® on cognitive function in patients with multiple sclerosis: A systematic review and meta-analysis. Mult Scler Relat Disord 2022; 68: 104173.
[http://dx.doi.org/10.1016/j.msard.2022.104173] [PMID: 36174323]

[118] Stasiulewicz A, Znajdek K, Grudzień M, Pawiński T, Sulkowska JI. A guide to targeting the endocannabinoid system in drug design. Int J Mol Sci 2020; 21(8): 2778. [http://dx.doi.org/10.3390/ijms21082778] [PMID: 32316328]

[119] Brown J, Winterstein A. Potential adverse drug events and drug–drug interactions with medical and consumer cannabidiol (CBD) use. J Clin Med 2019; 8(7): 989. [http://dx.doi.org/10.3390/jcm8070989] [PMID: 31288397]

[120] Tudorancea IM, Ciorpac M, Stanciu GD, *et al.* The therapeutic potential of the endocannabinoid system in age-related diseases. Biomedicines 2022; 10(10): 2492. [http://dx.doi.org/10.3390/biomedicines10102492] [PMID: 36289755]

[121] Manzanares J, Julian M, Carrascosa A. Role of the cannabinoid system in pain control and therapeutic implications for the management of acute and chronic pain episodes. CN 2006; 4: 239-57. [http://dx.doi.org/10.2174/157015906778019527]

[122] Pacher P, Kunos G. Modulating the endocannabinoid system in human health and disease – successes and failures. FEBS J 2013; 280(9): 1918-43. [http://dx.doi.org/10.1111/febs.12260] [PMID: 23551849]

[123] Pacher P, Bátkai S, Kunos G. The endocannabinoid system as an emerging target of pharmacotherapy. Pharmacol Rev 2006; 58(3): 389-462. [http://dx.doi.org/10.1124/pr.58.3.2] [PMID: 16968947]

[124] Viveros M, Marco E, File S. Endocannabinoid system and stress and anxiety responses. Pharmacol Biochem Behav 2005; 81(2): 331-42. [http://dx.doi.org/10.1016/j.pbb.2005.01.029] [PMID: 15927244]

[125] Vasincu A, Rusu RN, Ababei DC, *et al.* Exploring the therapeutic potential of cannabinoid receptor antagonists in inflammation, diabetes mellitus, and obesity. Biomedicines 2023; 11(6): 1667. [http://dx.doi.org/10.3390/biomedicines11061667] [PMID: 37371762]

CHAPTER 6

Investigating Botanical Bioactives: Innovative Strategies for Treating Systemic Lupus Erythematosus

Parul Gupta[1], **Ashna Gupta**[1], **Sweta Kamboj**[1], **Shikha Kamboj**[1] and **Rohit Kamboj**[1,*]

Department of Pharmaceutics, Guru Gobind Singh College of Pharmacy, Yamunanagar 135001, Haryana, India

Abstract: Systemic Lupus Erythematosus (SLE) is an inflammatory illness characterised by chronic inflammation and multi-organ dysfunction. Secondary plant metabolites have received attention as potential innovative treatment agents. These metabolites provide a variety of pharmacological actions that are effective in managing SLE. These metabolites include polyphenols, alkaloids, terpenoids, and glycosides. While their immune-modulatory activities can address the immunological dysfunction characteristic of the disease, their anti-inflammatory qualities improve in lowering the chronic inflammation observed in SLE. These substances additionally show strong antioxidant activity, which reduces oxidative stress, a major factor in the pathogenesis of SLE. These natural compounds have been shown in numerous studies to have the capacity to suppress pro-inflammatory cytokines, control lymphocyte proliferation, and alter the function of various immune cells. Compared to traditional manufactured medications, secondary plant metabolites have a lower potential for side effects due to their natural origin. For SLE patients, ongoing research and clinical trials are crucial in determining the therapeutic potential of these natural substances and developing effective treatment strategies.

Keywords: Anti-inflammatory, Immunomodulatory, Natural therapy, Oxidative stress, Polyphenols, Secondary plant metabolites, Systemic lupus erythematosus.

INTRODUCTION

Systemic Lupus Erythematosus (SLE) is an autoimmune, multi-organ disease characterized by a range of clinical signs. Young women are more likely to have SLE. Compared to females, men are more likely to develop SLE (1:5–10) [1, 2]. External factors that commonly raise the risk of SLE include UV radiation, demethylating medications (Azacitidine, Decitabine), as well as viral infections

* **Corresponding author Rohit Kamboj:** Guru Gobind Singh College of Pharmacy, Yamunanagar 135001, Haryana, India; E-mail: rkamboj538@gmail.com

M.S. Ashawat, Aditi Kaushik, Akash Jain, Jasmine Chaudhary & Manish Kaushik (Eds.)
All rights reserved-© 2025 Bentham Science Publishers

(Epstein-Barr virus). SLE is more frequently linked to women because higher hormone concentrations, such as those found in prolactin and oestrogen, activate autoimmune characteristics. Both hormones boost plasma cell survival rates, which results in a high affinity for autoreactive B cells [3, 4]. Auto-antibodies and antibody-immune complexes are generated in SLE, leading to tissue injury and inflammation [5, 6]. Patients with SLE go through periods of remission and relapse [7]. The skin, kidneys, joints, heart, lungs, liver, *etc*., and blood vessels are among the organs that may be affected by SLE [8, 9]. Numerous indices, including the Systemic Lupus Erythematosus Disease Activity Index (SLEDAI), Safety of Oestrogens in Lupus Erythematosus National Assessment (SELENA), and British Isles Lupus Activity Group (BILAG) index, can be used to evaluate the state of the diseases because different organs are involved in SLE [10]. Genetic factors (the presence of genes that activate inflammation, genes that express toll-like receptors, and genes that are involved in the STAT signaling system) are the key etiological factors that cause SLE [11 - 13]. DNA repair genes, including TREX1, KLK1, and KLK3, have also been shown to be absent or to be hidden in the genetic architecture of SLE-responsive people [14 - 16]. The etiology of SLE is demonstrated in Fig. (**1**).

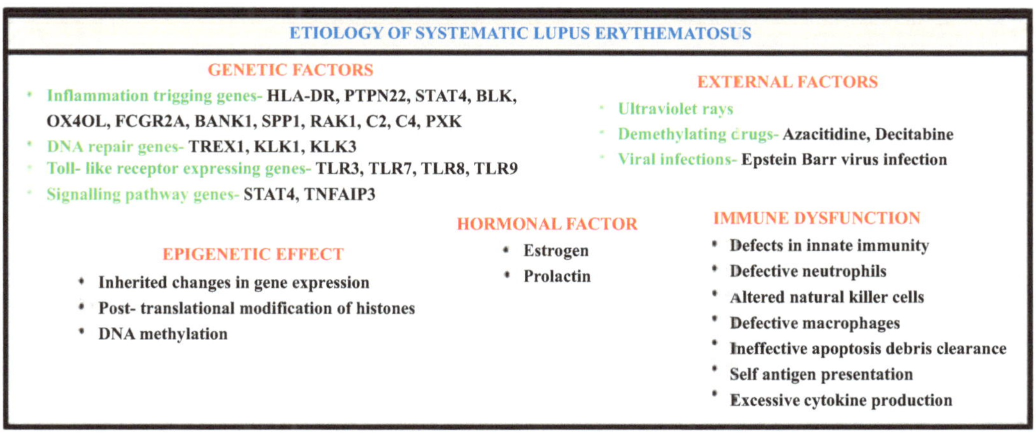

Fig. (1). The etiology of systematic lupus erythematosus.

Anti-double-stranded DNA (anti-dsDNA) antibodies play a crucial role in the pathogenesis of Sickle Cell Disease (SCD) and their levels are linked to disease activity. In other cases, therapy aims to restore normalcy in anti-dsDNA antibody levels [7]. Lupus nephritis causes kidney injury by inflammatory reactions triggered by increased B and T lymphocyte activity, autoantibody misproduction, immune complex accumulation in kidney tissue, and dysregulation of T-regulatory cells [17, 18]. Pharmaceuticals used to treat SLE include systemic lymph node irradiation therapy, nonsteroidal anti-inflammatory medications, antimalarial drugs, immunosuppressive drugs, glucocorticoids, and plasma treatment. In spite of this, SLE patients continue to have unacceptably high rates of morbidity and mortality [8, 19]. The recommended medications lower patients' quality of life and expose them to side effects [20]. Patients are encouraged to try complementary and alternative treatments, including acupuncture, moxibustion, herbal remedies, medicinal plants, phytochemicals, vitamins, and mineral supplements, as well as spiritual therapies like yoga. Additionally, a lot of work has gone into finding safe and efficient supplements and drugs for the condition that make use of both natural and synthetic derivatives of natural components. Using PubMed, the Cochrane Library, Web of Science, Scopus, the National Library of Medicine (NLM) catalogue, and Google Scholar, a thorough literature search was conducted. The American College of Rheumatology's (ACR) guidelines are now used to diagnose SLE. According to the ACR, a patient has lupus if they exhibit four of the eleven indications or symptoms shown in Fig. (**2**).

The American College of Rheumatology Criteria for Identifying Systemic Lupus Erythematosus

Skin criteria

Butterfly rash (lupus over the cheeks and nose)
Discoid rash (a thick, disk-like rash that scars, usually on sun-exposed areas)
Sun sensitivity (rash after being exposed to ultraviolet A and B light)
Oral ulcerations (recurrent sores in the mouth or nose)

Laboratory criteria

Blood abnormalities (hemolytic anemia, low white blood cell counts, low platelet counts)
Immunologic disorder (blood testing indicating either a positive LE preparation, anti-DNA, false-positive syphilis test or a positive anti-Sm)
Positive ANA blood test

Systemic criteria

Arthritis (inflammation of two peripheral joints with tenderness, swelling or fluid)
Serositis (inflammation of the lining of the lung (also called pleura) or the heart (also called the pericardium))
Kidney disorder (protein in urine samples or abnormal sediment in urine seen under the microscope)
Neurologic disorder (seizures or psychosis with no other explanation)

Fig. (2). The criteria for identifying systemic lupus erythematosus by the American College of Rheumatology.

Pathophysiology of SLE

SLE has a complicated pathophysiology, and our knowledge of it is always changing. When genetically vulnerable people are exposed to environmental stressors, their tolerance breaks down, which triggers the development of autoimmunity. The immune system is exposed to self-antigens as a result of cell damage brought on by infections and other environmental causes. This stimulation of T and B cells results in a chronic, self-directed immunological response that is self-sustaining. Organ damage is caused by complement activation, autoantibody synthesis, and cytokine release.

The pathophysiology of SLE involves both the immune system's adaptive and innate components. Either Toll-Like Receptors (TLRs) or other receptors are required for the activation of the innate immune system. The extracellular DNA and RNA of dying cells bind to the cell membrane-bound TLRs 2, 4, and 6, activating them. This triggers the transcription factors NF-κB, MAP kinases, and the Interferon Regulatory Factor (IRF-3), which in turn activate the cell membrane-bound TLRs and cause the generation of proinflammatory mediators like IFN-β. The generation of interferon-alpha and RNA-binding autoantibodies, such as those against Ro La, Sm, and RNP, is triggered by single-stranded RNA as well as demethylated DNA, which activates the endosomal TLRs (TLR7-9). Intracytoplasmic RNA (RIG-1, MDA-5) and DNA (IFI16, DAI) sensors initiate the TLR-independent pathway, which in turn activates NF-κB and IRF3. This activation can be caused by either foreign or self-DNA/RNA, including that from viruses. The pathophysiology of SLE has recently drawn more focus to NETosis. When neutrophils are stimulated by different agents, including cytokines, activated platelets, or vascular endothelial cells, they routinely discharge their nuclear aggregates into the extracellular space. These nuclear aggregates will subsequently trigger thrombosis and vascular injury, stimulate the dendritic cells to produce interferon-alpha, and act as self-antigens for T lymphocytes. The pathophysiology of SLE is significantly influenced by T- and B-lymphocytes. Antigen-presenting cells deliver apoptotic, along with damaged cell-derived antigens, to T-cells. In sickle cell disease (SLE), T-cells exhibit aberrant gene expression that results in the release of several cytokines. The generation of regulatory T-cells is changed as a result of these T-cells producing less IL-2.

Mononuclear cell production is enhanced by elevated IL-6, IL-10, IL-12, & IL-23, whereas T-cell production is enhanced by elevated IL-17 and IL-21. A higher level of interfern-γ results in faulty T-cell generation. T-cells stimulate autoreactive B-cells through the release of cytokines and CD40L, which results in the generation of autoantibodies, a defining feature of SLE. These B-cells are activated by toll-like receptors upon contact with DNA and RNA; the most common antigens causing B-cell activation are nucleic acid with protein-containing intranuclear complexes. These autoantibodies are harmful and affect cell function, resulting in apoptosis and the creation of cytokines and complement, including neutrophil activation, all of which damage organs [21, 22].

Furthermore, because there is a defect in the process that neutralises autoreactive B cells functionally, autoreactive B cells in SLE that are triggered by self-antigens are difficult to eradicate. By exposing T-cells to internalised soluble antigens, B-cells can also function as antigen-presenting cells, along with stimulating T-cells. As a result, an upward spiral is started in which T and B cells stimulate one another, increasing autoimmunity [23].

Natural Treatment of Systemic Lupus Erythematosus

Medicinal herbs play important roles in protecting humans from numerous harmful bacteria and diseases while minimizing the risk of adverse effects. Plant medications and dietary supplements are effective in the therapy of systemic lupus erythematosus. Prior to the 1200s, the medical literature used the Latin name lupus, which means wolf, to describe skin sores that consume the flesh, and physicians' resources to help individuals were restricted [24, 25]. The traditional understanding of how to treat this illness includes the use of multiple medicinal herbs or plant-based combinations. Studies on ethnobotany and ethnopharmacology show that *Cinchona spp.* [26]. and "Thanatka," which is formed of *Limonia acidissima* bark and *Hesperethusa crenulata* [27], have applications in dermatology, particularly in the management of lupus erythematosus. Additionally, systemic lupus erythematosus has been reported to be treated with sieketroos Arctopus species [28], *Juniperus* species [29], *Onopordum acanthium* [30], and *Centella asiatica* [31]. According to traditional Persian medicine practiced in Iran, the primary causes of nephritis—referred to as 'Varam-e-Kolye'—are infections and fever. For the treatment of lupus nephritis, or "Varam-e-Kolye," several medicinal plants have been suggested, including *Anethum graveolens L., Carum carvi L., Coriandrum sativum L., Cucurbita pepo L., Cydonia oblonga Mill., Ficus carica L., Linum usitatissimum L., Melissa officinalis L., Prunus amygdalus,* and *Ziziphus jujuba Mill.* These herbs have been shown in specific recent research to have nephroprotective and anti-inflammatory properties [32 - 34]. Changes in diet and lifestyle may help modify or eradicate the underlying cause of systemic lupus erythematosus through natural therapies. A number of medicinal plants are included in Table **1** for the treatment of systemic lupus erythematosus.

Table 1. Medicinal plants for the treatment of SLE.

Plant name	Biological name	family	Phytoconstituent	Part of the plant used	SLE activity	References
Turmeric	*Curcuma longa*	Zingiberaceae	Curcumin	rhizome	antioxidant and anti-inflammatory activity	[35]
Green tea	*Camellia sinensis*	Theaceae	Epigallocatechin gallate	leaves	immunomodulator, antiapoptosis agent, and anti-pyroptosis agent	[36]

(Table 1) cont.....

Plant name	Biological name	family	Phytoconstituent	Part of the plant used	SLE activity	References
Ginger	*Zingiber officinale*	Zingiberaceae	Gingerol	Rhizome	antioxidant and anti-inflammatory activity	[37]
Garlic	*Allium sativum*	Amaryllidaceae	Allicin	Bulb	anti-inflammatory, antioxidant, antimicrobial, antifungal, immunomodulatory, antiatherosclerotic, anti-hypertensive effects	[38]
Ashwagandha	*Withania somnifera*	Solanaceae	Withaferin A	Root	anti-inflammatory activity	[39]
Liquorice	*Glycyrrhiza glabra*	Fabaceae	Glycyrrhizin	Root	Immunostimulatory effects	[40]
Aloevera	*Aloe barbedensis miller*	Asphodelaceae	Aloin	Leaves	antioxidant, anti-inflammatory, antimicrobial	[41]
Cat's claw	*Uncaria tomentosa*	Rubiaceae	Oxindole alkaloids	Bark, roots	Anti- inflammatory	[42]
Ginseng	*Panax ginseng*	Araliaceae	Ginsenosides	Root	Immunoregulatory effect	[43]
Echinacea	*Echinacea purpurea*	Asteraceae	Alkamides	Root, aerial parts	Immunostimulatory effect	[44]
Evening primrose	*Oenothera biennis*	Onagraceae	Gamma linolenic acid	Seeds	Anti-inflammatory effect	[45]
Saffron	*Crocus sativus*	Iridaceae	Crocin	Stigma	anti-inflammatory, antioxidant, analgesic, antihypertensive	[46]
Milk thistle	*Silybum marianum*	Asteraceae	Silymarin	Seeds	Immunomodulatory effect	[47]
Neem	*Azadirachta indica*	Meliaceae	Azadirachtin	Leaves, bark	Anti-inflammatory, immunosuppressive effect	[48]
Gotu kola	*Centella asiatica*	Apiaceae	Asiaticoside	Leaves, stem	Anti-inflammatory effect	[49]

Natural Sources of Immunoregulatory Drug Candidates

Phytocompounds have been utilized for eons as safer immunomodulatory medicinal agents. By either reducing the activities of immune cells or limiting the synthesis of inflammatory cytokines, these phytoconstituents work as immunoregulatory medication candidates and preserve immunological homeostasis [28]. An antagonistic effect against oxidative stresses, which in turn produces free radicals that target cytokines and autoantibodies, is the primary mechanism by which a natural immunosuppressant works. Numerous plants, including *Acacia farnesiana, Allium sativum, Andrographis paniculata, Commelina benghalensis, Angelica glauca, Arundo donax, Camellia sinensis, Coriandrum sativum, Costus speciosus, Curcuma longa, Cymbopogon citratus, Dracocephalum rupestre, Malus domestica, Morinda citrifolia, Ocimum gratissimum, Paeonia lactiflora, Picrorhiza scrophulariiflora, Salvia miltiorrhiza,* and *Uncaria tomentosa,* among others, have been shown to exert such immunomodulation. One or more phytoconstituents in these plants possess distinct anti-inflammatory or anti-oxidant activities. In the case of SLE, these phytoconstituents may also serve as modulators of cytokine production and B-T cell co-stimulation, hence preventing autoantibody formation and immune response hyperactivation [50 - 53].

Plant Compounds as Intracellular Regulators of Signalling

It is widely known that some natural plant substances have significant anti-inflammatory activities by modulating the expression of several signalling protein kinases and cell cycle proteins involved in the creation of inflammatory cytokines and autoantibodies. *Curcuma longa* contains curcumin, an active phytoconstituent that inhibits TLR2 and NFκB transcription. These two mechanisms are critical in priming the plasma cytoid dendritic cell to present autoantigens, which induces the creation of autoantibodies. Curcumin has also been shown to decrease STAT3 expression, preventing the downstream activation of pro-inflammatory cytokines such as BCL6 and IL17 [28, 54]. *Tripterygium wilfordii* includes a diterpenoid epoxide, triptolide, which is known to block the transcription of IL-17 and STAT3 [28, 33]. Similarly, an alkaloid identified in *Berberis aristata*, berbamine, has been shown to reduce STAT3 expression while also inhibiting the production of interferons that cause an apoptotic cascade in SLE [55]. Several other plant species, such as *Andrographis paniculata, Argyrolobiumroseum, Artemisiavestita, Bupleurum falcatum, Campylotropishirtella, Clerodendron trichotomum, Dracocephalum kotschyi, Periploca sepium, and Salvia mirzayanii*, have also been found to play similar roles as intracellular signalling regulators, suggesting that they may be useful as natural remedies for SLE [28, 50, 56 - 58].

Natural Herbs for Symptomatic Management

Nonsteroidal Anti-Inflammatory Medicines (NSAIDS), corticosteroids, and antimalarial pharmaceuticals are among the conventional treatments for Systemic Lupus Erythematosus (SLE). Therapy approaches, however, have varying outcomes depending on patient profiles. In addition, the potential for organ toxicity makes all of these chemotherapeutic moieties hazardous for long-term use [59 - 61]. In these circumstances, the use of holistic medicines and natural plant products—as well as other alternative medicine treatments—has grown in popularity as an SLE therapeutic option. These multi-targeting holistic herbs ultimately offer symptomatic alleviation for SLE patients, who experience a range of clinical symptoms and opportunistic diseases [28, 62 - 64]. SLE's most common clinical manifestations are heart, brain, hematological, liver, mucosa, musculoskeletal, lung, and kidney diseases. Certain phytoconstituents, such as papaverine (*Papaver somniferum*), pseudoephedrine (*Ephedra sinica*), theophylline (*Camellia sinensis*), pyrocatechol (*Allium cepa, Achillea millefolium*), pyrogallol (*Anogeissus latifolia*), tyramine (*Crataegus laevigata*), and yohimbine (*Catharanthus roseus*), have been shown to alleviate symptoms associated with cardiovascular manifestations. Tangeretin, puerarin, naringenin, glabridin, arecoline, baicalin, ginkgolide, glabridin, naringenin, quercetin, rosmarinic acid, and tocopherol are examples of natural compounds with neurostimulant and cerebro-protective characteristics. Cyanocobalamin and folacin are hepatoprotective and hematopoietic therapies (found in *Aloe vera, Anacardium occidentale, Angelica sinensis, Arachis hypogaea, Avena sativa, Beta vulgaris, Brassicarapa, Medicagosativa, Panaxquinquefolius*, *etc*.). Renal and pulmonary infections can be treated using several herbs, including *Ephedra antisyphilitica, Alchemilla arvensis, Bixa orellana, Cimicifuga racemosa, Helianthus annuus, Ledum palustre, Piper longum*. Maculopapular cutaneous rashes can be treated with herbal remedies like *Achyranthes aspera, Allium cepa, Allium sativum, Aloe vera, Azadirachta indica, Bauhinia variegata, Beta vulgaris, Calendula officinalis, Camellia sinensis, Curcuma longa, Lawsonia inermis, Lycopersicon esculentum, Momordica charantia*, and *Rosmarinus officinalis.*

In-vitro Studies

The development of successful therapeutics for Systemic Lupus Erythematosus (SLE) is heavily dependent on *in vivo* investigations. These investigations, conducted on living organisms such as human volunteers and animal models, provide a comprehensive understanding of the pharmacological behavior, safety, efficacy, and biological mechanisms of potential therapies. *In vivo* studies, which closely resemble the intricate interactions found in the human body, provide essential data that informs clinical practices and directs the development of novel therapeutic options for SLE. These studies also enable researchers to assess how new medications impact disease progression as well as patient health. Some *in vitro* studies for the treatment of SLE are discussed in Table **2**.

Table 2. Phytoconstituents along with their mechanism of action in the treatment of SLE.

Phytoconstituent	Animal/Cell model/SLE population	Dose	Duration	Mechanism of action	Reference
Punicalagin	NZB/W F1 mice	1 and 3 mg/ kg	7 weeks	lessen proteinuria, renal ICAM-1 & VCAM-1 expression, and kidney damage and splenomegaly.	[65]
Sulforaphane	MRL/lpr mice	12.5 mg/kg	28 weeks	Improve the functioning of the kidney.	[66]
Oleuropein	BALB/c mice	100 mg/kg	24 weeks	reduced levels of prostaglandin E2 and serum plasma matrix metalloproteinase 3 as well as renal damage.	[67]
Curcumin	PBMCs	0.1 μg/ml	48 h	suppresses PYK2 expression and activation in PBMCs from LN patients as opposed to healthy individuals.	[68]
Curcumin	SLE patients with SLEDAI >3 and 25(OH)D level	60 mg daily	3 months	During therapy, there were no appreciable differences in the groups' SLEDAI reduction, IL-6 serum levels, or TGF-1 serum levels.	[69]
Resveratrol	PIL mice	50,75 mg/kg	7 months	Reduced immunoglobulin deposition, proteinuria, and glomerulonephritis.	[70]
Curcumin	NZB/W F1 mice	500 mg/kg	14 days	Renal damage and decreased spleen weight during 26 weeks of age. Decreased kidney damage at age 32 weeks.	[71]
Curcumin	MRL/lpr mice	200 mg/kg	8 weeks	Decreased spleen size, serum anti-ds DNA, renal inflammation, and proteinuria.	[72]
Apigennin	SNF1 mice	3,6,20 mg/kg	8 weeks	Inhibited and encouraged T and B cells, as well as APC, apoptosis.	[73]
Icariin	MLR/lpr mice	10 mg/kg	8 weeks	Reduced anti-DNA antibody levels in serum, immunological complex, and kidney disease.	[74]

(Table 2) cont.....

Phytoconstituent	Animal/Cell model/SLE population	Dose	Duration	Mechanism of action	Reference
Resveratrol	MRL/Mp-Faslpr mice	0.01% in ethanol	10 weeks	Elevated SIRT1 mRNA levels and decreased mRNA for CX3CL1 & vascular endothelial growth factors in the hippocampal regions.	[75]
Resveratrol	BALB/c mice	50 mg/kg 4 mg/kg	7 months	Decrease in the proportion of B & Th1 cells in G.	[76]
Apigenin	NZB and SWR mice	20 mg/kg	8 weeks	IFN-γ, IL-17, & COX-2 suppression.	[77]
Astilbin	MRL/lpr mice	20 mg/kg	7 months	Reduction of TNF-α, IL-1β, IL-17, IFN-γ, & IL-6.	[78]
Epigallocatechin Gallate	(NZB/W) F1 lupus-prone mice	120 mg/kg	5 months	Decreased activation of NF-κB, NLRP3, IL-1β, & IL-18.	[79]
SFN	MRL/lpr mice	82.9 μmol/kg	27 days	Reduce the proportions of neutrophils, dendritic cells, Tfh cells, and plasma cells.	[80]

Cell Senescence in SLE

Numerous stressors, such as oxidative damage, genetic instability, and chronic inflammation, may cause irreversible cell cycle stoppage or cell senescence. Senescence promotes tissue regeneration and lowers the risk of cancer, but its persistence may have unfavourable effects. The early senescence of immune cells, including T cells, B cells, and macrophages, is a hallmark of the pathophysiology of SLE [81].

Mechanisms of Cell Senescence in SLE

- **Oxidative Stress and DNA Damage:** High Reactive Oxygen Species (ROS) levels aggravate DNA damage, which is one of the main causes of cellular senescence in SLE. It has been shown that oxidative stress markers such as 8-hydroxy-2′-deoxyguanosine are higher in SLE patients.
- **Attrition of Telomeres:** Fast telomere shortening in SLE T cells leads to early senescence.
- **Chronic Inflammation:** By triggering a feedback loop that increases the release of growth factors and inflammatory cytokines, chronic inflammation in SLE makes senescence worse [82].

Senescence Associated with Secretory Phenotype

Senescent cells release a class of pro-inflammatory substances known as a Secretory Phenotype Associated with Senescence (SASP). These consist of cytokines (such as IL-6, IL-1β, and TNF-α), chemokines (like CCL2 and CXCL8), and Matrix Metalloproteinases (MMPs). According to Hernandez-Segura *et al.* (2018), SASP aggravates systemic inflammation in SLE, leading to tissue damage and immunological dysregulation [83].

Immune Cells and Senescence in SLE

Senescent T cells in SLE perform fewer proliferative and effector functions. According to Wen *et al.* (2020), they also generate pro-inflammatory cytokines, which encourage inflammation. Premature aging of B cells affects tolerance and antibody production, resulting in the development of autoimmune clones and autoantibodies. Cellular debris builds up and nuclear antigens are created when senescent macrophages are unable to adequately eliminate apoptotic cells, which triggers autoimmunity in the macrophages [84].

Autoantibodies in SLE

Immunoglobulins known as autoantibodies recognize and attach to the body's own proteins, RNA, and DNA. These antibodies are created as a result of inadequate immunological regulation in SLE and reduce self-tolerance. These autoantibodies function as direct mediators of illness and diagnostic markers, causing inflammation and organ damage [85].

Autoantibody Production Mechanisms

Numerous immune system disorders cause autoantibodies to manifest in SLE.

- **Immunological tolerance decline:**

B Cell Tolerance Defects: Throughout development, autoreactive B lymphocytes in healthy individuals are either deactivated or eliminated. Because SLE patients have limited tolerance, autoreactive B cells may keep proliferating and producing autoantibodies.

T cell dysregulation: When B cells generate dangerous autoantibodies in the presence of hyperactive helper T cells, namely T follicular helper cells, the ability of regulatory T cells (T_{regs}) to reduce autoreactive lymphocytes is often impaired.

- Apoptotic cell clearance: In SLE, impaired clearance of apoptotic cells leads to the accumulation of extracellular debris. This accumulation exposes the immune system to autoantigens such as DNA, histones, and ribonucleoproteins, triggering the production of autoantibodies. The phagocytic cells, particularly macrophages, exhibit reduced efficiency in removing this cellular debris, making these antigens more readily available and contributing to the pathogenesis of SLE. **Epitope spread and molecular mimicry:** Autoimmunity may result from infections and other environmental stressors that cause molecular mimicry, in which foreign antigens resemble self-antigens. An initial immune response to a single antigen might expand to identify many self-antigens, increasing the range of autoantibodies. This phenomenon is known as epitope spread [86].

Mechanisms Involving Autoantibody Production and Cellular Senescence

In SLE, cellular senescence and autoantibody production interact in a complicated way, resulting in the formation of a pro-inflammatory environment, immune cell activation, and autoantigen release.

- **Senescent Cell Autoantigens Extracellular Release of Nuclear Material:** Senescent cells' recurrent nuclear envelope instability results in the release of histones, chromatin fragments, and double-stranded DNA (dsDNA) into the surrounding environment. When the immune system recognizes these molecules as alien, it produces autoantibodies such as anti-dsDNA and anti-histone antibodies. Senescent cells produce nuclear antigen-containing microparticles that stimulate B-cell activation and dendritic cell antigen presentation.
- **Immune activation and SASP:** Senescent cells (SASP) release inflammatory cytokines and chemokines, which activate the immune system and increase the formation of autoantibodies. SASP cytokines, including IL-6 and IL-1β, increase B-cell survival, differentiation, and antibody production. As a result, autoreactive B cells develop, causing deadly autoantibodies. SASP factors improve dendritic cells' capacity to present antigens, allowing autoreactive T and B cells to encounter antigens originating from senescent cells. Promoting T-Cell Dysregulation: IL-6 and other SASP cytokines boost Th17 cell growth, which also impacts regulatory T cells (T_{regs}), producing an environment favourable for autoantibody formation.
- **Reduced senescent cell clearance:** Phagocytes, such as macrophages, are less efficient in removing senescent and apoptotic cells in SLE. The concentration of these cells increases antigen exposure and autoantibody synthesis [87,88].

Autoantibodies: Increase the Senescence of Cells

Autoantibodies may hasten senescence, whereas senescence encourages the generation of autoantibodies, resulting in a vicious cycle that lengthens the course of illness.

- **Inflammation and the formation of immune complexes:** Autoantibodies attach to self-antigens, generating immune complexes that accumulate in tissues and trigger the complement cascade. This causes oxidative stress, cellular damage, and chronic inflammation, which leads to senescence of the surrounding cells.
- **Autoantibodies induce direct cell injury:** Certain auto antibodies, such as anti-dsDNA antibodies, may enter cells and directly degrade DNA. This damage triggers the DNA Damage Response (DDR), one of the leading drivers of senescence.
- **Long-term SASP Exposure:** Autoantibody-induced inflammation exposes cells to SASP cytokines over time, causing paracrine signalling and senescence. TNF-α and IL-1β promote senescence in fibroblasts and endothelial cells [89,90].

CHALLENGES AND FUTURE PROSPECTS

There are many obstacles in the way of researching plant bioactives for the treatment of Systemic Lupus Erythematosus (SLE). The intrinsic complexity of botanical extracts, which are made up of several components that might interact in unforeseen ways, is a major obstacle. Extensive fractionation methods guided by bioassays and advanced analytical techniques are needed to identify the active ingredients accountable for the therapeutic effects [91]. Furthermore, differences in plant chemical composition might result from differences in harvesting time, location, and processing techniques, which can cause variations in safety and efficacy [92]. It is challenging to guarantee uniform dosing because of the diversity in botanical extract processing and quality control, which is exacerbated by a lack of standardisation [93].

Another key barrier is the lack of large-scale, carefully organised clinical trials to investigate the efficacy and safety of botanical bioactives in the treatment of SLE. The majority of preclinical research conducted to date has had small sample sizes and methodological faults [94]. Furthermore, regulatory frameworks for botanical drugs are usually less developed than those for conventional pharmaceuticals, and botanical products face significant regulatory challenges due to the rigorous standards for demonstrating safety and efficacy.

The use of botanical bioactives in the treatment of SLE appears to have a bright future despite these challenges. Plant extracts include complex interactions that can be better understood and bioactive chemicals can be found using advanced analytical techniques such as proteomics, metabolomics, and genomics [95]. Nanotechnology offers innovative delivery methods that has the potential to enhance the therapeutic benefits of botanical bioactives by enhancing their stability, bioavailability, and targeted distribution [96].

Treatment strategies for SLE that are more thorough and effective may arise from the synergistic effects of integrating botanical bioactives with conventional therapies in an integrated manner [97]. Advances in pharmacogenomics and personalized medicine have made it possible to tailor herbal medicines to the specific genetic profile of each patient, thereby improving their efficacy and mitigating their adverse effects [98]. Additionally, improved collaboration between modern scientists, regulatory bodies, and conventional medical practitioners can facilitate the integration of botanical bioactives into conventional medicine [99].

Accelerating research and development in this field necessitates additional money and cooperation from institutions and governments. Increased financing may help with the discovery of botanical bioactives for SLE and their therapeutic applications [100]. The promise of unique and successful botanical medicines in the treatment of SLE can be achieved by addressing these difficulties using cutting-edge research techniques, regulatory reforms, and integrative approaches.

CONCLUSION

In conclusion, the investigation of botanical bioactives for the treatment of Systemic Lupus Erythematosus (SLE) is highly promising and may open up new therapeutic paths. Because of their many active chemicals, plant extracts are complicated and require sophisticated analytical methods to identify their active ingredients. To provide consistent and dependable treatment effects, it is imperative to address the diversity in plant composition through strict standardisation. Botanical bioactives may supplement conventional therapeutic paradigms, notwithstanding the paucity of scientific trials in the current landscape. Integrating these bioactives into mainstream healthcare will need cooperative efforts by practitioners of traditional medicine, contemporary scientists, and regulatory agencies. The development of novel and successful herbal medicines for the management of SLE will ultimately depend on increased funding and institutional support for research and development.

LIST OF ABBREVIATIONS

SLE	Systemic Lupus Erythematosus
SLEDAI	Systemic Lupus Erythematosus Disease Activity Index
SELENA	Safety of Estrogens in Lupus Erythematosus National Assessment
BILAG	British Isles Lupus Activity Group
ACR	American College of Rheumatology
NETosis	Neutrophil Extracellular Trap Formation
TLR	Toll-Like Receptor
NF-κB	Nuclear Factor kappa B
MAP	Mitogen-Activated Protein
IRF	Interferon Regulatory Factor
RIG-I	Retinoic Acid-Inducible Gene I
MDA-5	Melanoma Differentiation-Associated Protein 5
IFI16	Interferon Gamma-Inducible Protein 16
DAI	DNA-Dependent Activator of Interferon Regulator
TLR7–9	Toll-Like Receptors 7 to 9
IL	Interleukin
TNF-α	Tumor Necrosis Factor Alpha
IFN-γ	Interferon Gamma
SIRT1	Sirtuin 1
PBMCs	Peripheral Blood Mononuclear Cells
ICAM-1	Intercellular Adhesion Molecule 1
VCAM-1	Vascular Cell Adhesion Molecule 1
PIL	Protein-Induced Lupus

REFERENCES

[1] Dörner T, Furie R. Novel paradigms in systemic lupus erythematosus. Lancet 2019; 393(10188): 2344-58.
[http://dx.doi.org/10.1016/S0140-6736(19)30546-X] [PMID: 31180031]

[2] Veeranki S, Choubey D. Systemic lupus erythematosus and increased risk to develop B cell malignancies: Role of the p200-family proteins. Immunol Lett 2010; 133(1): 1-5.
[http://dx.doi.org/10.1016/j.imlet.2010.06.008] [PMID: 20599558]

[3] Ballestar E, Esteller M, Richardson BC. The epigenetic face of systemic lupus erythematosus. J Immunol 2006; 176(12): 7143-7.
[http://dx.doi.org/10.4049/jimmunol.176.12.7143] [PMID: 16751355]

[4] Grimaldi CM. Sex and systemic lupus erythematosus: the role of the sex hormones estrogen and prolactin on the regulation of autoreactive B cells. Curr Opin Rheumatol 2006; 18(5): 456-61.
[http://dx.doi.org/10.1097/01.bor.0000240354.37927.dd] [PMID: 16896282]

[5] Lightfoot YL, Blanco LP, Kaplan MJ. Metabolic abnormalities and oxidative stress in lupus. Curr Opin Rheumatol 2017; 29(5): 442-9.

[http://dx.doi.org/10.1097/BOR.0000000000000413] [PMID: 28639951]

[6] Bertsias GK, Pamfil C, Fanouriakis A, Boumpas DT. Diagnostic criteria for systemic lupus erythematosus: has the time come?. Nat Rev Rheumatol 2013; 9(11): 687-94. [http://dx.doi.org/10.1038/nrrheum.2013.103] [PMID: 23838616]

[7] Bootsma H, Spronk P, de Boer G, *et al.* Prevention of relapses in systemic lupus erythematosus. Lancet 1995; 345(8965): 1595-9. [http://dx.doi.org/10.1016/S0140-6736(95)90114-0] [PMID: 7783536]

[8] Loram LC, Culp ME, Connolly-Strong EC, Sturgill-Koszycki S. Melanocortin peptides: potential targets in systemic lupus erythematosus. Inflammation 2015; 38(1): 260-71. [http://dx.doi.org/10.1007/s10753-014-0029-5] [PMID: 25323206]

[9] Fanouriakis A, Tziolos N, Bertsias G, Boumpas DT. Update on the diagnosis and management of systemic lupus erythematosus. Ann Rheum Dis 2021; 80(1): 14-25. [http://dx.doi.org/10.1136/annrheumdis-2020-218272] [PMID: 33051219]

[10] Mikdashi J, Nived O. Measuring disease activity in adults with systemic lupus erythematosus: the challenges of administrative burden and responsiveness to patient concerns in clinical research. Arthritis Res Ther 2015; 17(1): 183. [http://dx.doi.org/10.1186/s13075-015-0702-6] [PMID: 26189728]

[11] Sarzi-Puttini P, Atzeni F, Iaccarino L, Doria A. Environment and systemic lupus erythematosus: An overview. Autoimmunity 2005; 38(7): 465-72. [http://dx.doi.org/10.1080/08916930500285394] [PMID: 16373251]

[12] Mok CC, Lau CS. Pathogenesis of systemic lupus erythematosus. J Clin Pathol 2003; 56(7): 481-90. [http://dx.doi.org/10.1136/jcp.56.7.481] [PMID: 12835292]

[13] Webber D, Cao J, Dominguez D, *et al.* Association of systemic lupus erythematosus (SLE) genetic susceptibility loci with lupus nephritis in childhood-onset and adult-onset SLE. Rheumatology (Oxford) 2020; 59(1): 90-8. [http://dx.doi.org/10.1093/rheumatology/kez220] [PMID: 31236574]

[14] Munroe ME, James JA. Genetics of lupus nephritis: Clinical implications. Semin Nephrol 2015; 35(5): 396-409. [http://dx.doi.org/10.1016/j.semnephrol.2015.08.002] [PMID: 26573543]

[15] Bertsias GK, Ioannidis JPA, Aringer M, *et al.* EULAR recommendations for the management of systemic lupus erythematosus with neuropsychiatric manifestations: report of a task force of the EULAR standing committee for clinical affairs. Ann Rheum Dis 2010; 69(12): 2074-82. [http://dx.doi.org/10.1136/ard.2010.130476] [PMID: 20724309]

[16] Belot A, Rice GI, Omarjee SO, *et al.* Contribution of rare and predicted pathogenic gene variants to childhood-onset lupus: a large, genetic panel analysis of British and French cohorts. Lancet Rheumatol 2020; 2(2): e99-e109. [http://dx.doi.org/10.1016/S2665-9913(19)30142-0] [PMID: 38263665]

[17] Almaani S, Meara A, Rovin BH. Update on lupus nephritis. Clin J Am Soc Nephrol 2017; 12(5): 825-35. [http://dx.doi.org/10.2215/CJN.05780616] [PMID: 27821390]

[18] Hoover PJ, Costenbader KH. Insights into the epidemiology and management of lupus nephritis from the US rheumatologist's perspective. Kidney Int 2016; 90(3): 487-92. [http://dx.doi.org/10.1016/j.kint.2016.03.042] [PMID: 27344205]

[19] Wallace DJ. The evolution of drug discovery in systemic lupus erythematosus. Nat Rev Rheumatol 2015; 11(10): 616-20. [http://dx.doi.org/10.1038/nrrheum.2015.86] [PMID: 26122951]

[20] Basta F, Fasola F, Triantafyllias K, Schwarting A. Systemic lupus erythematosus (SLE) therapy: The old and the new. Rheumatol Ther 2020; 7(3): 433-46.

[http://dx.doi.org/10.1007/s40744-020-00212-9] [PMID: 32488652]

[21] Tayem MG, Shahin L, Shook J, Kesselman MM. A review of cardiac manifestations in patients with systemic lupus erythematosus and antiphospholipid syndrome with focus on endocarditis. Cureus 2022; 14(1): e21698.
[http://dx.doi.org/10.7759/cureus.21698] [PMID: 35242470]

[22] Scheen M, Adedjouma A, Esteve E, *et al.* Kidney disease in antiphospholipid antibody syndrome: Risk factors, pathophysiology and management. Autoimmun Rev 2022; 21(5): 103072.
[http://dx.doi.org/10.1016/j.autrev.2022.103072] [PMID: 35217200]

[23] Takeshima Y, Iwasaki Y, Nakano M, *et al.* Immune cell multiomics analysis reveals contribution of oxidative phosphorylation to B-cell functions and organ damage of lupus. Ann Rheum Dis 2022; 81(6): 845-53.
[http://dx.doi.org/10.1136/annrheumdis-2021-221464] [PMID: 35236659]

[24] Sun XG, Fu XQ, Cai HB, *et al.* Proteomic analysis of protective effects of polysaccharides from Salvia miltiorrhiza against immunological liver injury in mice. Phytother Res 2011; 25(7): 1087-94.
[http://dx.doi.org/10.1002/ptr.3487] [PMID: 21480413]

[25] Sheng Y, Li L, Holmgren K, Pero RW. DNA repair enhancement of aqueous extracts of Uncaria tomentosa in a human volunteer study. Phytomedicine 2001; 8(4): 275-82.
[http://dx.doi.org/10.1078/0944-7113-00045] [PMID: 11515717]

[26] Reis SRIN, Valente LMM, Sampaio AL, *et al.* Immunomodulating and antiviral activities of Uncaria tomentosa on human monocytes infected with Dengue Virus-2. Int Immunopharmacol 2008; 8(3): 468-76.
[http://dx.doi.org/10.1016/j.intimp.2007.11.010] [PMID: 18279801]

[27] Chandrashekara PM, Venkatesh YP. Immunostimulatory properties of fructans derived from raw garlic (Allium sativum L.). Bioactive Carbohydrates and Dietary Fibre 2016; 8(2): 65-70.
[http://dx.doi.org/10.1016/j.bcdf.2016.11.003]

[28] Amirghofran Z. Herbal medicines for immunosuppression. Iran J Allergy Asthma Immunol 2012; 11(2): 111-9.
[PMID: 22761185]

[29] Ishida M, Nishi K, Kunihiro N, Onda H, Nishimoto S, Sugahara T. Immunostimulatory effect of aqueous extract of *Coriandrum sativum* L. seed on macrophages. J Sci Food Agric 2017; 97(14): 4727-36.
[http://dx.doi.org/10.1002/jsfa.8341] [PMID: 28369918]

[30] Chauhan PS, Gupta KK, Bani S. The immunosuppressive effects of Agyrolobium roseum and pinitol in experimental animals. Int Immunopharmacol 2011; 11(2): 286-91.
[http://dx.doi.org/10.1016/j.intimp.2010.11.028] [PMID: 21156221]

[31] Rahayu RP, Prasetyo RA, Purwanto DA, Kresnoadi U, Iskandar RPD, Rubianto M. The immunomodulatory effect of green tea (*Camellia sinensis*) leaves extract on immunocompromised Wistar rats infected by *Candida albicans*.. Vet World 2018; 11(6): 765-70.
[http://dx.doi.org/10.14202/vetworld.2018.765-770] [PMID: 30034167]

[32] Bukoye O, Musbau A. Immune modulation potentials of aqueous extract of Andrographis paniculata leaves in male rat. Researcher 2011; 3(3): 48-57.

[33] Wan YG, Che XY, Sun W, *et al.* Low-dose of multi-glycoside of Tripterygium wilfordii Hook. f., a natural regulator of TGF-β1/Smad signaling activity improves adriamycin-induced glomerulosclerosis *in vivo*. J Ethnopharmacol 2014; 151(3): 1079-89.
[http://dx.doi.org/10.1016/j.jep.2013.12.005] [PMID: 24362077]

[34] Zhu YN, Zhao WM, Yang YF, *et al.* Periplocoside E, an effective compound from *Periploca sepium* Bge, inhibited T cell activation *in vitro* and *in vivo*. J Pharmacol Exp Ther 2006; 316(2): 662-9.
[http://dx.doi.org/10.1124/jpet.105.093732] [PMID: 16204471]

[35] Momtazi-Borojeni AA, Haftcheshmeh SM, Esmaeili SA, Johnston TP, Abdollahi E, Sahebkar A. Curcumin: A natural modulator of immune cells in systemic lupus erythematosus. Autoimmun Rev 2018; 17(2): 125-35.
[http://dx.doi.org/10.1016/j.autrev.2017.11.016] [PMID: 29180127]

[36] Mawarti H, Nugraha J, Purwanto DA, Soeroso J. Identifying and revealing active compound from green tea (*Camellia sinensis*) for curing systemic lupus erythematosus by acting as CASPASE 1 inhibitor. Med-Leg Update 2020; 20(2): 323-9.
[http://dx.doi.org/10.37506/mlu.v20i3.1439]

[37] Maharani P, Mulia AS, Wulandari D, Veninda HR, Pandapotan FA. Plants as candidates for herbal treatment of SLE (Systemic Lupus Erythematosus). Cerdika. Jurnal Ilmiah Indonesia 2023; 3(5): 458-68.
[http://dx.doi.org/10.59141/cerdika.v3i5.600]

[38] Pasdaran A, Hassani B, Tavakoli A, Kozuharova E, Hamedi A. A review of the potential benefits of herbal medicines, small molecules of natural sources, and supplements for health promotion in lupus conditions. Life (Basel) 2023; 13(7): 1589.
[http://dx.doi.org/10.3390/life13071589] [PMID: 37511964]

[39] Minhas U, Minz R, Bhatnagar A. Prophylactic effect of *Withania somnifera* on inflammation in a non-autoimmune prone murine model of lupus. Drug Discov Ther 2011; 5(4): 195-201.
[http://dx.doi.org/10.5582/ddt.2011.v5.4.195] [PMID: 22466301]

[40] Damle M. Glycyrrhiza glabra (Liquorice)—a potent medicinal herb. Int J Herb Med 2014; 2(2): 132-6.

[41] Boudreau MD, Beland FA. An evaluation of the biological and toxicological properties of *Aloe barbadensis* (miller), *Aloe vera.* J Environ Sci Health Part C Environ Carcinog Ecotoxicol Rev 2006; 24(1): 103-54.
[http://dx.doi.org/10.1080/10590500600614303] [PMID: 16690538]

[42] Erowele GI, Kalejaiye AO. Pharmacology and therapeutic uses of cat's claw. Am J Health Syst Pharm 2009; 66(11): 992-5.
[http://dx.doi.org/10.2146/ajhp080443] [PMID: 19451609]

[43] Yu X, Zhang N, Lin W, *et al.* Regulatory effects of four ginsenoside monomers in humoral immunity of systemic lupus erythematosus. Exp Ther Med 2018; 15(2): 2097-103.
[PMID: 29434811]

[44] Fugh-Berman A. Echinacea for the prevention and treatment of upper respiratory infections. Seminars in Integrative Medicine 2003; 1(2): 106-11.
[http://dx.doi.org/10.1016/S1543-1150(03)00012-7]

[45] Belch JJF, Hill A. Evening primrose oil and borage oil in rheumatologic conditions. Am J Clin Nutr 2000; 71(1) (Suppl.): 352S-6S.
[http://dx.doi.org/10.1093/ajcn/71.1.352S] [PMID: 10617996]

[46] Chrastina M, Dráfi F, Pružinská K, *et al. Crocus sativus L.* extract (saffron) effectively reduces arthritic and inflammatory parameters in monotherapy and in combination with methotrexate in adjuvant arthritis. Nutrients 2023; 15(19): 4108.
[http://dx.doi.org/10.3390/nu15194108] [PMID: 37836391]

[47] M Vila L, Lebrón-Torres LF. Efficacy of milk thistle in a patient with systemic lupus erythematosus presenting with autoimmune hepatitis. International Journal of Clinical Studies and Medical Case Reports 2023; 29(1): 15-20.
[http://dx.doi.org/10.46998/IJCMCR.2023.29.000701]

[48] Gupta AT. Tinospora cordifolia can cure systemic lupus erythematosus. Int J Pharmacogn. 2019 Jul 31;6(7):237–52.
[http://dx.doi.org/10.13040/IJPSR.0975-8232.IJP.6(7).237-52]

[49] Zhang Y, Yang Z, Cock IE. *Centella asiatica (L.)* Urban leaf extracts inhibit the growth of bacterial

triggers of selected autoimmune inflammatory diseases and potentiate the activity of conventional antibiotics. Pharmacogn Commun 2020; 10(3): 119-29.
[http://dx.doi.org/10.5530/pc.2020.3.24]

[50] Ziaei A, Hoppstädter J, Kiemer AK, Ramezani M, Amirghofran Z, Diesel B. Inhibitory effects of teuclatriol, a sesquiterpene from salvia mirzayanii, on nuclear factor-κB activation and expression of inflammatory mediators. J Ethnopharmacol 2015; 160: 94-100.
[http://dx.doi.org/10.1016/j.jep.2014.10.041] [PMID: 25446581]

[51] Upadhyay RK. Nutraceutical, pharmaceutical and therapeutic uses of *Allium cepa*: A review. International Journal of Green Pharmacy 2016; 10: S46-64.

[52] Kala C, Ali SS, Khan NA. Immunostimulatory potential of n-butanolic fraction of hydroalcoholic extract of *Costus speciosus Koen*. Rhizome. Int J Pharm Sci Res 2015; 6(7): 2886-92.
[http://dx.doi.org/10.13040/IJPSR.0975-8232.6(7).2886-92]

[53] Thangam R, Sathuvan M, Poongodi A, *et al.* Activation of intrinsic apoptotic signaling pathway in cancer cells by Cymbopogon citratus polysaccharide fractions. Carbohydr Polym 2014; 107: 138-50.
[http://dx.doi.org/10.1016/j.carbpol.2014.02.039] [PMID: 24702929]

[54] Gandhi M, Shree R. Immuno-modulatory effect of turmeric (*Curcuma longa*) and Aloe vera on cultured polymorphonuclear cells (PMN) and adherent mononuclear cells. Webmedcentral 2016; 7(4): 2-7.

[55] Nam S, Xie J, Perkins A, *et al.* Novel synthetic derivatives of the natural product berbamine inhibit Jak2/Stat3 signaling and induce apoptosis of human melanoma cells. Mol Oncol 2012; 6(5): 484-93.
[http://dx.doi.org/10.1016/j.molonc.2012.05.002] [PMID: 22717603]

[56] Yin Y, Gong FY, Wu XX, *et al.* Anti-inflammatory and immunosuppressive effect of flavones isolated from *Artemisia vestita*. J Ethnopharmacol 2008; 120(1): 1-6.
[http://dx.doi.org/10.1016/j.jep.2008.07.029] [PMID: 18721870]

[57] Sani TA, Mohammadpour E, Mohammadi A, *et al.* Cytotoxic and apoptogenic properties of *Dracocephalum kotschyi* aerial part different fractions on CALU-6 and MEHR-80 lung cancer cell lines. Farmacia 2017; 65(2): 189-99.

[58] Faham N, Javidnia K, Bahmani M, Amirghofran Z. Calycopterin, an immunoinhibitory compound from the extract of *Dracocephalum kotschyi*. Phytother Res 2008; 22(9): 1154-8.
[http://dx.doi.org/10.1002/ptr.2382] [PMID: 18683896]

[59] Wang GJ, Sweet DE, Reger SI, Thompson RC. Fat-cell changes as a mechanism of avascular necrosis of the femoral head in cortisone-treated rabbits. J Bone Joint Surg Am 1977; 59(6): 729-35.
[http://dx.doi.org/10.2106/00004623-197759060-00003] [PMID: 908695]

[60] Richards RN. Side effects of short-term oral corticosteroids. J Cutan Med Surg 2008; 12(2): 77-81.
[http://dx.doi.org/10.2310/7750.2008.07029] [PMID: 18346404]

[61] Østensen M, Villiger PM. Nonsteroidal anti-inflammatory drugs in systemic lupus erythematosus. Lupus 2001; 10(3): 135-9.
[http://dx.doi.org/10.1191/096120301668183556] [PMID: 11315341]

[62] Dasgupta A, Hammett-Stabler CA. Herbal Supplements: Efficacy, Toxicity, Interactions with Western Drugs and Effects on Clinical Laboratory Tests. 1st ed. Hoboken, NJ: John Wiley & Sons 2011; pp. 135-54.

[63] Haija AJ, Schulz SW. The role and effect of complementary and alternative medicine in systemic lupus erythematosus. Rheum Dis Clin North Am 2011; 37(1): 47-62.
[http://dx.doi.org/10.1016/j.rdc.2010.11.005] [PMID: 21220085]

[64] Jiao B, Gao J. Intensive research on the prospective use of complementary and alternative medicine to treat systemic lupus erythematosus. Drug Discov Ther 2013; 7(4): 167-71.
[http://dx.doi.org/10.5582/ddt.2013.v7.4.167] [PMID: 24071580]

[65] Seo Y, Mun CH, Park SH, *et al.* Punicalagin ameliorates lupus nephritis *via* inhibition of PAR2. Int J Mol Sci 2020; 21(14): 4975.
[http://dx.doi.org/10.3390/ijms21144975] [PMID: 32674502]

[66] Jiang T, Tian F, Zheng H, *et al.* Nrf2 suppresses lupus nephritis through inhibition of oxidative injury and the NF-κB-mediated inflammatory response. Kidney Int 2014; 85(2): 333-43.
[http://dx.doi.org/10.1038/ki.2013.343] [PMID: 24025640]

[67] Castejon ML, Sánchez-Hidalgo M, Aparicio-Soto M, *et al.* Dietary oleuropein and its new acyl-derivate attenuate murine lupus nephritis through HO-1/Nrf2 activation and suppressing JAK/STAT, NF-κB, MAPK and NLRP3 inflammasome signaling pathways. J Nutr Biochem 2019; 74: 108229.
[http://dx.doi.org/10.1016/j.jnutbio.2019.108229] [PMID: 31698204]

[68] Wang M, Zhou G, Lv J, Zeng P, Guo C, Wang Q. Curcumin modulation of the activation of PYK2 in peripheral blood mononuclear cells from patients with lupus nephritis. Reumatologia 2017; 55(6): 269-75.
[http://dx.doi.org/10.5114/reum.2017.72623] [PMID: 29491534]

[69] Khajehdehi P, Zanjaninejad B, Aflaki E, *et al.* Oral supplementation of turmeric decreases proteinuria, hematuria, and systolic blood pressure in patients suffering from relapsing or refractory lupus nephritis: a randomized and placebo-controlled study. J Ren Nutr 2012; 22(1): 50-7.
[http://dx.doi.org/10.1053/j.jrn.2011.03.002] [PMID: 21742514]

[70] Wang ZL, Luo XF, Li MT, *et al.* Resveratrol possesses protective effects in a pristane-induced lupus mouse model. PLoS One 2014; 9(12): e114792.
[http://dx.doi.org/10.1371/journal.pone.0114792] [PMID: 25501752]

[71] Dent EL, Taylor EB, Turbeville HR, Ryan MJ. Curcumin attenuates autoimmunity and renal injury in an experimental model of systemic lupus erythematosus. Physiol Rep 2020; 8(13): e14501.
[http://dx.doi.org/10.14814/phy2.14501] [PMID: 32652896]

[72] Zhao J, Wang J, Zhou M, Li M, Li M, Tan H. Curcumin attenuates murine lupus *via* inhibiting NLRP3 inflammasome. Int Immunopharmacol 2019; 69: 213-6.
[http://dx.doi.org/10.1016/j.intimp.2019.01.046] [PMID: 30738291]

[73] Kang HK, Ecklund D, Liu M, Datta SK. Apigenin, a non-mutagenic dietary flavonoid, suppresses lupus by inhibiting autoantigen presentation for expansion of autoreactive Th1 and Th17 cells. Arthritis Res Ther 2009; 11(2): R59.
[http://dx.doi.org/10.1186/ar2682] [PMID: 19405952]

[74] Su B, Ye H, You X, Ni H, Chen X, Li L. Icariin alleviates murine lupus nephritis *via* inhibiting NF-κB activation pathway and NLRP3 inflammasome. Life Sci 2018; 208: 26-32.
[http://dx.doi.org/10.1016/j.lfs.2018.07.009] [PMID: 30146016]

[75] Jhou JP, Chen SJ, Huang HY, Lin WW, Huang DY, Tzeng SJ. Upregulation of FcγRIIB by resveratrol *via* NF-κB activation reduces B-cell numbers and ameliorates lupus. Exp Mol Med 2017; 49(9): e381.
[http://dx.doi.org/10.1038/emm.2017.144] [PMID: 28960214]

[76] Oliveira ALB, Monteiro VVS, Navegantes-Lima KC, et al. Resveratrol modulates immune responses and ameliorates progression of systemic autoimmune diseases: A mini-review. Nutrients 2017; 9(12): 1306.
[http://dx.doi.org/10.3390/nu9121306]

[77] Kasiri N, Rahmati M, Ahmadi L, Eskandari N. Apigenin, a plant-derived flavone, attenuates autoimmune responses by modulating pro-inflammatory cytokines and T cell proliferation. Inflammopharmacology 2018; 26(5): 1359–1373.
[http://dx.doi.org/10.1007/s10787-018-0531-8]

[78] Tsai PY, Ka SM, Chang JM, *et al.* Epigallocatechin-3-gallate prevents lupus nephritis development in mice *via* enhancing the Nrf2 antioxidant pathway and inhibiting NLRP3 inflammasome activation. Free Radic Biol Med 2011; 51(3): 744-54.

[http://dx.doi.org/10.1016/j.freeradbiomed.2011.05.016] [PMID: 21641991]

[79] Guo L, Liu W, Lu T, *et al.* Decrease of functional activated T and B cells and treatment of glomerulonephitis in lupus-prone mice using a natural flavonoid astilbin. PLoS One 2015; 10(4): e0124002.
[http://dx.doi.org/10.1371/journal.pone.0124002] [PMID: 25867237]

[80] Du P, Zhang W, Cui H, *et al.* Sulforaphane ameliorates the severity of psoriasis and SLE by modulating effector cells and reducing oxidative stress. Front Pharmacol 2022; 13: 805508.
[http://dx.doi.org/10.3389/fphar.2022.805508] [PMID: 35126161]

[81] Gu Z, Cao X, Jiang J, *et al.* Upregulation of p16INK4A promotes cellular senescence of bone marrow-derived mesenchymal stem cells from systemic lupus erythematosus patients. Cell Signal 2012; 24(12): 2307-14.
[http://dx.doi.org/10.1016/j.cellsig.2012.07.012] [PMID: 22820504]

[82] Tsai CY, Shen CY, Liao HT, *et al.* Molecular and cellular bases of immunosenescence, inflammation, and cardiovascular complications mimicking "inflammaging" in patients with systemic lupus erythematosus. Int J Mol Sci 2019; 20(16): 3878.
[http://dx.doi.org/10.3390/ijms20163878] [PMID: 31395799]

[83] Gao L, Bird AK, Meednu N, *et al.* Bone marrow–derived mesenchymal stem cells from patients with systemic lupus erythematosus have a senescence-associated secretory phenotype mediated by a mitochondrial antiviral signaling protein–interferon-β feedback loop. Arthritis Rheumatol 2017; 69(8): 1623-35.
[http://dx.doi.org/10.1002/art.40142] [PMID: 28471483]

[84] Cunha ALS, Perazzio SF. Effects of immune exhaustion and senescence of innate immunity in autoimmune disorders. Braz J Med Biol Res 2024; 57: e13225.
[http://dx.doi.org/10.1590/1414-431x2024e13225] [PMID: 38896644]

[85] Dema B, Charles N. Autoantibodies in SLE: specificities, isotypes and receptors. Antibodies (Basel) 2016; 5(1): 2.
[http://dx.doi.org/10.3390/antib5010002] [PMID: 31557984]

[86] Han S, Zhuang H, Shumyak S, Yang L, Reeves WH. Mechanisms of autoantibody production in systemic lupus erythematosus. Front Immunol 2015; 6: 228.
[http://dx.doi.org/10.3389/fimmu.2015.00228] [PMID: 26029213]

[87] Lu Y, Ruan Y, Hong P, *et al.* T-cell senescence: A crucial player in autoimmune diseases. Clin Immunol 2023; 248: 109202.
[http://dx.doi.org/10.1016/j.clim.2022.109202] [PMID: 36470338]

[88] Ray D, Yung R. Immune senescence, epigenetics and autoimmunity. Clin Immunol 2018; 196: 59-63.
[http://dx.doi.org/10.1016/j.clim.2018.04.002] [PMID: 29654845]

[89] van den Hoogen L, Sims G, van Roon J, Fritsch-Stork R. Aging and systemic lupus erythematosus-immunosenescence and beyond. Curr Aging Sci 2015; 8(2): 158-77.
[http://dx.doi.org/10.2174/1874609808666150727111904] [PMID: 26212055]

[90] López P, Rodríguez-Carrio J, Martínez-Zapico A, Caminal-Montero L, Suarez A. Senescent profile of angiogenic T cells from systemic lupus erythematosus patients. J Leukoc Biol 2016; 99(3): 405-12.
[http://dx.doi.org/10.1189/jlb.5HI0215-042R] [PMID: 26232454]

[91] Fiehn O. Metabolomics—the link between genotypes and phenotypes. Functional Genomics 2002; pp. 155-71.

[92] Williams RJ, Spencer JPE, Rice-Evans C. Flavonoids: antioxidants or signalling molecules?. Free Radic Biol Med 2004; 36(7): 838-49.
[http://dx.doi.org/10.1016/j.freeradbiomed.2004.01.001] [PMID: 15019969]

[93] Martin-Mercado TM. An investigation of the role of precision medicine in the treatment of systemic lupus erythematosus. Doctoral dissertation, Rutgers The State University of New Jersey, Rutgers

School of Health Professions

[94] Ahmad I, Aqil F, Ahmad F, Owais M. Herbal medicines: prospects and constraints. Modern Phytomedicine. Turning Medicinal Plants into Drugs 2006; pp. 59-77. [http://dx.doi.org/10.1002/9783527609987.ch3]

[95] Dixon RA, Strack D. Phytochemistry meets genome analysis, and beyond. Phytochemistry 2003; 62(6): 815-6. [http://dx.doi.org/10.1016/S0031-9422(02)00712-4] [PMID: 12590109]

[96] Sharma R, Prajapati PK. Predictive, preventive and personalized medicine: leads from Ayurvedic concept of Prakriti (human constitution). Curr Pharmacol Rep 2020; 6(6): 441-50. [http://dx.doi.org/10.1007/s40495-020-00244-3]

[97] Mills SY, Bone K. The essential guide to herbal safety Elsevier Health Sciences; 2004 Dec 23

[98] Shastry BS. Pharmacogenetics and the concept of individualized medicine. Pharmacogenomics J 2006; 6(1): 16-21. [http://dx.doi.org/10.1038/sj.tpj.6500338] [PMID: 16302022]

[99] Fabricant DS, Farnsworth NR. The value of plants used in traditional medicine for drug discovery. Environ Health Perspect 2001; 109(Suppl 1) (Suppl. 1): 69-75. [http://dx.doi.org/10.1289/ehp.01109s169] [PMID: 11250806]

[100] Foster-Duette A. Integrating complementary and alternative medicine into private insurance vs. Medicare and Medicaid: history, trends, current status and areas for improvement. Doctoral dissertation, California State University, Northridge

CHAPTER 7

Advancements in Immunology: Comprehensive Insights into Autoimmune Disorders, Diagnostic Innovations, and Emerging Therapeutic Strategies.

Ekambaram Gayathiri[1], **Palanisamy Prakash**[2], **Ramachandran Kaliaperumal**[3], **Suganya Kannan**[4], **Poorna Chandrika Sabapathy**[5], **Asbar Banu Bazeer**[6], **Kirtik Ramadoss**[6], **Sharangouda J. Patil**[7] and **Prithiviraj Nagarajan**[6,*]

[1] *Department of Plant Biology and Plant Biotechnology, Guru Nanak College (Autonomous), Chennai 600042, India*

[2] *Department of Botany, Periyar University, Periyar Palkalai Nagar, Salem 636011, Tamil Nadu, India*

[3] *Department of Biochemistry, Sri Manakula Vinayagar Medical College and Hospital, Madagadipet, Kalitheerthalkuppam, Puducherry 605107, India*

[4] *Central Research Laboratory for Biomedical Research and Molecular Biology, Vinayaka Mission's Medical College and Hospital, Vinayaka Mission's Research Foundation, Karaikal, Puducherry 609609, India*

[5] *Directorate of Medical Research, Research and Innovation Lab, Aarupadai Veedu Medical College & Hospital, Vinayaka Mission, India*

[6] *Department of Medical Biotechnology, Aarupadai Veedu Medical College & Hospital, Vinayaka Mission's Research Foundation (Deemed to be University), Kirumampakkam, Puducherry 607403, India*

[7] *Department of Zoology, NMKRV College for Women, Bengaluru 560011, Karnataka, India*

Abstract: Autoimmune diseases are among the most challenging conditions to manage in healthcare practice because of the chronic and often multifactorial nature of their pathophysiology. This chapter focuses mainly on autoimmune disorders and begins by establishing the context of the immune system, as well as its components, with a description of its functions, antigen presentation, clonal selection, memory cells, and the key mechanisms of immune responses. Moving on, it discusses autoimmune disorders, outlining their classification and employing the pathophysiology, molecules involved, and genetic factors, including HLA genes and gene mutations. Diagnostic procedures involving hematological examination, radiological imaging, and fine-needle aspiration cytology are employed to portray the modern techniques used in the

* **Corresponding author Prithiviraj Nagarajan:** Department of Medical Biotechnology, Aarupadai Veedu Medical College & Hospital, Vinayaka Mission's Research Foundation (Deemed to be University), Kirumampakkam, Puducherry 607403, India; E-mail: prithivinaga@gmail.com

M.S. Ashawat, Aditi Kaushik, Akash Jain, Jasmine Chaudhary & Manish Kaushik (Eds.)
All rights reserved-© 2025 Bentham Science Publishers

diagnosis of autoimmune disorders. An assessment of pharmacological and non-pharmacological treatment options currently available examines the former in terms of corticosteroids, immunosuppressing agents, biologics, and small-molecule inhibitors, while the latter includes lifestyle interventions and complementary medicine. This chapter also focuses on advanced research and new treatment directions, such as gene therapy, monoclonal antibodies, repurposing drug approaches, malaria transcription intervention factor targeting, immune checkpoint blockage, autophagy regulation, and biodegradable nanoparticles to build up antigen-specific tolerance. New treatment regimens are characterized by pharmacodynamics, evidence-based, side effects or complications, and improved benefits compared with earlier interventions. The chapter concludes with a summary of the key points, emphasizing the importance of advancing our understanding and treatment of autoimmune disorders through ongoing research and innovation.

Keywords: Autoimmune disorders, Biodegradable nanoparticles, Cytology, Gene therapy, Hematology, Immune cells, Immune response, Immunology, Monoclonal antibodies, Small-molecule inhibitors.

INTRODUCTION

The immune system is one of the most intricate and constantly changing systems of the body that helps defend against pathogens, illnesses, and other foreign substances. It is involved in the regulation of homeostasis through the ability to differentiate between self and non-self and their subsequent management to either eliminate or neutralize threats [1]. The immune system is broadly categorized into two major categories, namely the innate immune system and the adaptive immune system. All these systems have individual but closely related functions in protecting the body against pathogens such as bacteria, viruses, fungi, and parasites, as well as identifying and eliminating cancer cells [2]. The main task of the immune system is to protect the integrity of an organism and its health by distinguishing between self and non-self entities and not harming the host's tissues. This is a very fine equilibrium between the innate and adaptive immune systems. The innate immune system is the first defense mechanism that is rapid and provides a general response to pathogens. Some of these are mechanical barriers, such as the skin and mucous membranes, and cellular defenses, such as phagocytes and natural killer cells [3]. In contrast, the adaptive immune system requires a more focused and specific response that involves the activation of lymphocytes, including B and T cells, which enables them to deal with the same pathogen in the future in a more efficient way [4].

Types and Roles of the Immune System

The immune system is the body's defense mechanism against diseases, illnesses, and foreign substances that invade the body.

The two types of immune responses are:

- The Innate immune system
- Adaptive immune system.

Innate Immune System

Innate immunity is considered the first line of defense that helps the body protect itself against pathogens. This system is non-specific, meaning that it operates in response to all pathogens, without the possibility of remembering specific pathogens.

The Innate Immune System Comprises Several Key Mechanisms and Components

Physical Barriers

The first line of defense includes anatomical barriers such as the skin and mucosal surfaces. These barriers function as the first line of defense, preventing pathogens from entering the body. The skin is a protective barrier that is hard and does not allow penetration, whereas mucous membranes trap and eliminate pathogens using mucus and cilia.

Phagocytic Cells

Macrophages and neutrophils are important components of the innate immunity. These cells are known as phagocytes, which engorge and destroy pathogens through a process known as phagocytosis. When a pathogen is consumed, it is engulfed by the cell as a phagosome, which then fuses with a lysosome, thus enzymatically destroying the pathogen [5].

Natural Killer Cells

These cells are very significant in the identification and elimination of infected or cancerous cells. Natural Killer (NK) cells are lymphocytes that eliminate target cells through apoptosis or programmed cell death by using cytotoxic granules containing perforin and granzymes. This mechanism is efficient for the removal of cells affected by infection or neoplastic diseases.

Inflammation is one of the basic mechanisms of innate immunity. Inflammatory mediators such as cytokines and chemokines are produced in damaged or infected tissues. These mediators dilate blood vessels and make the blood vessel walls more permeable, allowing immune cells to travel to the infected or injured area. Immune cells that are attracted to the area include neutrophils and macrophages, which help eliminate pathogens and facilitate tissue repair.

Adaptive Immune System

Adaptive immunity is a body's advanced and targeted method of dealing with pathogens. Adaptive immunity is significantly different from innate immunity because it can recognize and remember past encounters with pathogens, allowing for more efficient responses in the future.

The adaptive immune system comprises several key components.

B Cells

B cells are involved in humoral immunity, which is an antibody-mediated defense mechanism. B cells can recognize antigens and subsequently mature into plasma cells that synthesize antibodies. It attaches to antigens on the surface of pathogens and either immobilizes them or marks their destruction by other immune cells. This process is important for identifying and eliminating pathogens in bodily fluids.

T Cells

T cells are essential for cellular immunity. These cells help the activation of other immune cells by secreting cytokines that boost the immune system. Regulatory T cells are involved in self-tolerance and immune suppression, whereas cytotoxic T cells (T_c cells) kill infected or cancerous cells by recognizing antigens on the surface of these cells. T cells can engage antigens with the assistance of MHC (Major Histocompatibility Complex) molecules to guarantee the targeting of pathogens or even abnormal cells.

Memory Cells

The adaptive immune system has the unique characteristic of creating memory cells. B and T cells have the potential to become memory cells following initial contact with pathogens. These memory cells remain in the body and provide a quick and effective response the next time the same pathogen is detected. This immunological memory is the foundation for a vaccine in which the body is introduced to a nonpathogenic form of the pathogen to produce memory cells to fight off the pathogen without causing the disease [6].

The immune system plays a critical role in fighting infections and other diseases. Understanding the roles of the immune system enables the development of medications and strategies for combating numerous immune system disorders.

The area of research in this field remains rich and continues to provide a better understanding of the immune response and its possible developments [7].

Antigen Presentation

The immune response is dependent on the presentation of antigenic peptides by MHC molecules to T cells, which is a vital process. This process assists in the identification of pathogens and abnormal cells in the body through the immune system. New data on antigen presentation has brought attention to the fact that there are many aspects and variations in the process.

Mechanisms of Antigen Presentation

Based on the route of antigen presentation, there are two main pathways: MHC class I and II. MHC class I molecules present endogenous antigens, which are primarily intracellular pathogens such as viruses, to CD8+ cytotoxic T cells. In contrast, exogenous antigens that are typically taken up from the extracellular environment are presented by MHC class II molecules to CD4+ T helper cells [8].

MHC Class I Pathway

- **Proteasomal Degradation:** The Proteins synthesized within the cell are broken down into peptides by proteasomes.
- **Peptide Transport:** They are transported into the Endoplasmic Reticulum (ER) by Transporters associated with Antigen Processing (TAP).
- **Peptide Loading:** In the ER, however, peptides bind to MHC class I.
- **Surface Expression:** Peptide-MHC class I complexes are then transported to the cell surface for recognition by CD8+ T cells [9].

MHC Class II Pathway

- **Antigen Uptake:** External antigens are engulfed by antigen-presenting cells, including dendritic cells, macrophages, and B cells.
- **Proteolytic Processing:** This antigen is broken down in endosomes.
- **Peptide Loading:** The final peptides are transported to the endosomal compartments, where they bind to MHC class II molecules.
- **Surface Expression:** Peptide-MHC class II complexes are transported to the cell surface to be recognized by CD4+ T cells [10].

Emerging Themes and Advances in Antigen Presentation

Recent studies have shed light on the role of antigen presentation in the immune system and its effect on disease development. One significant advancement in this area is our understanding of how autophagy contributes to the efficient presentation of antigens to the immune system. Cellular degradation, also called autophagy, involves the processing of endogenous antigens for the presentation of MHC class II molecules. This process is beneficial in cross-presentation, where exogenous antigens are presented through MHC class I molecules, forming a link between innate and adaptive immunity [11]. Other developments include the recognition of what is known as "cryptic" peptides. These peptides originate from non-coding regions of the genome or from frames other than the normal ones, thereby increasing the spectrum of antigens that are capable of being presented to the immune system. Consequently, this discovery has implications for the study of autoimmunity and tumor immunity and may be helpful in the development of cancer therapies. The development in antigen presentation is important for clinical applications, especially in cancer immunotherapy, because of the understanding of the antigen presentation mechanisms. This provides the potential for designing effective cancer vaccines and adoptive T cell therapies. The improvement in mass spectrometry and computational modeling has improved the recognition of tumor-associated antigens, which in turn has resulted in improved immunotherapies [12].

Clonal Selection

Clonal selection is a critical theory in immunology that explains how specific lymphocytes are selected for replication, depending on their ability to identify an antigen. This mechanism implies that the immune system can generate a specific and strong response to pathogens. Recent studies have shed further light on various aspects of clonal selection and have underlined its relevance in natural and artificial immune systems.

Mechanisms of Clonal Selection

The Clonal Selection Theory states that each lymphocyte has a unique receptor for an antigen. When in contact with a particular antigen, a lymphocyte becomes active, resulting in the replication and transformation of lymphocytes into effectors and memories. This process involved several key steps.

- **Antigen Recognition:** Naïve B and T cells, each with a unique receptor, are present in the bloodstream. When the receptor of the lymphocyte crosses a particular antigen, it binds to it, which triggers lymphocyte activation.
- **Clonal Expansion:** The Activated lymphocytes begin to divide, resulting in a group of cells that are all clones; each clone is specific for recognizing a particular antigen.
- **Differentiation:** These clonal cells further develop into two categories: effector cells, which contribute to the immune response, and memory cells, which remain resident in the body to provide a quick response to the NEXT antigen encounter [13].

Recent Advances

Current trends have further enriched our knowledge of clonal selection, particularly regarding the use of artificial immune systems and optimization algorithms. The process used by the immune system for defense, which is clonal selection, has been adopted in the development of Clonal Selection Algorithms (CSA) for use in optimization, machine learning, and other areas. A key use of CSAs is to solve challenging optimization problems. These algorithms are based on the natural process of clonal selection, where solutions are chosen based on their fitness, cloned, mutated, and then the best-performing solutions are selected. This repeating process improves the optimization, and based on a recent study, it has proven to be better than conventional algorithms in some cases [14]. One emerging area is the enhancement of CSAs to increase productivity and usefulness. For example, adaptive clonal selection algorithms have been proposed to fine-tune certain factors, such as mutation rates and clone sizes, to improve convergence speed and solution quality [15]. These adaptive algorithms overcome some of the challenges associated with traditional CSAs, such as early convergence and the requirement of tuning many parameters.

Applications and Implications

In addition to immunology and other scientific and engineering disciplines, clonal selection principles are widely used and essential. For instance, in cancer research, knowledge of clonal selection aids the understanding of tumor progression and the acquisition of therapy resistance. This phenomenon enables cancer cells to adapt to the pressures resulting from treatment, leading to the development of resistant clones. Single-cell genomics has been used to study the clonality of tumors, tumor evolution, and spatial and temporal heterogeneity [16]. In computational biology, CSAs have been applied to pattern matching, data mining, and optimization problems. It has been stated that such algorithms are well suited to solving complex real-world problems because they mimic the immune system, improve computational power, and generate effective solutions [17].

Nevertheless, specific problems remain open to the analysis and application of clonal selection. A major problem is that current models are not as specific or reproducible as they should be to imitate the biological mechanisms of clonal selection. Furthermore, the performance of CSAs has been demonstrated; however, they are often sensitive to the problem at hand and the chosen parameters. Further research is required to enhance the design of similar algorithms, which could prove to have higher versatility in other applications. In addition, combining clonal selection with other biological and computational concepts, such as gene expression programming and evolutionary strategies, results in more effective combined approaches. Such a combination of methods can provide the best advantages of the considered methodologies for solving complex tasks [18].

Memory Cells

Memory cells are a key component of adaptive immunity as they mediate long-term immunity and a rapid response to reexposure to the same antigen. These cells include memory B cells and memory T cells, which are involved in immune memory. New discoveries in immunology have elaborated on the formation, regulation, and role of these cells, which are critical elements in the management of diseases and the development of vaccines.

Formation of Memory Cells

Memory B and T cells are produced during the primary immune response to the antigens. Upon encountering an antigen, naïve B and T cells clonally expand and create effector cells to deal with the infection. Some of these effector cells transform into memory cells that are long-lived and linger in the body, even after the pathogen is eliminated, for quick action the next time the body encounters it [19]. Memory B cells are found in secondary lymphoid tissues and the bone marrow, and re-exposure to the antigen can quickly produce high-affinity antibodies. Memory T cells are present in the blood, found in various tissues, and are activated when the antigen of the pathogen is encountered again [20].

New Findings in Memory B Cells

Memory B cells are a subset of B cells involved in the immune response and comprise a diverse population, including subsets that produce IgG+, IgA+, and IgM+ antibodies. One of the most interesting subpopulations is IgM+ memory B cells, which constitute a large part of memory B cells and, upon restimulation with an antigen, can undergo an additional round of SHR and affinity maturation [21]. Recent studies have also shown that TLR signaling is instrumental in the early recall of memory B cells to produce antibodies against recurrent infections.

New Developments in Memory T Cells

There are three subsets of Memory T cells: central memory T cells (T_{CM}), Effector Memory T cells (T_{EM}), and tissue-resident memory T cells (T_{RM}). T_{CM} cells travel through secondary lymphoid tissues and have a high potential for expansion when antigens are reencountered. T_{EM} cells circulate in peripheral tissues and provide immediate effector functions, whereas T_{RM} cells dwell in tissues and are essential for tissue immunity [22]. Specifically, T_{RM} cells have been postulated to provide a better defense against specific infections and tumors because of their location at the portals of pathogen entry [23]. Other studies have also identified the presence of innate memory T cells, including memory $\gamma\delta$ T cells and Natural Killer (NK) cells, with characteristics of memory T cells. These cells can rapidly and effectively respond to recurrent infections and connect inherent and acquired immunity [24]. The knowledge of memory cell biology has a significant impact on immunotherapy and vaccine development. Therefore, the generation of effective and durable memory T cell responses has become a major goal in cancer immunotherapy. T_{CM} cells especially hold much potential in this regard as they can expand and further differentiate into effector T cells when restimulated with tumor antigens [25]. Thus, vaccine development aims to induce memory B and T cells with long-lasting functionality. Vaccines that can generate T_{RM} cells provide better protection against mucosal pathogens because they require a quicker immune response in the affected area [26]. However, there are still some issues concerning memory cells and their research and application. Another primary focus is to determine the surface markers for different memory cell subsets that can be used to monitor their life span and function in patients. In addition, the processes of memory cell generation and survival, including cytokines, antigenic load, and microenvironment, require further characterization [27]. The integration of Memory Cell Biology with other aspects of the immune response, including the Microbiota and Epigenetics, to boost memory may be helpful. Further studies should be conducted on the use of memory cells in the treatment of chronic infections and autoimmune diseases, as modifying memory responses may be beneficial [28].

Major Aspects of the Immune Reactions

The immune response is one of the most important and elaborate defense mechanisms of an organism, enabling it to prevent diseases, infections, and other adverse stimuli. It comprises a series of well-organized processes that entail the identification of pathogens, defense against pathogens, and their eradication. They can be divided into two types, innate and adaptive immunity, which have different functions and subunits. Recent research has been conducted on these processes, which have proven to be intricate and interactive.

Innate Immune Responses

The innate immune system is the first defense mechanism against pathogens and encompasses several cellular and molecular components. The key components of the innate immune response include the following.

- **Pattern Recognition Receptors [PRRs]:** PRRs, such as Toll-Like Receptors (TLRs), identify PAMPs that are found in the pathogen. TLRs are vital for the identification of microbial pathogens and the initiation of an inflammatory response. They engage in several cascades that result in the synthesis of cytokines and other mediators, which are useful for removing pathogens and organizing adaptive immunity [29].

- **Cytokines and Chemokines:** These molecules are crucial for the immune response, given that they control immune cell functions. Chemokines, interleukins, and interferons are proteins that are released during infection and play a role in the immune response. Chemokines facilitate the movement of immune cells to the site of infection, thus enabling the movement of neutrophils, macrophages, and other effector cells.
- **Phagocytosis:** Phagocytic cells, including macrophages and neutrophils, swallow and destroy the pathogens. This process is beneficial for eradicating infections and displaying antigens in the adaptive immune cells. Opsonization is a process by which pathogens are targeted for destruction by antibodies and complement proteins, resulting in improved phagocytosis.

Adaptive Immune Responses

Adaptive immunity is more efficient and involves lymphocyte involvement. It offers lifelong protection and memory, which helps combat pathogens. Key mechanisms include:

- **Antigen Presentation:** Dendritic cells and other Antigen-Presenting Cells (APCs) present antigens to T cells in association with MHC molecules. This interaction is important for T-cell activation and the initiation of adaptive immunity [10].
- **Clonal Selection:** T and B cells that are specific to a given antigen activate clonal expansion and differentiation. This process creates a group of effector cells capable of fighting infection as well as memory cells that provide long-term protection [9].
- **Humoral and Cell-Mediated Immunity:** B cells synthesize antibodies that prevent pathogens from infecting cells and target them for destruction by other immune cells. T-cells, particularly cytotoxic T-cells, lyse infected cells. Cytokines released by helper T cells support the activation and function of B cells and cytotoxic T cells [30].

Regulatory Mechanisms and Homeostasis

The immune system also has its own checks and balance mechanisms to ensure that the immune response is not over-exaggerated and that it causes harm to the body through autoimmunity or chronic inflammation.

The key regulatory elements include the following.

- **Regulatory T Cells (T_{regs}):** T_{regs} regulate the immune response and maintain the immune system by attacking the body's tissues and causing autoimmune diseases. It regulates the immune response and ensures that it does not overreact or threaten the body [31].
- **Immune Checkpoints:** There are molecules such as CTLA-4 and PD-1, which are immune checkpoints that suppress T cell activity and avoid overactivation of the immune response. These checkpoints are critical for immune control and are considered therapeutic targets for cancer immunotherapy because they improve the ability of the immune system to fight cancer [32].
- **Feedback Mechanisms:** The immune system has many negative feedback mechanisms that are used to stop the response once all pathogens have been cleared. For example, a decrease in antigen load results in a decrease in immune cell activation, and these cells either die or become memory cells [33].

New Findings and Evaluation of the Existing Literature

New knowledge regarding the mechanisms and pathways of immune reactions has been reported in the field of immunology. For instance, the role of the microbiome in immune system development is increasingly being studied. Research has shown that members of the commensal microbiota regulate the establishment and function of both innate and adaptive immunity, thus modulating the immune balance and immunopathies [34]. In addition, developments and improvements in systems immunology have offered a more comprehensive view of how the body's immune system works through the integration of information from various cellular and molecular levels. This approach has enhanced the capacity of scientists to estimate vaccine efficacy and comprehend the processes that occur in the immune system during infections and vaccinations [35]. Despite these developments, the following issues remain. One critical aspect is the identification of the processes that regulate immune tolerance and autoimmunity. Although the roles of regulatory T cells and immune checkpoints cannot be overemphasized, more studies are needed to understand the molecular pathways and genetic factors involved in these processes [36].

AUTOIMMUNE DISORDERS

Autoimmune diseases constitute one of the major disease categories in which the immune system targets the tissues in the body. This phenomenon occurs because the body develops tolerance to self-antigens and continuous tissue inflammation beyond normal levels. These disorders affect the functioning of organs and systems of the body in different ways and in different extremities (Fig. **1**).

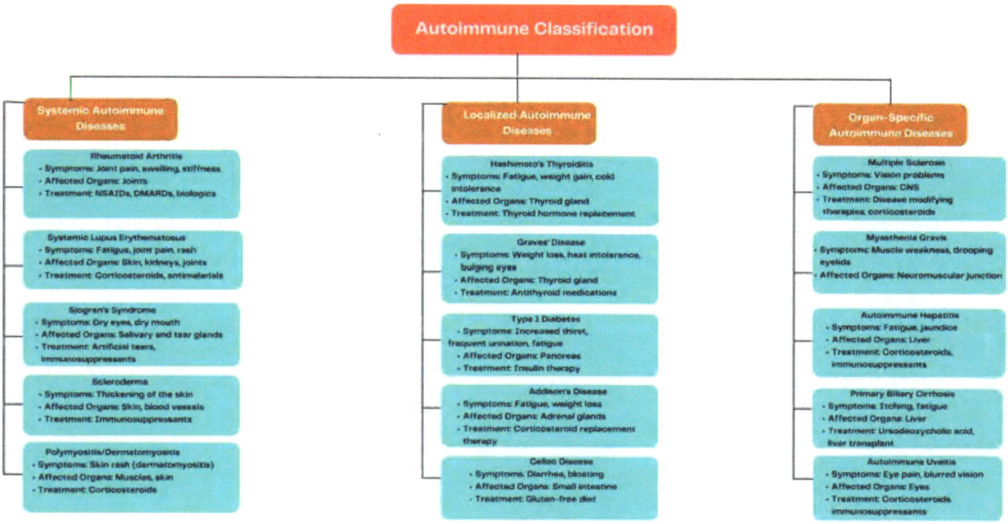

Fig. (1). Classification of Autoimmune Disorders.

Classification

Autoimmune diseases can be classified in different ways (Table **1**).

Table 1. Classification of autoimmune disorders with genes involved and mechanisms.

Autoimmune Disorder	Classification	Genes Involved	Mechanism	References
Rheumatoid Arthritis (RA)	Systemic Autoimmune	PTPN22, HLA-DRB1	T-cell activation, B-cell activation	[37]
Systemic Lupus Erythematosus (SLE)	Systemic Autoimmune	PTPN22, HLA-DRB1, IRF5	Immune complex deposition, B-cell hyperactivity	[38]
Type 1 Diabetes (T1D)	Endocrine Autoimmune	HLA-DR3/DR4, INS, PTPN22	T-cell-mediated beta-cell destruction	[39]
Multiple Sclerosis (MS)	Neurological Autoimmune	HLA-DRB1, IL2RA, IL7R	T-cell-mediated myelin destruction	[40]
Crohn's Disease (CD)	Gastrointestinal Autoimmune	NOD2, ATG16L1, IL23R	Dysregulated intestinal immune response	[41]
Celiac Disease (CeD)	Gastrointestinal Autoimmune	HLA-DQ2/DQ8, IL2, IL21	T-cell-mediated response to gluten	[42]
Psoriasis	Cutaneous Autoimmune	HLA-C, IL12B, IL23R	Keratinocyte proliferation, T-cell-mediated inflammation	[43]

(Table 1) cont.....

Autoimmune Disorder	Classification	Genes Involved	Mechanism	References
Hashimoto's Thyroiditis	Endocrine Autoimmune	HLA-DR3, CTLA4, PTPN22	T-cell-mediated thyroid follicular cell destruction	[44]
Ankylosing Spondylitis (AS)	Musculoskeletal Autoimmune	HLA-B27, ERAP1, IL23R	Inflammation of the axial skeleton, T-cell mediated	[45]
Sjögren's Syndrome (SS)	Systemic Autoimmune	HLA-DRB1, STAT4, IRF5	Lymphocytic infiltration of exocrine glands	[46]

Classical Classification

Organ-Specific Autoimmune Diseases

i. **Autoimmune Thyroid Diseases:** These include Hashimoto's thyroiditis and Graves' disease. Hashimoto's thyroiditis is an inflammatory disease resulting from the infiltration of T lymphocytes into the thyroid tissue, with subsequent destruction of the thyroid gland and the development of hypothyroidism. Graves' disease involves autoantibodies that act on the thyroid gland, leading to hyperthyroidism [47].
ii. **Type 1 Diabetes Mellitus:** This Type 1 diabetes is characterized by the destruction of insulin-producing beta cells in the pancreas, which leads to insulin deficiency and hyperglycemia. It is linked to autoantibodies against islet cell antigens [48].
iii. **Multiple Sclerosis (MS):** MS is an inflammatory demyelinating disease of the CNS in which there is immune-mediated damage to the myelin sheath of nerve fibres. Myelin basic protein is an autoantigen in MS, and autoantibodies and autoreactive T cell responses to the same protein are postulated in the disease [49].

Systemic Autoimmune Diseases

i. **Systemic Lupus Erythematosus (SLE):** SLE is defined as the production of autoantibodies against nuclear components, which results in inflammation and damage to several organs, such as the skin, kidneys, and joints [50].
ii. **Rheumatoid Arthritis (RA):** RA mainly affects the joints, causing them to become inflamed, swollen, and the synovial membrane thickens, leading to joint destruction. RF (Rheumatoid Factor) and ACPA (Anti-Citrullinated Protein Antibodies) are autoantibodies that are usually present in the sera of patients with RA and are commonly observed in the diagnosis of the disease [51].

iii. **Systemic Sclerosis (SSc):** SSc is characterized by excessive fibrosis of the skin and internal organs, vasculitis, and immune activation. Anti-topoisomerase I antibodies, which are nuclear antigens, are present in patients [52].

Emerging Classification Systems

The knowledge of immunological regulations and genetic differences in inherited autoimmune diseases is expected to enhance the development of more significant subclasses. Together with the genotypes, molecular types, and clinical diagnoses, they improve comprehension of ailments and patients.

Genetic and Molecular Classification

Immunological Disease Continuum: This concept categorizes diseases into two groups —Autoinflammatory and Autoimmune —according to the mechanism of the immune response. Autoinflammatory diseases are caused by dysregulation of innate immunity, whereas autoimmune diseases are caused by dysregulation of adaptive immunity. Some diseases present characteristics of both autoinflammation and autoimmunity, such as Crohn's disease [53].

Systems-Based Classification: The discovery of molecular pathways in systems biology has led to classifications that encompass numerous pathways involved in the development of diseases, including genetic susceptibility, environmental factors, and the immune system [54].

Clinical and Serological Classifications

Autoimmune Syndromes: This approach categorizes related diseases based on their frequent occurrence in patients, genetic and immune system links. For instance, autoimmune thyroid diseases coexist with other autoimmune diseases such as type 1 diabetes and SLE [55].

Epigenetic Influences: Research has also shown that epigenetic changes, including DNA methylation and histone modification, play a crucial role in autoimmune diseases. These changes affect gene regulation and the immune system, thus modulating disease risk and advancement [56].

Comorbidity and Data Mining-based Classification

Comorbidity Patterns: It is estimated that one in four patients with one autoimmune disease will have other related autoimmune diseases. Data mining procedures have been applied to identify potential comorbid autoimmune diseases using co-citation analysis in PubMed. This approach groups autoimmune diseases by systems such as gastrointestinal, neuronal, cutaneous, and musculoskeletal [57].

Molecular Taxonomy

Molecular Features and Pathogenesis: This is because information regarding the molecular mechanisms of systemic autoimmune diseases, in conjunction with the application of bioinformatics tools, can enable the redefinition of the diseases. This can help in the identification of novel biomarkers for patient stratification and prognosis, thereby influencing clinical trial design and the development of molecular targeting therapies [58].

Pathophysiology of Autoimmune Disorders

To understand the pathophysiology of autoimmune disorders, it is necessary to examine how the immune system fails and the molecular processes that lead to these diseases. New findings in genetics, epigenetics, and immunology have shed light on how these processes are highly regulated and influenced by the environment. Further investigation in these fields is crucial for the identification of novel treatment strategies and the enhancement of care for patients with autoimmune disorders.

Immune System Malfunctions

Autoimmune diseases result from immune system dysfunction, which mainly results from the loss of self-tolerance and can involve both innate and adaptive immunity. Examples include Toll-Like Receptors (TLRs), which are components of innate immunity and may contribute to autoimmunity by recognizing self-molecules as pathogens. TLR2 and TLR4 are involved in the development of many autoimmune diseases, including rheumatoid arthritis, systemic lupus erythematosus, and multiple sclerosis. When activated, these receptors engage adaptors, such as MyD88 and TRIF, leading to the progression of inflammatory pathways that exacerbate autoimmunity. Immune checkpoints that are important for immune regulation include PD-1 and CTLA-4. Abnormalities in these pathways can lead to autoimmunity. Current research has focused on the function of these checkpoints in diseases such as type 1 diabetes and SLE [59]. Other factors that regulate the immune response are regulatory T cells (T_{regs}). Tregs are known to control excessive immune reactions in a healthy human body and to prevent the development of autoimmune diseases. In autoimmune diseases, the efficiency and overall count of Tregs are usually impaired, resulting in the development of inflammation and tissue lesions. This is the case in diseases such as rheumatoid arthritis and type 1 diabetes, where Treg-mediated suppression is absent [60]. Cytotoxic T-Lymphocyte-Associated protein 4 (CTLA-4) is another important regulator of the immune response. CTLA-4 gene polymorphisms have been associated with several autoimmune diseases, underscoring the role of CTLA-4 in immune tolerance [61]. Changes in DNA methylation and histone modifications, which affect gene expression and immune cell activity, have also been reported. For instance, hypomethylation of DNA in T cells results in overexpression of genes related to autoimmunity, as in the case of SLE [56]. The immune system is significantly affected by the presence of the human microbiome. Dysbiosis of the microbiome can lead to the recruitment of autoreactive immune cells. Some probiotics have been found to induce autoimmunity either through molecular mimicry of autoantigens or by altering self-antigens [62].

Molecular Mechanisms

Autoimmune diseases occur when the immune system mistakenly attacks the body's own cells. The molecular mechanisms underlying this process include mimicry, epitope spreading, and bystander activation. Molecular mimicry is a process by which immune systems that target microbial antigens also target self-antigens, thereby causing autoimmunity. This has been described, for instance, in cases of Guillain-Barré syndrome, where antibodies against *Campylobacter jejuni* lipooligosaccharides are targeted at peripheral nerve gangliosides [63]. Autoimmune diseases can be induced by infection in several ways, including molecular mimicry, epitope spreading, and bystander activation. Epstein–Barr Virus [EBV] has been suggested to cause multiple sclerosis and systemic lupus erythematosus [64].

Epitope spreading is a process by which the immune system moves from one epitope to several epitopes on the same or different proteins. This mechanism is relevant in SLE, in which the initial targeted antigens are nucleosomal components, with the immune response spreading to other nuclear antigens, which is detrimental to patient health [65]. Bystander activation is a process that occurs when immune cells are activated in any given tissue and are associated with inflammation, but may result in the activation of autoreactive T cells. This mechanism is frequently observed in viral infections, when the inflammatory microenvironment can stimulate T cells that can react with self-antigens and may cause autoimmune diseases [66]. Changes in self-proteins through post-translational modifications, including citrullination or glycosylation, generate neoantigens that can be recognized by the immune system. This is evident in rheumatoid arthritis, in which citrullinated proteins are the main autoantigens [67]. Genetic factors have a major influence on susceptibility to autoimmune diseases. The HLA region is one of the most important genetic factors involved in antigen presentation and immune reactions. Specific alleles like HLA-DRB1*04:01 have been found to be closely related to rheumatoid arthritis [61].

These findings have increased our awareness of the role of epigenetic modifications in controlling autoimmune processes. Epigenetic modifications such as DNA methylation, histone modification, and microRNA (miRNA) can modify gene expression, but not DNA, which may affect the activity of immune cells and thus play a role in the appearance and evolution of autoimmune disorders. For instance, in SLE, T cells exhibit hypomethylation of DNA, resulting in the activation of genes that cause autoimmunity [56]. MicroRNAs have also been established to participate in the development of autoimmune diseases due to their regulation of genes controlling immune response. Dysregulated miRNAs have also been shown to cause hyperactivation of immune cells and production of autoantibodies as a result of immune complex-mediated diseases such as rheumatoid arthritis and multiple sclerosis [68]. Therefore, it is important to acknowledge that genetic susceptibility, along with infections and pollutants, is the leading cause of autoimmune diseases. Molecular mimicry and bystander activation can induce autoimmunity in the context of infection (Fig. **2**). In addition, other environmental factors, such as cigarette smoke and ultraviolet light, can cause oxidative stress and inflammation, which in turn increase autoimmune reactions [69, 70].

Genetic Factors in Autoimmune Diseases

Autoimmune diseases are induced by a combination of genes, environment, and the immune system. Therefore, genetic factors in autoimmune diseases are both HLA-linked and non-HLA-linked and include point mutations. Understanding these susceptibilities is important for designing therapies and enhancing patient prognoses. Such diseases remain a subject of active research that aims to reveal all the genetic and molecular factors involved in their development, which means that only tailored approaches make sense in terms of treatment and prevention. Genetic factors are considered important, and Human Leukocyte Antigen (HLA) genes are known to be major determinants of the disease. Furthermore, specific gene mutations in Crohn's disease, such as NOD2, are critical in the development of autoimmune diseases.

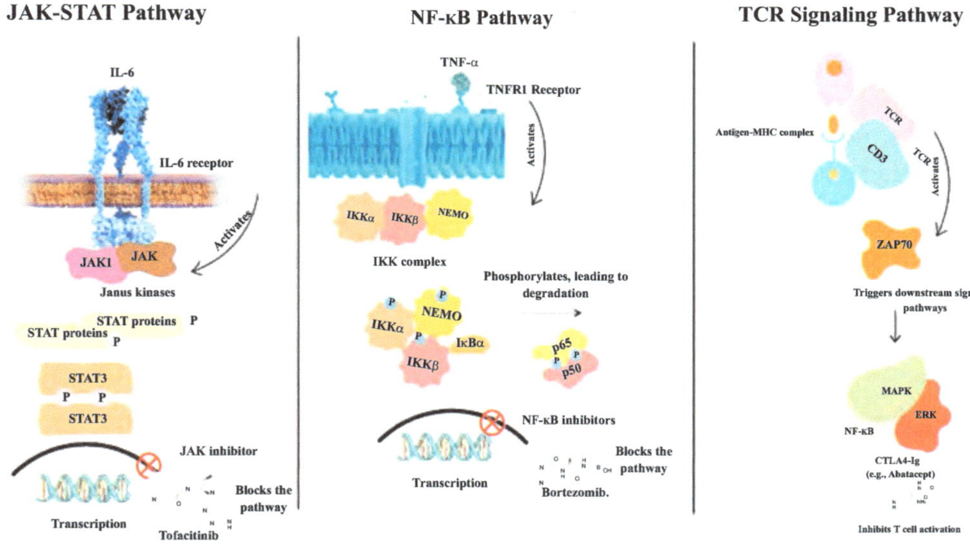

Fig. (2). Three cellular signaling pathways in molecular management of autoimmune diseases.

HLA Genes

The HLA complex is located on chromosome 6 and consists of genes that encode proteins that are critical to the immune system, especially in antigen presentation. Allelic differences in HLA genes are significant determinants of vulnerability to autoimmune disease. For instance, HLA-B27 is closely associated with ankylosing spondylitis, HLA-DRB1 alleles with rheumatoid arthritis, and multiple sclerosis [71]. HLA class II molecules such as HLA-DR, HLA-DQ, and HLA-DP are involved in antigen presentation to CD4+ T lymphocytes. Specific alleles such as HLA-DRB103: HLA-DQB1:01 and HLA-DRB104:01 are associated with diseases, such as SLE and type 1 diabetes, respectively. These alleles increase disease risk by altering the immune system's recognition of self-antigens [72]. The existing literature also shows that there are significant epistatic effects among the HLA genes. For example, the DRB104:01-DQB103:02 haplotype is one of the highest-risk combinations for numerous autoimmune diseases, including rheumatoid arthritis and type 1 diabetes. Thus, these interactions highlight the polygenic nature of these diseases [73]. Epigenetic changes can also influence HLA gene expression and function. Epigenetic changes in DNA methylation and histone modifications of the HLA locus have been implicated in the predisposition to autoimmune diseases [74]. Notably, the frequency of HLA alleles differs across populations, which in turn affects the incidence and risk of disease. For example, the HLA-DRB1*13 allele is less prevalent in autoimmune diseases in different ethnic populations, underlining the necessity of ethnogeographical genetic research [75].

Gene Mutations

NOD2 has been identified as having a very high association with Crohn's disease, an inflammatory bowel disease. NOD2 polymorphisms have been identified as genetic factors that contribute to susceptibility to Crohn's, particularly in pediatric patients. There is evidence that NOD2 polymorphisms are related to the CD-like phenotype, growth retardation, and arthropathy in patients with Very Early Onset Inflammatory Bowel Disease (VEO-IBD) [76]. In addition, NOD2 is related to other intracellular pathways, including the inhibitor of apoptosis (IAP) family, including cIAP1, cIAP2, and XIAP, which strengthens the relationship between NOD2 and IBD [77]. Surprisingly, NOD2 is associated with CD, and other genetic factors are involved in the development of this disease. For example, mutations in the MEFV gene, which are related to Familial Mediterranean Fever (FMF), have been considered in relation to IBD; however, no direct link with IBD phenotypic traits has been reported [78, 79]. This emphasizes that there is no single cause of IBD; rather, several genes and environmental factors lead to IBD [80]. NOD2 encodes a protein involved in the recognition of bacteria and defensive measures against them. Specific gene alterations, such as R702W, G908R, and L1007fs, affect NOD2, thus increasing the risk of developing Crohn's disease. PTPN22 encodes a tyrosine phosphatase involved in the regulation of T-cell receptor activation and has been associated with RA, T1DM, and SLE. The R620W polymorphism in PTPN22 is a well-established risk factor that affects immune cell activation and increases the risk of autoimmunity [81]. CTLA4 encodes a protein that controls T-cell activation in the immune system. The variants of CTLA4 are linked to autoimmune disorders, including type 1 diabetes, Graves' disease, and Hashimoto's thyroiditis. These variants alter the function of CTLA4, thereby increasing T-cell activation and causing autoimmunity [82]. One of the genes linked to MS and type 1 diabetes is IL2RA, which encodes a protein known as the alpha chain of the interleukin-2 receptor. Genetic polymorphisms of IL2RA are involved in the modulation of Tregs, which are vital for immune system homeostasis [83]. Thus, the role of genetic factors in autoimmune diseases cannot be overlooked. However, the environment, which includes infections and pollutants, also plays an important role. For example, viral infections cause autoimmunity through molecular mimicry, epitope spreading, and bystander activation, particularly in genetically predisposed populations [84].

DIAGNOSTIC INNOVATIONS

Hematological Examination

Autoimmune diseases are diagnosed and managed *via* hematological examinations. Due to recent advancements in diagnostic tools and technologies, these examinations have become more precise and rapid, and include multiparametric immunoassays, CyTOF, and proteomic biomarkers. Future research in this area is important to improve the quality of patient care and refine treatment plans.

Multiparametric Immunoassays

Multivariate immunoassays are widely used for the diagnosis of autoimmune diseases. These tests can detect multiple autoantibodies simultaneously and are therefore more accurate and efficient. However, it is essential to understand the working of these assays and their strengths and weaknesses in clinical settings [85]. Multiparametric immunoassays are especially helpful in cases where several autoantibodies have to be identified simultaneously, such as in SLE and RA. Research indicates that these assays enhance the diagnosis of autoimmune diseases by offering a holistic view of the autoantibodies present in the patient's body [85]. Multiparametric autoantibody tests have been proposed to increase the specificity of immunological diagnosis and shorten diagnostic time. These tests not only facilitate diagnosis but also help determine the risk of disease onset, phenotype, and prognosis of the patient. They can identify which patients will benefit from specific treatments, making personalized medicine possible [86].

Indirect Immunofluorescence (IIF)

Indirect immunofluorescence is considered the gold standard for detecting autoantibodies because of its high diagnostic sensitivity. Owing to technological advancements, it has been automated and standardized to a greater degree, making it suitable for standard applications [87].

Antigen Microarrays

Autoantibodies targeting a broad spectrum of antigens can be detected using antigen microarrays. This technology provides better diagnostic efficiency and the ability to categorize patients into different phenotypic groups [88]. For instance, a study on autoimmune peripheral neuropathies established that antigen microarrays differentiated a wide range of antiganglioside autoantibodies that are useful in diagnosing disorders such as Guillain-Barré syndrome [89].

CytoBead Assay

CytoBead Assay is a sensitive screening test followed by a specific confirmation test in the same reaction mixture, which reduces the time required for serological diagnosis of autoimmune diseases. This new method is suitable for the identification of multiple autoantibodies that exist in the blood, such as

Antinuclear Antibodies [ANAs], which enhance the effectiveness of diagnostic measures [90].

Automated Multiparametric Line Immunoassay

Automated multiparametric line immunoassays are useful for identifying autoantibodies. These assays have high sensitivity and specificity and can therefore be used in routine clinical practice. These tests enable the identification of multiple autoantibodies in the same serum with great convenience and at a lower cost than the traditional methods [91].

Recombinant Cell-Based Immunofluorescence

Recombinant cell-based immunofluorescence assays and multiparameter analysis in BIOCHIP mosaics are valuable for the simultaneous detection of autoantibodies in autoimmune encephalitis. This method improves the quick release of diagnostic results, which is vital for proper treatment [92].

Multifunctional Analysis by Spot Immunoassay

The SeraSpot® ANA assay enables the identification of several autoantibodies related to CTDs in a single test. This assay has demonstrated high diagnostic specificity and favorable likelihood ratios, making it a helpful tool in the diagnosis of CTDs [93].

Multiparametric Autoantibody Profiling

Multiparametric autoantibody profiling is already used to generate detailed autoantibody profiles in patients with diseases such as Systemic Sclerosis (SSc). This is helpful in the early diagnosis and subtype classification of SSc, thereby improving patient management [94].

Multiplex Technologies in Systemic Autoimmune Diseases

Some modern diagnostic techniques that are currently in use include line immunoassays, bead-based immunoassays, and microarrays, which have been established to accurately identify different disease biomarkers. These technologies provide better analytical capabilities, speed, and a smaller footprint and are useful for the diagnosis of autoimmune diseases [95].

Standardization and Diagnostic Consistency International Consensus on ANA Patterns [ICAP]

The ICAP project is intended to standardize ANA testing and has the potential to increase diagnostic consistency across laboratories (Table **2**). Standardization of ANA pattern reporting increases the value of these tests in patient care [96].

Table 2. Diagnostic procedures in autoimmune diseases.

Diagnostic Method	Description	Autoimmune Diseases	Advantages	References
Enzyme-Linked Immunosorbent Assay (ELISA)	Detects specific autoantibodies by binding them to antigens coated on a solid surface and measuring bound antibodies.	Autoimmune blistering skin diseases, SLE, RA	High sensitivity and specificity, quantitative measurement	[105]
Indirect Immunofluorescence (IIF)	Uses fluorescently labeled antibodies to detect autoantibodies in patient serum binding to antigens in tissue sections.	SLE, RA, Sjögren's Syndrome, autoimmune hepatitis	Visualizes antibody binding patterns, with high diagnostic accuracy	[65]
Multiplex Autoantibody Assays	Simultaneously measures multiple autoantibodies using antigen microarrays or bead-based systems.	Various autoimmune diseases	High throughput, reduced sample volume, comprehensive profiling	[88]
Next-Generation Sequencing (NGS)	Analyzes genetic variants and transcriptomics in autoimmune diseases.	Connective tissue diseases, various autoimmune conditions	Comprehensive genetic analysis identifies novel variants	[106]
Polymerase Chain Reaction (PCR)	Amplifies specific DNA sequences associated with genetic susceptibility to autoimmune diseases.	RA, T1D, MS	High sensitivity, rapid results, applicable to small tissue samples	[107]
Positron Emission Tomography (PET)	Uses radioactive tracers to visualize metabolic activity in tissues, highlighting inflammation.	RA, SLE, vasculitis	High sensitivity for active inflammation, non-invasive imaging	[108]
Magnetic Resonance Imaging (MRI)	Provides detailed images of soft tissues, identifying structural abnormalities and inflammation.	MS, RA, ankylosing spondylitis	High resolution, non-invasive, aids CNS and joint assessment	[109]

(Table 2) cont.....

Diagnostic Method	Description	Autoimmune Diseases	Advantages	References
Confocal Microscopy	Enhances traditional immunofluorescence by providing higher resolution images and three-dimensional reconstruction.	Autoimmune blistering skin diseases	Superior imaging quality, detailed visualization of immune deposits	[110]
Mass Spectrometry (MS)	Analyzes protein and peptide profiles in serum to identify biomarkers and autoantigens.	SLE, RA, Sjögren's Syndrome	High sensitivity and specificity in identifying novel biomarkers	[109]
Autoantibody Microarrays	Uses microarray technology to detect multiple autoantibodies in a single assay.	Various autoimmune diseases	High throughput, reduced reagent costs, comprehensive profiling	[111]

Cytometry by Time-of-Flight (CyTOF)

CyTOF is a hybrid of flow cytometry and mass spectrometry that enables the comprehensive characterization of immune cells with minimal constraints of fluorophores. This technology provides information on the activation and function of immune cells [97].

Proteomic Biomarkers

In recent years, proteomic technologies have contributed to the identification of potential biomarkers of autoimmune diseases. These biomarkers can aid in the diagnosis, classification, and treatment of diseases. New techniques currently being used include mass spectrometry and protein microarrays [98].

Multiplex Diagnostic Technologies

New multiplex diagnostic techniques have been used to identify multiple autoantibodies and to help identify patients with multiple autoimmune conditions. Such technologies enhance the ability to diagnose autoimmune diseases [99].

Autoantibodies as Predictive Markers

Autoantibodies appear before the onset of clinical manifestations and can serve as early predictors of autoimmune diseases. This is because early detection can assist in preventive measures and enhance disease management [100].

Liver Function test and Immunophenotyping

Standard diagnostic procedures include complete blood count with differential, metabolic panel, inflammatory markers, and flow cytometry for the diagnosis and management of autoimmune diseases. These tests offer an overall picture of the patient's immune system and disease activity [101].

Blood Cytology and Autoimmune Hematological Diseases

A puncture smear or blood cytology is useful in the diagnosis of autoimmune hematologic diseases such as autoimmune hemolytic anemia and immune thrombocytopenia. These conditions are relatively difficult to diagnose because they manifest symptoms similar to those of other hematologic diseases [102].

Laboratory Examinations in Children with Rheumatic Diseases

In children, laboratory parameters such as ESR, CRP, and specific autoantibodies must be used to diagnose and monitor rheumatic diseases. These tests assist in determining the current status of the disease and the effectiveness of its management [103, 104].

Radiological Imaging

Magnetic resonance imaging, positron emission tomography/computed tomography, ultrasound, and Computed Tomography (CT) have gradually become the primary diagnostic and monitoring modalities for autoimmune diseases. New developments have enhanced diagnosis, thereby enhancing disease management. The development of new radiopharmaceuticals and advancements in imaging technologies are creating the possibility of developing more effective and individualized treatments.

Magnetic Resonance Imaging (MRI)

MRI is most useful in the diagnosis of central nervous system involvement in autoimmune diseases such as multiple sclerosis. It has high-resolution images that show lesions and inflammation in the brain and spinal cord. Recent studies support the use of MRI in increasing the specificity of the diagnosis of different autoimmune diseases by detecting specific imaging findings [112]. In addition, advanced MRI techniques such as DWI and DCE-MRI provide both functional and anatomical information, which can reveal the presence of small amounts of active disease at an early stage [113].

Tomography, such as Positron Emission Tomography (PET) and the Combination of PET with Computed Tomography (PET/CT).

PET and PET/CT are exceptional for identifying the spread of autoimmune diseases to other parts of the body. They enable a whole-body scan, which helps localize inflammation and assess changes in disease activity in conditions such as rheumatoid arthritis and systemic lupus erythematosus. Research has shown that FDG-PET/CT is useful for identifying areas of ongoing inflammation based on increased glucose metabolism [114]. In addition, PET/CT imaging is highly sensitive for the identification of basic cellular factors in the pathological process involving both innate and adaptive immunity, which makes it crucial for the development of personalized medicine for the treatment of autoimmune diseases [115].

Ultrasound

To a great extent, musculoskeletal involvement in autoimmune diseases is assessed using ultrasound. It is most effective for the evaluation of joint inflammation in rheumatoid arthritis and the identification of salivary gland lesions in Sjögren's syndrome. High-frequency ultrasound can aid in the visualization of shallow structures and can be useful for early diagnosis and treatment [116]. Techniques such as Doppler and Contrast-Enhanced Ultrasound (CEU_S) increase blood flow and tissue perfusion information, and improve diagnostic potential [117].

Computed Tomography [CT]

Computed Tomography (CT) is useful for diagnosing pulmonary involvement in autoimmune diseases, including systemic sclerosis and rheumatoid arthritis-associated interstitial lung disease. It provides a detailed cross-sectional view of the lung, which aids in the diagnosis and characterization of lung diseases [118]. In addition, PET/CT co-registration enhances diagnostic precision by integrating metabolic and anatomical information, providing a holistic assessment of the disease [119].

Nuclear Medicine Imaging

All nuclear medicine procedures, including SPECT and PET, are characterized by high sensitivity and specificity for inflammation. Radiolabeled probes can provide a precise description of the site and level of inflammation in autoimmune diseases [115]. Recent developments have focused on the application of (18F)-FDG PET/CT for evaluating disease activity in entities such as systemic lupus erythematosus and Sjögren's syndrome, which provides a comprehensive picture of the disease burden and aids timely management [120].

Fine-Needle Aspiration Cytology (FNAC) in Autoimmune Diseases

Fine-Needle Aspiration Cytology (FNAC) is a diagnostic procedure that involves the use of a thin needle to obtain a sample of cells from a patient's body for the analysis of autoimmune disorders. It has become a valuable instrument for diagnosing and managing such diseases because it provides fast and precise examination of samples containing cells.

Diagnostic Accuracy and Applications

FNAC aids in the diagnosis of lymphadenopathy secondary to autoimmune diseases, such as Sjögren's syndrome and systemic lupus erythematosus. This process helps in the assessment of lymph node structure and the recognition of certain cell populations, which is beneficial for diagnosis [121]. In addition, FNAC is useful in the assessment of thyroid nodules and the nature of lesions in conditions such as Hashimoto's thyroiditis and Graves' disease. The incorporation of molecular studies into FNAC samples has improved diagnostic productivity, enabling proper risk stratification and management [122]. FNAC, which is frequently observed in patients with Sjögren's syndrome, is widely used in the diagnostic assessment of salivary gland diseases. It assists in distinguishing between malignant and benign tumors, which is helpful for patient management. Research has also indicated that FNAC is effective in the diagnosis of salivary gland pathologies [116]. The addition of FNAC with flow cytometry and immunophenotyping has increased the diagnostic yield of lymphoproliferative disorders. It is particularly suitable for the diagnosis of lymphoma and other hematologic disorders observed in autoimmune diseases. This enables the specification of cell surface marker information, which is paramount for the identification and management of conditions [123]. The use of FNAC is in the assessment of synovial fluid from joints involved in rheumatoid arthritis. This is useful for identifying inflammatory cells and immune complexes that are relevant for diagnosing or assessing disease progression. It is a less invasive approach than surgical biopsy, making it a gentler option for patients [124].

FNAC is also employed in children, for instance, to identify neuroblastic tumors, offering rapid and precise diagnosis with minimal discomfort to the child. This enables early and correct intervention under these conditions [125]. Modern techniques for FNAC include molecular diagnostic methods such as Next-Generation Sequencing (NGS) and Polymerase Chain Reaction (PCR). These methods increase the sensitivity of FNAC by identifying genetic alterations and molecular markers of autoimmune diseases [122]. Over the years, other methods, such as immunocytochemistry, flow cytometry, and molecular cytology, have increased the sensitivity and specificity of FNAC. These advancements have enabled the identification of cellular specimen details and have aided in the diagnosis of complex autoimmune diseases [123]. FNAC is inexpensive, simple, and safer than other invasive diagnostic procedures in areas with limited resources. This minimizes the need for more intrusive measures, such as surgical biopsies, and enables the diagnosis and development of a treatment plan within a short timeframe [126]. Nevertheless, there are some drawbacks to FNAC: the efficacy of FNAC is solely dependent on the expertise of the practitioner conducting the aspiration, as well as the quality of the sample acquired. Methods to enhance the diagnostic performance of the procedure include standardization of the procedure and enhanced training [127].

AUTOIMMUNE DISEASES- AVAILABLE TREATMENT REGIMENS

Pharmacological Treatments

Pharmacological therapies play a critical role in the treatment of autoimmune diseases, as they help alleviate symptoms, decrease inflammation, and alter the course of the disease. These include corticosteroids, immunosuppressive agents, biologics, and small-molecule inhibitors.

Corticosteroids

Corticosteroids are a type of medication used to reduce inflammation in the body, especially in autoimmune disorders. These processes decrease the immune system activity and inflammation. Corticosteroids have anti-inflammatory action due to the suppression of cytokine synthesis and reduction in the activity of immune cells. They are also useful in the control of exacerbation of autoimmune diseases, such as rheumatoid arthritis and lupus [128]. Corticosteroids are widely used in the management and treatment of symptoms and their remission in autoimmune diseases such as SLE and multiple sclerosis [128]. Some undesirable effects of corticosteroids include osteoporosis, hyperglycemia, and increased vulnerability to infections when used over the long term. Therefore, they are administered together with other drugs to reduce these side effects [129]. Thus, the key point is to control the dosage of corticosteroids in the treatment of patients, as they are effective and can have adverse effects. Termination methods are used to slowly decrease dosage and avoid unpleasant consequences [130]. Corticosteroids are usually administered along with DMARDs or biologics to improve treatment effectiveness and reduce steroid dosage [130]. Contemporary studies have aimed at identifying corticosteroid-sparing drugs to decrease the side effects of long-term corticosteroid therapy [131]. Current research is being conducted to determine the effectiveness of corticosteroids in new combinations, as well as different doses, to enhance treatment outcomes and reduce risks [132]. Current research on corticosteroids is directed towards the creation of delivery systems that minimize the overall systemic absorption and thus the adverse effects [128].

Immunosuppressing Agents

These drugs are used to manage autoimmune diseases by suppressing the immune system. Thereby preventing them from attacking the body tissues. Immunosuppressants affect the immune response in different ways, including T-cell activation and cytokine synthesis. Frequently used agents include methotrexate, azathioprine, and mycophenolate mofetil [133]. Methotrexate is one of the most commonly used drugs for rheumatoid arthritis and has demonstrated great capacity to decrease disease activity and prevent joint deterioration [134]. The use of immunosuppressants is associated with side effects including increased susceptibility to infections, liver toxicity, and gastrointestinal complications. These risks should be checked on a frequent basis in order to control them [133]. The concomitant use of immunosuppressants with biologics or corticosteroids can improve treatment results and decrease the required dosages of medicines, thus decreasing adverse effects [49]. New immunosuppressive drugs are being discovered, some of which include JAK inhibitors that target particular pathways of the immune system, indicating that there are other improved ways of treating the disease with fewer side effects [49]. Current research is assessing the effectiveness of newly developed immunosuppressive drugs for the management of various autoimmune diseases. These studies are important in the current world to evaluate the effectiveness of these drugs in practice [135]. Therefore, it is imperative to understand the pharmacokinetics of immunosuppressive drugs to adapt them to appropriate dosing schedules, thereby enhancing patient outcomes [49]. Future research should aim to create individualized strategies for immunosuppressive treatment depending on the patient's disease parameters and features [135].

Biologics

Biologics are medications produced from biological sources that act on specific segments of the immune system. They are used to treat numerous autoimmune disorders by blocking certain mechanisms that are fundamental to the immune system. Biologics work on proteins that are part of the immune system, including tumor necrosis factor-alpha, interleukin-6, and B cells. Some of these include infliximab, etanercept, and rituximab [136]. Biologics have proven beneficial in the treatment of rheumatoid arthritis, psoriatic arthritis, and Crohn's disease. They can cause remission, control manifestations, and increase patient survival and well-being [136]. The possible side effects of biological agents include infusion reactions, higher susceptibility to infections, and a risk of malignancy. These risks must be closely monitored for effective management [136]. Biologics are sometimes administered alongside DMARDs or corticosteroids to improve the treatment effects and minimize the dosage of the two drugs [136]. Recent biologics that target other pathways are under development, such as IL-17 and IL-23 inhibitors, to expand treatment options for autoimmune diseases [137]. Many active clinical trials have compared the efficacy and safety of new biologics in the treatment of different autoimmune diseases. These trials are important for the development of new treatments in clinical practice [136]. The pharmacokinetics and pharmacodynamics of biologics are essential for determining optimal dosing regimens and improving patient conditions [49]. Future research will be directed towards the creation of more precise biologics with fewer adverse effects and to identify new applications for the presently available biologics [137].

Small Molecule Inhibitors

Small-molecule inhibitors are drugs that inhibit the activity of certain enzymes or pathways of the immune response. They are an option for biologics and can be administered orally. Small-molecule inhibitors modulate specific enzymes or pathways related to immune processes. These include Janus Kinase (JAK) inhibitors and S1P receptor modulators. JAK inhibitors such as tofacitinib have been found to be highly effective in managing rheumatoid arthritis and psoriatic arthritis because they help decrease the level of inflammation and disease activity [134]. Side effects of small-molecule inhibitors include gastrointestinal symptoms, hepatotoxicity, and increased susceptibility to infections. Therefore, it is crucial to observe and control these side effects [49], and the co-administration of small-molecule inhibitors with other agents or biological drugs can improve the treatment effect and lower the total doses of the drugs needed [136]. New small-molecule inhibitors that affect different pathways, such as BTK inhibitors, are being introduced in the market for the management of autoimmune diseases [135]. Several phase II and III clinical trials have assessed the effectiveness and safety of new small-molecule inhibitors for several autoimmune disorders. It is through trials that new therapies have been introduced into clinical practice [136]. Knowledge of the basic principles of pharmacokinetics and pharmacodynamics of small-molecule inhibitors is important for the development of dosing schedules and better treatment outcomes [49]. Future work is needed to identify more specific small molecules that can create fewer side effects and have other uses for existing drugs [135].

- **Small Molecule Inhibitors:** JAK inhibitors, which are small-molecule inhibitors, differ in their safety from large molecules. Some of the most frequent adverse effects include infections, hypercholesterolemia, and elevated liver enzymes. As with other biological products, thrombosis has also been reported as an adverse effect. Therefore, patients' conditions and risk factors should be carefully considered [138].

- **Immune checkpoint inhibitors:** Immune checkpoint inhibitors are used for cancer treatment and autoimmune diseases. They may cause immune-related Adverse Events (irAEs), which result from the heightened immune response. These irAEs can affect any organ in the body, including the skin, GIT, liver, and endocrine glands, and may require immunosuppressive therapy [139].
- **Long-Term Safety:** In today's world, where new therapies are being developed, post-marketing safety data are useful for evaluating the safety of long-term therapies. Specifically, biologics and small-molecule inhibitors have been noted to have a build-up of toxicity over time, which includes malignancies and cardiovascular diseases. Thus, the significance of monitoring and risk mitigation strategies [140].
- **Patient-Specific Factors:** Certain patient characteristics, such as age, comorbidities, and genetic predispositions, may intensify some outcomes. New approaches in patient management, including pharmacogenetic testing, are being employed to identify patients who are likely to experience complications and to adjust treatment plans to minimize adverse effects [141].

Non-pharmacologic Interventions in Autoimmune Diseases

Lifestyle Interventions

It is important to note that lifestyle changes are a vital part of autoimmune disease management, usually in conjunction with drug use. Some of the interventions include changes in diet, physical activity, stress reduction, and better sleep, all of which help in the fight against inflammation. Diet has been shown to have a significant effect on the management of autoimmune diseases. Specific diets that are low in inflammation, such as the Mediterranean diet, have been shown to decrease disease activity and alleviate symptoms in patients with rheumatoid arthritis and lupus. These diets are based on the consumption of fruits, vegetables, whole-grain products, and healthy fats, avoiding processed foods and red meat [130]. A meta-synthesis of qualitative research has also highlighted the efficacy of certain nutrients, such as omega-3 fatty acids and probiotics, in influencing immune function and dampening inflammation [142]. Exercise is recommended for patients with autoimmune diseases, as it increases the capacity of the heart, builds muscle, and reduces fatigue. Aerobic activities, such as walking and swimming, have been shown to decrease symptoms and enhance the quality of life in patients with multiple sclerosis and rheumatoid arthritis [142]. A meta-analysis of several studies confirmed that low-impact aerobic exercise is most effective in decreasing fatigue and increasing physical functioning [143]. The assessment of stress in individuals with autoimmune conditions has been found to worsen these conditions. Mindfulness, relaxation, and cognitive techniques, such as cognitive-behavioral therapy, have been proven effective in reducing stress levels and improving disease outcomes. A research review revealed that MBSR helps reduce disease activity and enhances psychological health in patients with different autoimmune diseases [134]. Sleep disturbances are also frequent in patients with autoimmune diseases and can contribute to the worsening of the condition. Consistency in sleep schedules, creating a comfortable sleep environment, and avoiding substances that can stimulate the body before bedtime can help improve sleep hygiene, thereby enhancing the quality of sleep and overall health of an individual [144]. According to research, it has been proven that if patients with rheumatoid arthritis follow the principles of sleep hygiene, pain and fatigue levels decrease [135]. Adhering to a healthy weight is important for the management of autoimmune diseases. Obesity increases the level of inflammation and can worsen symptoms of the patient's condition. Diet and exercise can help individuals lose weight, which can decrease disease activity and increase the patient's quality of life [145].

Complementary Medicine

Complementary medicine includes several therapies that can be combined with conventional therapies to control autoimmune diseases. Other alternatives include herbal medicine, acupuncture, chiropractic, and dietary supplements. Several herbs have shown promise in the treatment of autoimmune diseases. For instance, curcumin, a component of turmeric, has anti-inflammatory properties that can assist in decreasing the symptoms of rheumatoid arthritis and inflammatory bowel disease. Studies have established the effectiveness of curcumin in relieving pain and inflammation, as analyzed in a trial conducted by Long *et al.* [146]. Acupuncture is used to alleviate pain and enhance the standard of living of patients with autoimmune disorders. A review identified that acupuncture can be useful in treating pain and improving the functioning of patients with rheumatoid arthritis and lupus by altering the inflammatory processes and increasing the levels of endorphins [147]. Chiropractic is a branch of health care that is concerned with the diagnosis and treatment of conditions related to mechanical dysfunction of the musculoskeletal system. However, there is little evidence that some autoimmune disease sufferers claim spinal manipulation, while other chiropractic interventions help them [148]. Popular supplements used for autoimmune diseases include omega-3 fatty acids, vitamin D, and probiotics. Omega-3 fatty acids have anti-inflammatory effects and can decrease the disease activity in rheumatoid arthritis and lupus. Vitamin D is critical for immunity, and its deficiency may affect the immune system in autoimmune diseases [149]. Complementary therapies, such as yoga and tai chi, have also been known to have a positive impact on the physical and mental well-being of patients with autoimmune diseases. These practices involve movement of the body and the incorporation of breathing and relaxation methods, which decrease stress and increase flexibility and wellness [150]. The gut microbiome is closely related to immune functions. Probiotics may assist in restoring the balance of gut flora, thereby decreasing inflammation and disease activity in autoimmune diseases. Some probiotics have been proven to help decrease the signs and symptoms of patients with inflammatory bowel disease and other autoimmune diseases [151]. Autoimmune diseases are a group of conditions in which the body's defense system mistakenly attacks and damages healthy tissues. Massage therapy can help decrease pain and enhance relaxation in patients with these diseases. According to the literature, massage therapy alleviates stress, boosts circulation, and improves general health [152]. Biofeedback helps people regulate their physiological processes using instruments that provide information on the activity of certain body parameters. Autoimmune diseases can help in symptom control by decreasing stress and increasing relaxation [153]. Hydrotherapy is a form of treatment that utilizes water to manage pain. It may include warm water aerobics, which assists in decreasing joint pain and enhancing flexibility in patients with rheumatoid arthritis and other autoimmune diseases [154]. Some specific nutrients, including antioxidants and polyphenols, have been found to have the potential to help manage autoimmune diseases. These compounds can influence immunity and diminish oxidative stress, which plays a role in autoimmune diseases [145].

EMERGING THERAPEUTIC STRATEGIES (TABLE 3)

Gene Therapy

Gene therapy is the most recent technique used to manage autoimmune diseases and to alter or regulate genetic and immunological defects. Recent developments in gene therapy have provided new ways to deal with multifaceted autoimmune diseases through the re-establishment of immune tolerance and modulation of the pathological immune response. Gene therapy is the process of transferring genes into patient cells to supplement or replace defective genes or regulate the immune system. This can be achieved through delivery vectors, such as viral and non-viral systems, to transfer genes that have a therapeutic role in releasing anti-inflammatory cytokines or shutting down pro-inflammatory pathways [155]. It has been used in the management of autoimmune disorders such as rheumatoid arthritis, multiple sclerosis, and systemic lupus erythematosus. In rheumatoid arthritis, gene therapy can be used to supply anti-inflammatory cytokines to joint tissues, thus managing inflammation and joint destruction [156]. Lentiviral vectors and Adeno-Associated Viruses (AAV) are widely employed in gene therapy because of their high levels of gene transfer and long-term gene expression. These vectors have been used to transfer genes encoding cytokine inhibitors and other regulatory proteins in the management of immune-mediated diseases [157]. For non-viral vectors, liposomes and nanoparticles are less prone to cause insertional mutagenesis and immune responses than viral vectors. These vectors have been studied for their ability to transfer genes that have a therapeutic effect while producing few adverse effects [158]. Many clinical trials are currently being conducted to assess the risks and benefits of gene therapy in the management of autoimmune diseases. For instance, a phase one study of gene therapy in RA patients, wherein the IL-1 receptor antagonist was used, has been found to be effective in reducing inflammation and disease [156]. Gene therapy can be employed to control the immune response by either increasing the generation of Tregs or by producing anti-inflammatory cytokines. This approach was designed to reactivate immune tolerance, thus avoiding autoimmune aggression against self-tissues [159]. Co-administration of gene therapy with other treatments, including biologics or small-molecule inhibitors, may increase the therapeutic effect and decrease the amount of gene therapy, biologics, or small-molecule inhibitors. This strategy is being pursued to capitalize on the combined effects and enhance patient care [160]. Gene therapies are regulated to ensure the highest standards of safety and efficacy and therefore require significant data. Therefore, improving regulatory science and harmonizing gene therapy trial guidelines is a key factor for the effective implementation of these therapies in clinical settings [157]. Nonetheless, Gene therapy faces key challenges that must be addressed, such as the delivery of genes to the target tissue, long-term gene expression, and selective switching of genes. Scientists are still developing efficient gene delivery systems to increase the selectivity of gene therapy for autoimmune diseases [161]. Future research should focus on creating new tools for genetic modification, including the CRISPR/Cas9 system, to cure genetic disorders at a molecular level. These technologies can offer even more efficient and long-lasting treatments for autoimmune diseases through genome manipulation [158].

Monoclonal Antibodies

Molecular medicine has brought about significant changes in the treatment of autoimmune diseases by introducing monoclonal antibodies as targeted and specific therapies against immune mediators in the disease process. These biological agents are far superior to commonly used non-specific immunosuppressive medications. These are administered along with other therapies, such as methotrexate or corticosteroids, to improve clinical outcomes and decrease disease activity. Combination treatment can function as an additive and enhance the quality of life of patients [162]. Monoclonal antibodies are considered safe; however, some side effects include infusion reactions, increased susceptibility to infections, and an increased risk of malignancies. Thus, the identification and control of these risks are crucial for protecting patients [163]. Autoimmune diseases are treated with monoclonal antibodies developed to attack certain antigens. These include antagonizing pro-inflammatory cytokines, reducing the number of pathogenic B cells, and inhibiting T cell activation. This feature enhances the potential for detailed control of the immune system with minimal side effects [136]. It is also used in the management of autoimmune diseases such as rheumatoid arthritis, multiple sclerosis, and Crohn's disease. For instance, infliximab, an anti-TNF-α monoclonal antibody, has been reported to be effective in managing inflammation and maintaining remission in patients with Crohn's disease [136]. The drugs used target Tumor Necrosis Factor-alpha (TNF-alpha) and include infliximab and adalimumab, which are monoclonal antibodies. These therapies have significantly improved the treatment of diseases, such as rheumatoid arthritis and ankylosing spondylitis, by reducing inflammation and preventing joint damage [162]. It is an anti-CD20 monoclonal antibody that depletes B cells and is used in the management of rheumatoid arthritis and systemic lupus erythematosus. Rituximab acts on B cells by targeting the CD20 protein, thereby decreasing the formation of autoantibodies and altering the immune response [163]. Tocilizumab is an interleukin-6 receptor antagonist used to treat rheumatoid arthritis and juvenile idiopathic arthritis. Tocilizumab works by inhibiting the action of IL-6, thereby decreasing inflammation levels and slowing joint deterioration. It has been established to be useful, especially in patients in whom other standard DMARDs have failed [164]. Abatacept is a fusion protein of CTLA-4Ig that inhibits T cell activation by preventing the co-stimulatory signal required for T cell activation. This therapy is used to treat rheumatoid arthritis and has the potential to control T-cell activity in other autoimmune diseases [165]. Currently, continuous research is being conducted to develop new monoclonal antibodies that can target various cytokines and immune cells implicated in autoimmune diseases. The objective of these efforts was to develop a safer and better treatment regimen [136].

Repurposing Drugs Approach

Drug repurposing involves identifying new therapeutic uses of existing drugs, offering a cost-effective and time-efficient strategy for the development of new drugs. This approach can significantly minimize the time and expense of drug discovery, as the safety of these drugs has previously been proven. This method has been used more frequently in autoimmune diseases, providing new therapeutic possibilities for already-known substances. Drug repurposing is defined as the process of identifying drugs available on the market for treating diseases other than those for which they were initially developed. This process builds on prior information regarding drug safety and pharmacodynamics to rapidly advance promising treatments in clinical trials [166]. Most early drug repurposing was performed based on chance or when a drug used for one disease was found to be effective for another. For instance, methotrexate, which was initially used for cancer treatment, was found to be useful in the treatment of rheumatoid arthritis because of its immunosuppressant effects [167]. Other drugs, such as hydroxychloroquine, which was initially used to treat malaria, have been found helpful in the management of autoimmune diseases such as lupus and rheumatoid arthritis because of their immunomodulatory properties [168, 169]. Currently, drug repurposing is based on computer modeling and analysis of large datasets to identify drugs with potential. Methods such as machine learning and network biology use big data to identify new drug-disease connections [170, 171]. Some drugs have also been used for the treatment of autoimmune diseases since they were originally developed for other conditions. For instance, thalidomide, which was initially used as a sedative, is now being used for the treatment of multiple myeloma and some autoimmune diseases owing to its anti-inflammatory effects [172]. However, drug repurposing has some issues, such as the requirement of new clinical trials to prove the effectiveness of the drug in the new indication, side effects of the drug when used for other purposes, and a lack of incentive for pharmaceutical companies to invest resources in products whose patents have expired [166, 173].

Malaria Transcription Factor Targeting

Malarial transcription factors can be considered as novel therapeutic targets for the treatment of autoimmune diseases. Transcription factors regulate genes involved in the immune system and their functions. Thus, these proteins can be used to control the immune system and decrease inflammation in autoimmune diseases [174]. Recent studies have identified certain transcription factors involved in the development of autoimmune diseases. For instance, the transcription factor NF-κB, which is implicated in inflammatory processes, has been targeted in numerous therapeutic approaches [175]. Malaria drugs that target transcription factors of the disease may be useful in the treatment of autoimmune diseases. For example, if the transcription factor AP-1, which plays a role in T-cell activation, is targeted, it can be useful for managing immune responses in diseases such as multiple sclerosis and lupus [176]. Currently, several studies are being conducted to determine the effectiveness of transcription factor inhibitors in autoimmune diseases. These trials are crucial for evaluating the safety and efficacy of new strategies [177]. This is because transcription factors regulate the expression of many genes and hence are difficult to target. This can cause what is known as off-target effects on gene expression and cellular activities. Scientists are currently trying to develop new inhibitors with fewer side effects. The process of creating transcription factor inhibitors involves the identification of compounds that can target these proteins and block their actions. These include high-throughput screening and computational modeling to identify potential drugs [178]. New transcription factors involved in autoimmune diseases can be used to aid in the development of other treatments. New transcription factors are still being investigated for their potential to combat these diseases, and combining transcription factor inhibitors with other therapies, such as biologics or small-molecule inhibitors, may enhance the results and reduce disease activity. This approach was investigated in several clinical studies. Current research employs precision medicine to develop therapeutic strategies for targeting transcription factors according to patient needs. Given the particular transcription factor underlying a patient's disease, management can be performed to enhance the effectiveness of treatment [179].

Immune Checkpoint Blockage

Immune Checkpoint Blockage [ICB] is a novel treatment paradigm for autoimmune diseases that aims to harness a patient's immune system to eradicate disease-associated cells. A new generation of treatments has introduced the possibility of using Immune Checkpoint Inhibitors (ICIs), including anti-CTLA-4, anti-PD-1, and anti-PD-L1 antibodies. These inhibitors function by limiting proteins that deactivate T cells, resulting in stronger immune responses against autoimmune diseases. Several studies have supported the use of ICIs in various autoimmune diseases such as multiple sclerosis, rheumatoid arthritis, and lupus. For example, PD-1 blockade has been reported to alleviate disease activity and prevent relapse in animal models of MS [180]. In addition, CTLA-4 inhibitors have shown promising efficacy in managing Systemic Lupus Erythematosus (SLE) through the regulation of T cell activation and increased tolerance. Nevertheless, there are several difficulties associated with using ICIs for the treatment of autoimmune diseases. The issue of irAEs persists. Therefore, patient selection and monitoring are crucial [181]. Some emerging research has examined combination strategies, including the use of ICI with standard immunosuppressive agents to prevent these adverse effects and improve treatment results [182]. Furthermore, current studies are focused on understanding the biomarkers that can help determine a patient's response to ICI treatment, thus enabling the enhancement of treatment plans and reducing side effects [59, 181].

Autophagy Regulation

Autophagy is an important process in cellular housekeeping and the recycling of cellular macromolecules. Autophagy in autoimmune diseases is involved in the control of immunological processes, which may contribute to the development of various diseases, including SLE, RA, and MS. Previous studies have also established a role for autophagy in the regulation of inflammation and autoimmunity. For instance, autophagy-related gene polymorphisms have been associated with the risk of autoimmune diseases, implying that dysregulation of autophagy pathways can lead to disease progression [183]. Hence, the regulation of autophagy provides a novel potential strategy for the treatment of autoimmune diseases. Drugs that can promote or suppress autophagy have been tested in preclinical models. For instance, chloroquine, an autophagy inhibitor, has been helpful in controlling the symptoms of lupus and RA by regulating the activity of immune cells as well as the levels of cytokines [184]. In contrast, drugs promoting autophagy, such as rapamycin, have been applied to increase the levels of autophagy and alleviate the disease course in an animal model of MS, namely EAE [185]. In addition to creating targeted therapies, much attention is being paid to the interaction between autophagy and other cellular processes such as apoptosis and inflammation. Recent studies have also attempted to apply nanomedicine to improve the targeting of autophagy-modulating agents to the affected tissues to enhance therapeutic outcomes while reducing adverse effects [186].

Biodegradable Nanoparticles

Biodegradable Nanoparticles (BNPs) are a modern potential solution for the treatment of autoimmune diseases. These nanoparticles can be designed to transport drugs to specific target cells, thereby increasing the effectiveness and minimizing the toxicity of the treatments. Recent studies have revealed that BNPs can control the immune system and generate tolerance in autoimmune diseases (Table **3**). For instance, biodegradable Polylactic-co-Glycolic Acid (PLGA) nanoparticles have been utilized to target antigens to immune cells, thereby inducing antigen-specific tolerance and regulatory responses and preventing autoimmune diseases [187]. This strategy has been advantageous in models of multiple sclerosis, whereby PLGA nanoparticles containing antigens were used to prevent and treat the relapsing-remitting form of the disease by decreasing inflammatory T cell infiltration in the CNS [188]. In addition, BNPs can be engineered to encapsulate various therapeutic substances such as small molecules, peptides, and nucleic acids. The surfaces of BNPs can be functionalized for better targeting and internalization in specific cell types. For instance, nanoparticles encapsulating antigens relevant to a particular disease and immunomodulatory molecules can be used to treat autoimmune diseases such as rheumatoid arthritis and systemic lupus erythematosus by controlling the activation of dendritic cells and T cells [63, 189]. Furthermore, the advancement in biodegradable nanoparticles, which can operate on cellular pathways such as autophagy and apoptosis, has created new ways of treatment. These nanoparticles can increase or decrease certain cellular functions, making it easier to control the type of treatment administered to the patient [190].

Table 3. New approaches to the treatment of autoimmune diseases.

Therapeutic Strategy	Focus Areas	Potential Benefits	Applications	References
Biological and Small Molecule Therapeutics	Biologics and Small Molecules	Enhanced Treatment Efficacy	Autoimmune Diseases	[191]
Targeting TNF-α, IL-6, CD20, CD80/86	Specific Immune Targets	Reduced Inflammation	Various Autoimmune Conditions	[191]
Gene Therapy	Genetic Interventions	Personalized Medicine	Autoimmune Disorders	[160]
Targeted approach for autoimmune disorders	Specific Targeting	Precise Immune Modulation	Specific Autoimmune Diseases	[160]
Interference with pathogenic processes	Pathogenic Process Interference	Disease Process Disruption	Multiple Autoimmune Conditions	[160]
Experimental models: diabetes, Rheumatoid arthritis, Multiple sclerosis	Animal Models	Insight into Disease Mechanisms	Diabetes, RA, MS	[160]
BAFF Inhibitors	B Cell Survival and Activity	Alleviation of Symptoms	Autoimmune Disease Symptoms	[192]
Immunometabolism	Metabolic Changes in Immune Cells	New Therapeutic Targets	Various Autoimmune Conditions	[193]

EFFICACY OF NEW THERAPEUTIC APPROACH

Pharmacodynamics

Pharmacodynamics (PD) is a science that deals with the interaction of drugs with the body, especially concerning receptor binding, post-receptor actions, and the consequences of drug therapy in terms of efficacy and toxicity. Therefore, the pharmacodynamics of new treatment regimens for autoimmune diseases are of great importance in managing patients and reducing adverse effects. New developments in this field have provided important information regarding the PD of biologics and small-molecule inhibitors used for autoimmune rheumatic diseases. The pharmacodynamics of biological agents, such as monoclonal antibodies, have been well understood. These agents focus on the cytokines or cell surface receptors implicated in autoimmune diseases, modulating the expression of their respective cytokines. For instance, the PD of TNF inhibitors, such as infliximab and adalimumab, has been confirmed, as these drugs decrease inflammation by neutralizing TNF-α, a significant cytokine in the inflammatory process. Another class of drugs with pharmacodynamic profiles is small-molecule inhibitors, including Janus Kinase (JAK) inhibitors. These inhibitors block pathways crucial for the initiation and development of immune cell activities. The PD properties of JAK inhibitors, such as tofacitinib, have shown that they have the potential to control the immune system, thereby decreasing disease activity in conditions such as rheumatoid arthritis [194]. Drug-target binding is a significant area of pharmacodynamics. The binding affinities and kinetics of new biologics have been investigated to understand their effectiveness and duration in the body. For instance, rituximab, a monoclonal antibody targeting CD20, exhibits high binding affinity and long-lasting receptor occupancy, which is associated with a prolonged effect on B-cell reduction and clinical benefit in autoimmune diseases, including systemic lupus erythematosus [163]. The identification of this relationship is vital for identifying the correct dosage schedule. In pharmacodynamic analyses, increased doses of biologics do not always produce an improved therapeutic response because of receptor saturation and a higher likelihood of adverse events. This shows the need to determine the correct dose to achieve the desired therapeutic effect without causing harm [195]. Quantitative models of the pharmacodynamics of new drugs have been proposed to evaluate their therapeutic and toxic effects. These models encompass information on drug-receptor binding, signal transduction pathways, and the cellular manifestations of drug action. These models are useful for designing and fine-tuning new therapeutic strategies [196].

Evidence Base

New treatment strategies for autoimmune diseases involve controlled trials, observational studies, and systematic reviews. These sources illustrate the effectiveness and safety of new therapies, which are beneficial for the practice and management of patients. RCTs are considered to be the best approach for assessing the effects of treatment and safety. Recent trials have shown that new biologics and small-molecule inhibitors manage many autoimmune diseases. For example, large-scale RCTs have supported the use of tocilizumab, an IL-6 receptor antagonist, in the treatment of rheumatoid arthritis, which promises to produce desired changes in the clinical and radiographic status of patients [164]. Real-world research complements RCT evidence by providing information on the success and risks of interventions in everyday practice. They frequently provide insights into the effectiveness and duration of treatment as well as differences in patient responses. For instance, in rheumatoid arthritis, real-life evidence of the effectiveness of TNF inhibitors has been reported to be durable, and the safety profile remains favorable in the long term [197]. Meta-analyses and systematic reviews compile data from multiple studies and provide a general idea regarding treatment outcomes. The use of biological therapies for SLE has been recently reviewed in a meta-analysis, which showed that belimumab is effective in controlling disease activity and flare-ups, and should be considered a standard of care [198]. Advanced trials and other new concepts are being gradually introduced to improve the efficiency and informational value of clinical studies. These designs enable modification of the trial protocol after the presentation of the intermediate results, thus enhancing the chances of finding the correct treatments. For instance, adaptive trials have been applied in rheumatoid arthritis to compare several biological therapies simultaneously, improve the efficiency of resource allocation, and accelerate the search for successful treatments [199].

Side Effects or Complications

The present study aimed to identify the possible side effects or complications of new regimens to enhance patient safety and therapeutic outcomes. Recent studies have identified the risks of using biologics, small-molecule inhibitors, and other new-generation therapies for autoimmune diseases. Biologics have side effects as they are very effective in managing targeted diseases. For example, TNF inhibitors may increase susceptibility to infections, such as tuberculosis and other opportunistic infections, because of their immunosuppressive action. In addition, infusion reactions and the formation of antibodies against biological agents can occur, which may decrease the effectiveness of treatment [200].

CONCLUSION

Autoimmune diseases are characterized by several factors that make diagnosis, management, and treatment difficult due to their chronic nature. Understanding of the immune system has been enhanced by immunological advancements such as antigen presentation, clonal selection, memory cells, and the general mechanisms of immune responses. This conceptual framework forms the basis of the development of novel methods for diagnosis, treatment, and future therapies. New methods for diagnosing autoimmune diseases include the use of radiology and fine-needle aspiration cytology. These technologies enable the identification of the disease and provide a detailed description of its mechanism, allowing for effective management and potential cure at an early stage. Other diagnostic procedures that are also significant in autoimmune diseases include hematological examinations to evaluate hematological alterations in these diseases. Autoimmune diseases are treated in various ways, ranging from the use of general medications to more targeted and complex approaches. Corticosteroids and immunosuppressants have not been altered. However, biologics and small-molecule inhibitors are current treatments for autoimmune diseases. These new agents have higher efficacy, safety, and patient outcomes than those of earlier management interventions. New treatment approaches include gene therapy, immune checkpoint inhibitors, autophagy modulators, and biodegradable nanoparticles. Gene therapy involves altering the genetic makeup to correct defects and control the immune system at the molecular level, thereby offering a potential treatment for autoimmune diseases. Immune checkpoint inhibitors and autophagy modulators are novel strategies for controlling the immune system and restoring immune tolerance. Some nanoparticles in the body that are degradable and involved in drug delivery can enhance the effectiveness of drug treatments. The efficacy of new treatment regimens has been assessed in controlled clinical trials and real-world practice, thereby increasing the evidence supporting these new approaches. Pharmacodynamic research has provided information on how new treatments work, the best schedules for their administration, and safety over time. Several studies on comparative effectiveness have established that biologics and small-molecule inhibitors yield better results than conventional therapies, thereby positively impacting patients. In conclusion, diagnostic tools and new therapeutic options currently being developed for autoimmune diseases are revolutionizing the current field and providing light for patients. Future research and clinical trials will further refine these strategies, making it possible to develop a treatment tailored to the individual and most effective for the patient. Advancements in technology and exploration of the immune system will continue, leading to improved patient care for autoimmune diseases.

ACKNOWLEDGEMENTS

The authors extend their sincere gratitude to Aarupadai Veedu Medical College and Hospital, Puducherry, and Guru Nanak College for their encouragement and support.

REFERENCES

[1] Chaplin DD. Overview of the immune response. J Allergy Clin Immunol 2010; 125(2) (Suppl. 2): S3-S23.
[http://dx.doi.org/10.1016/j.jaci.2009.12.980] [PMID: 20176265]

[2] Medzhitov R. Recognition of microorganisms and activation of the immune response. Nature 2007; 449(7164): 819-26.
[http://dx.doi.org/10.1038/nature06246] [PMID: 17943118]

[3] Delves PJ, Roitt IM. The immune system. First of two parts. N Engl J Med 2000; 343(1): 37-49.
[http://dx.doi.org/10.1056/NEJM200007063430107] [PMID: 10882768]

[4] Kavathas PB, Krause PJ, Ruddle NH. Organization and Cells of the Immune System. In: Krause PJ, Kavathas PB, Ruddle NH, Eds. Immunoepidemiology. Cham: Springer International Publishing 2019; pp. 21-38.
[http://dx.doi.org/10.1007/978-3-030-25553-4_2]

[5] Kimbrell DA, Beutler B. The evolution and genetics of innate immunity. Nat Rev Genet 2001; 2(4): 256-67.
[http://dx.doi.org/10.1038/35066006] [PMID: 11283698]

[6] Poletaev AB. The main principles of adaptive immune system function: self-recognition, self-interaction, and self-maintenance. Physiologic Autoimmunity and Preventive Medicine. Bentham Science Publishers 2013; pp. 3-20.
[http://dx.doi.org/10.2174/9781608057245113010004]

[7] Calder PC, Kew S. The immune system: a target for functional foods?. Br J Nutr 2002; 88(S2) (Suppl. 2): S165-76.
[http://dx.doi.org/10.1079/BJN2002682] [PMID: 12495459]

[8] Amigorena S. Antigen presentation: from cell biology to physiology. Immunol Rev 2016; 272(1): 5-7.
[http://dx.doi.org/10.1111/imr.12436] [PMID: 27319337]

[9] Jensen PE. Recent advances in antigen processing and presentation. Nat Immunol 2007; 8(10): 1041-8.
[http://dx.doi.org/10.1038/ni1516] [PMID: 17878914]

[10] Vyas JM, Van der Veen AG, Ploegh HL. The known unknowns of antigen processing and presentation. Nat Rev Immunol 2008; 8(8): 607-18.
[http://dx.doi.org/10.1038/nri2368] [PMID: 18641646]

[11] Van Kaer L, Parekh VV, Postoak JL, Wu L. Role of autophagy in MHC class I-restricted antigen presentation. Mol Immunol 2019; 113: 2-5.
[http://dx.doi.org/10.1016/j.molimm.2017.10.021] [PMID: 29126597]

[12] Gfeller D, Bassani-Sternberg M. Predicting antigen presentation—what could we learn from a million peptides?. Front Immunol 2018; 9: 1716.
[http://dx.doi.org/10.3389/fimmu.2018.01716] [PMID: 30090105]

[13] Silverstein AM. The Clonal Selection Theory: what it really is and why modern challenges are misplaced. Nat Immunol 2002; 3(9): 793-6.
[http://dx.doi.org/10.1038/ni0902-793] [PMID: 12205463]

[14] Luo W, Lin X. Recent advances in clonal selection algorithms and applications In: 2017 IEEE Symposium Series on Computational Intelligence. SSCI 2017; pp. 1-8.https://ieeexplore.ieee.org/document/8285340
[http://dx.doi.org/10.1109/SSCI.2017.8285340]

[15] Garrett SM. Parameter-free, adaptive clonal selection 2004.https://ieeexplore.ieee.org/document/1330978/authors#authors
[http://dx.doi.org/10.1109/CEC.2004.1330978]

[16] Morita K, Wang F, Jahn K, *et al.* Clonal evolution of acute myeloid leukemia revealed by high-throughput single-cell genomics. Nat Commun 2020; 11(1): 5327.
[http://dx.doi.org/10.1038/s41467-020-19119-8] [PMID: 33087716]

[17] de Castro LN, Von Zuben FJ. Learning and optimization using the clonal selection principle. IEEE Trans Evol Comput 2002; 6(3): 239-51.
[http://dx.doi.org/10.1109/TEVC.2002.1011539]

[18] Karakasis VK, Stafylopatis A. Data Mining based on gene expression programming and clonal selection In: 2006 IEEE International Conference on Evolutionary Computation. 2006; pp. 514-21. Internet
[http://dx.doi.org/10.1109/CEC.2006.1688353]

[19] Lanzavecchia A, Sallusto F. Human B cell memory. Curr Opin Immunol 2009; 21(3): 298-304.
[http://dx.doi.org/10.1016/j.coi.2009.05.019] [PMID: 19497721]

[20] Seifert M, Küppers R. Human memory B cells. Leukemia 2016; 30(12): 2283-92.
[http://dx.doi.org/10.1038/leu.2016.226] [PMID: 27499139]

[21] Tangye SG, Tarlinton DM. Memory B cells: Effectors of long-lived immune responses. Eur J Immunol 2009; 39(8): 2065-75. [http://dx.doi.org/10.1002/eji.200939531] [PMID: 19637202]

[22] Mueller SN, Mackay LK. Tissue-resident memory T cells: local specialists in immune defence. Nat Rev Immunol 2016; 16(2): 79-89. [http://dx.doi.org/10.1038/nri.2015.3] [PMID: 26688350]

[23] Shin H, Iwasaki A. Tissue-resident memory T cells. Immunol Rev 2013; 255(1): 165-81. [http://dx.doi.org/10.1111/imr.12087] [PMID: 23947354]

[24] Sun JC, Ugolini S, Vivier E. Immunological memory within the innate immune system. EMBO J 2014; 33(12): 1295-303. [http://dx.doi.org/10.1002/embj.201387651] [PMID: 24674969]

[25] Liu Q, Sun Z, Chen L. Memory T cells: strategies for optimizing tumor immunotherapy. Protein Cell 2020; 11(8): 549-64. [http://dx.doi.org/10.1007/s13238-020-00707-9] [PMID: 32221812]

[26] Muruganandah V, Sathkumara HD, Navarro S, Kupz A. A systematic review: The role of resident memory T cells in infectious diseases and their relevance for vaccine development. Front Immunol 2018; 9: 1574. [http://dx.doi.org/10.3389/fimmu.2018.01574] [PMID: 30038624]

[27] Reading JL, Gálvez-Cancino F, Swanton C, Lladser A, Peggs KS, Quezada SA. The function and dysfunction of memory CD 8 $^{+}$ T cells in tumor immunity. Immunol Rev 2018; 283(1): 194-212. [http://dx.doi.org/10.1111/imr.12657] [PMID: 29664561]

[28] Ratajczak W, Niedźwiedzka-Rystwej P, Tokarz-Deptuła B, Deptuła W. Immunological memory cells. Cent Eur J Immunol 2018; 43(2): 194-203. [http://dx.doi.org/10.5114/ceji.2018.77390] [PMID: 30135633]

[29] Iwasaki A, Medzhitov R. Toll-like receptor control of the adaptive immune responses. Nat Immunol 2004; 5(10): 987-95. [http://dx.doi.org/10.1038/ni1112] [PMID: 15454922]

[30] Blanden RV. T cell response to viral and bacterial infection. Immunol Rev 1974; 19(1): 56-88. [http://dx.doi.org/10.1111/j.1600-065X.1974.tb00128.x] [PMID: 4152201]

[31] Parijs LV, Abbas AK. Homeostasis and self-tolerance in the immune system: turning lymphocytes off. Science 1998; 280(5361): 243-8. [http://dx.doi.org/10.1126/science.280.5361.243] [PMID: 9535647]

[32] Hawlisch H, Köhl J. Complement and Toll-like receptors: Key regulators of adaptive immune responses. Mol Immunol 2006; 43(1-2): 13-21. [http://dx.doi.org/10.1016/j.molimm.2005.06.028] [PMID: 16019071]

[33] Jaroszewski J, Ahmed A, Sell KW. Mechanism for regulation of immune responses. J Theor Biol 1976; 57(1): 121-9. [http://dx.doi.org/10.1016/S0022-5193(76)80008-2] [PMID: 60508]

[34] Furman D, Davis MM. New approaches to understanding the immune response to vaccination and infection. Vaccine 2015; 33(40): 5271-81. [http://dx.doi.org/10.1016/j.vaccine.2015.06.117] [PMID: 26232539]

[35] Winslow GM, Bitsaktsis C. Immunity to the ehrlichiae: new tools and recent developments. Curr Opin Infect Dis 2005; 18(3): 217-21. [http://dx.doi.org/10.1097/01.qco.0000168381.86024.cf] [PMID: 15864098]

[36] Torres-Aguilar H, Sosa-Luis SA, Aguilar-Ruiz SR. Infections as triggers of flares in systemic autoimmune diseases: novel innate immunity mechanisms. Curr Opin Rheumatol 2019; 31(5): 525-31. [http://dx.doi.org/10.1097/BOR.0000000000000630] [PMID: 31135383]

[37] Wang L, Wang FS, Gershwin ME. Human autoimmune diseases: a comprehensive update. J Intern Med 2015; 278(4): 369-95.
[http://dx.doi.org/10.1111/joim.12395] [PMID: 26212387]

[38] Delgado-Vega A, Sánchez E, Löfgren S, Castillejo-López C, Alarcón-Riquelme ME. Recent findings on genetics of systemic autoimmune diseases. Curr Opin Immunol 2010; 22(6): 698-705.
[http://dx.doi.org/10.1016/j.coi.2010.09.002] [PMID: 20933377]

[39] Burrack AL, Martinov T, Fife BT. T cell-mediated beta cell destruction: Autoimmunity and alloimmunity in the context of type 1 diabetes. Front Endocrinol (Lausanne) 2017; 8: 343.
[http://dx.doi.org/10.3389/fendo.2017.00343] [PMID: 29259578]

[40] Richard-Miceli C, Criswell LA. Emerging patterns of genetic overlap across autoimmune disorders. Genome Med 2012; 4(1): 6.
[http://dx.doi.org/10.1186/gm305] [PMID: 22284131]

[41] Naser SA, Arce M, Khaja A, *et al.* Role of *ATG16L*, *NOD2* and *IL23R* in Crohn's disease pathogenesis. World J Gastroenterol 2012; 18(5): 412-24.
[http://dx.doi.org/10.3748/wjg.v18.i5.412] [PMID: 22346247]

[42] Pozo-Rubio T, Olivares M, Nova E, *et al.* Immune development and intestinal microbiota in celiac disease. Clin Dev Immunol 2012; 2012: 1-12.
[http://dx.doi.org/10.1155/2012/654143] [PMID: 23008734]

[43] Nair RP, Ruether A, Stuart PE, *et al.* Polymorphisms of the IL12B and IL23R genes are associated with psoriasis. J Invest Dermatol 2008; 128(7): 1653-61.
[http://dx.doi.org/10.1038/sj.jid.5701255] [PMID: 18219280]

[44] Chistiakov DA. Immunogenetics of Hashimoto's thyroiditis. J Autoimmune Dis 2005; 2(1): 1.
[http://dx.doi.org/10.1186/1740-2557-2-1] [PMID: 15762980]

[45] Lettre G, Rioux JD. Autoimmune diseases: insights from genome-wide association studies. Hum Mol Genet 2008; 17(R2): R116-21.
[http://dx.doi.org/10.1093/hmg/ddn246] [PMID: 18852199]

[46] Cadena-Sandoval D, Montúfar-Robles I, Elda Barbosa-Cobos R, *et al.* Interactions between TNFAIP3, PTPN22, and TRAF1-C5 gene polymorphisms in patients with primary Sjögren's syndrome. Arch Rheumatol 2024; 39(1): 60-70.
[http://dx.doi.org/10.46497/ArchRheumatol.2024.10108] [PMID: 38774701]

[47] Vanderpump MPJ, Tunbridge WMG. Epidemiology and prevention of clinical and subclinical hypothyroidism. Thyroid 2002; 12(10): 839-47.
[http://dx.doi.org/10.1089/105072502761016458] [PMID: 12487765]

[48] Atkinson MA, Eisenbarth GS, Michels AW. Type 1 diabetes. Lancet 2014; 383(9911): 69-82.
[http://dx.doi.org/10.1016/S0140-6736(13)60591-7] [PMID: 23890997]

[49] Barten LJ, Allington DR, Procacci KA, Rivey MP. New approaches in the management of multiple sclerosis. Drug Des Devel Ther 2010; 4: 343-66.
[PMID: 21151622]

[50] Tsokos GC. Systemic lupus erythematosus. N Engl J Med 2011; 365(22): 2110-21.
[http://dx.doi.org/10.1056/NEJMra1100359] [PMID: 22129255]

[51] Smolen JS, Aletaha D, McInnes IB. Rheumatoid arthritis. Lancet 2016; 388(10055): 2023-38.
[http://dx.doi.org/10.1016/S0140-6736(16)30173-8] [PMID: 27156434]

[52] A G, Ev A, T K. Scleroderma. N Engl J Med 2009; 360(19) https://pubmed.ncbi.nlm.nih.gov/19420368/ [Internet].

[53] McGonagle D, Aziz A, Dickie LJ, McDermott MF. An integrated classification of pediatric inflammatory diseases, based on the concepts of autoinflammation and the immunological disease continuum. Pediatr Res 2009; 65(5 Part 2): 38R-45R.

[http://dx.doi.org/10.1203/PDR.0b013e31819dbd0a] [PMID: 19190531]

[54] Savic S, Caseley EA, McDermott MF. Moving towards a systems-based classification of innate immune-mediated diseases. Nat Rev Rheumatol 2020; 16(4): 222-37. [http://dx.doi.org/10.1038/s41584-020-0377-5] [PMID: 32107482]

[55] Humbert P, Dupond JL. [Multiple autoimmune syndromes]. Ann Med Interne (Paris) 1988; 139(3): 159-68. [PMID: 3059902]

[56] Wang Z, Chang C, Lu Q. Epigenetics of CD4+ T cells in autoimmune diseases. Curr Opin Rheumatol 2017; 29(4): 361-8. [http://dx.doi.org/10.1097/BOR.0000000000000393] [PMID: 28362657]

[57] Samuels H, Malov M, Saha Detroja T, *et al.* Autoimmune disease classification based on pubMed text mining. J Clin Med 2022; 11(15): 4345. [http://dx.doi.org/10.3390/jcm11154345] [PMID: 35893435]

[58] Barturen G, Beretta L, Cervera R, Van Vollenhoven R, Alarcón-Riquelme ME. Moving towards a molecular taxonomy of autoimmune rheumatic diseases. Nat Rev Rheumatol 2018; 14(2): 75-93. [http://dx.doi.org/10.1038/nrrheum.2017.220] [PMID: 29362467]

[59] Pardoll DM. The blockade of immune checkpoints in cancer immunotherapy. Nat Rev Cancer 2012; 12(4): 252-64. [http://dx.doi.org/10.1038/nrc3239] [PMID: 22437870]

[60] Choileain NN, Redmond HP. Regulatory T-cells and autoimmunity. J Surg Res 2006; 130(1): 124-35. [http://dx.doi.org/10.1016/j.jss.2005.07.033] [PMID: 16154142]

[61] Simmonds MJ, Gough SCL. Genetic insights into disease mechanisms of autoimmunity. Br Med Bull 2005; 71(1): 93-113. [http://dx.doi.org/10.1093/bmb/ldh032] [PMID: 15701924]

[62] Dehner C, Fine R, Kriegel MA. The microbiome in systemic autoimmune disease: mechanistic insights from recent studies. Curr Opin Rheumatol 2019; 31(2): 201-7. [http://dx.doi.org/10.1097/BOR.0000000000000574] [PMID: 30624285]

[63] Getts DR, Chastain EML, Terry RL, Miller SD. Virus infection, antiviral immunity, and autoimmunity. Immunol Rev 2013; 255(1): 197-209. [http://dx.doi.org/10.1111/imr.12091] [PMID: 23947356]

[64] Smatti MK, Cyprian FS, Nasrallah GK, Al Thani AA, Almishal RO, Yassine HM. Viruses and autoimmunity: A review on the potential interaction and molecular mechanisms. Viruses 2019; 11(8): 762. [http://dx.doi.org/10.3390/v11080762] [PMID: 31430946]

[65] Mahler M, Bentow C, Serra J, Fritzler MJ. Detection of autoantibodies using chemiluminescence technologies. Immunopharmacol Immunotoxicol 2016; 38(1): 14-20. [http://dx.doi.org/10.3109/08923973.2015.1077461] [PMID: 26525648]

[66] Sfriso P, Ghirardello A, Botsios C, *et al.* Infections and autoimmunity: the multifaceted relationship. J Leukoc Biol 2009; 87(3): 385-95. [http://dx.doi.org/10.1189/jlb.0709517] [PMID: 20015961]

[67] Haro I, Sanmartí R, Gómara MJ. Implications of post-translational modifications in autoimmunity with emphasis on citrullination, homocitrullination and acetylation for the pathogenesis, diagnosis and prognosis of rheumatoid arthritis. Int J Mol Sci 2022; 23(24): 15803. [http://dx.doi.org/10.3390/ijms232415803] [PMID: 36555449]

[68] Hu R, Wallace J, Dahlem TJ, Grunwald DJ, O'Connell RM. Targeting human microRNA genes using engineered Tal-effector nucleases (TALENs). PLoS One 2013; 8(5): e63074. [http://dx.doi.org/10.1371/journal.pone.0063074] [PMID: 23667577]

[69] Sakkas LI, Bogdanos DP. Infections as a cause of autoimmune rheumatic diseases. Auto Immun Highlights 2016; 7(1): 13.
[http://dx.doi.org/10.1007/s13317-016-0086-x] [PMID: 27629582]

[70] F S, K R, K R. The role of viral infections in the onset of autoimmune diseases. Viruses 2023; 15(3)https://pubmed.ncbi.nlm.nih.gov/36992490/ [Internet].

[71] Thorsby E, Lie BA. HLA associated genetic predisposition to autoimmune diseases: Genes involved and possible mechanisms. Transpl Immunol 2005; 14(3-4): 175-82.
[http://dx.doi.org/10.1016/j.trim.2005.03.021] [PMID: 15982560]

[72] Cruz-Tapias P, Pérez-Fernández OM, Rojas-Villarraga A, Rodríguez-Rodríguez A, Arango MT, Anaya JM. Shared HLA class II in six autoimmune diseases in latin America: A Meta-Analysis. Autoimmune Dis 2012; 2012: 1-10.
[http://dx.doi.org/10.1155/2012/569728] [PMID: 22577522]

[73] Ritari J, Koskela S, Hyvärinen K. FinnGen, Partanen J. Phenome-wide HLA association study of Finnish biobank participants reveals infection-autoimmune disease links and modifier effects between HLA genes and alleles. medRxiv 2020; 2020.10.26.20219899. https://www.medrxiv.org/content/10.1101/2020.10.26.20219899v1 Internet

[74] Johansson T, Yohannes DA, Koskela S, Partanen J, Saavalainen P. HLA RNA sequencing with unique molecular identifiers reveals high allele-specific variability in mRNA expression. Front Immunol 2021; 12: 629059.
[http://dx.doi.org/10.3389/fimmu.2021.629059] [PMID: 33717155]

[75] Ceccarelli F, Agmon-Levin N, Perricone C. Genetic factors of autoimmune diseases. J Immunol Res 2016; 2016: 1-2.
[http://dx.doi.org/10.1155/2016/3476023] [PMID: 26925423]

[76] Watson A, Forbes Satter L, Reiland Sauceda A, Kellermayer R, Karam LB. *NOD2* polymorphisms may direct a crohn disease phenotype in patients with very early-onset inflammatory bowel disease. J Pediatr Gastroenterol Nutr 2023; 77(6): 748-52.
[http://dx.doi.org/10.1097/MPG.0000000000003846] [PMID: 37229767]

[77] Pedersen J, LaCasse EC, Seidelin JB, Coskun M, Nielsen OH. Inhibitors of apoptosis (IAPs) regulate intestinal immunity and inflammatory bowel disease (IBD) inflammation. Trends Mol Med 2014; 20(11): 652-65.
[http://dx.doi.org/10.1016/j.molmed.2014.09.006] [PMID: 25282548]

[78] Abu Shtaya A, Orenstein N, Bazak L, Lidzbarsky G, Kalis ML, Amarilyo G, *et al.* High frequency of MEFV disease-causing variants in children with very-early-onset inflammatory bowel disease. Pediatr Res 2024.
[PMID: 38734812]

[79] Yurtcu E, Gokcan H, Yilmaz U, Sahin FI. Detection of MEFV gene mutations in patients with inflammatory bowel disease. Genet Test Mol Biomarkers 2009; 13(1): 87-90.
[http://dx.doi.org/10.1089/gtmb.2008.0094] [PMID: 19309279]

[80] Sullivan KE, Conrad M, Kelsen JR. Very early-onset inflammatory bowel disease: an integrated approach. Curr Opin Allergy Clin Immunol 2018; 18(6): 459-69.
[http://dx.doi.org/10.1097/ACI.0000000000000484] [PMID: 30299395]

[81] Matzaraki V, Kumar V, Wijmenga C, Zhernakova A. The MHC locus and genetic susceptibility to autoimmune and infectious diseases. Genome Biol 2017; 18(1): 76.
[http://dx.doi.org/10.1186/s13059-017-1207-1] [PMID: 28449694]

[82] Einarsdottir E, Söderström I, Löfgren-Burström A, *et al.* The CTLA4 region as a general autoimmunity factor: An extended pedigree provides evidence for synergy with the HLA locus in the etiology of type 1 diabetes mellitus, Hashimoto's thyroiditis and Graves' disease. Eur J Hum Genet 2003; 11(1): 81-4.

[http://dx.doi.org/10.1038/sj.ejhg.5200903] [PMID: 12529710]

[83] Parnell GP, Booth DR. The multiple sclerosis (MS) genetic risk factors indicate both acquired and innate immune cell subsets contribute to MS pathogenesis and identify novel therapeutic opportunities. Front Immunol 2017; 8: 425.
[http://dx.doi.org/10.3389/fimmu.2017.00425] [PMID: 28458668]

[84] Russell JT, Roesch LFW, Ördberg M, *et al.* Genetic risk for autoimmunity is associated with distinct changes in the human gut microbiome. Nat Commun 2019; 10(1): 3621.
[http://dx.doi.org/10.1038/s41467-019-11460-x] [PMID: 31399563]

[85] Damoiseaux J. Multiparametric autoimmune diagnostics: recent advances. Pathol Lab Med Int 2016; 8: 15-25.
[http://dx.doi.org/10.2147/PLMI.S56781]

[86] Cinquanta L, Infantino M, Bizzaro N. Detecting autoantibodies by multiparametric assays: Impact on prevention, diagnosis, monitoring, and personalized therapy in autoimmune diseases. J Appl Lab Med 2022; 7(1): 137-50.
[http://dx.doi.org/10.1093/jalm/jfab132] [PMID: 34996071]

[87] Tozzoli R, D'Aurizio F, Villalta D, Bizzaro N. Automation, consolidation, and integration in autoimmune diagnostics. Auto Immun Highlights 2015; 6(1-2): 1-6.
[http://dx.doi.org/10.1007/s13317-015-0067-5] [PMID: 26138781]

[88] Burbelo PD, O'Hanlon TP. New autoantibody detection technologies yield novel insights into autoimmune disease. Curr Opin Rheumatol 2014; 26(6): 717-23.
[http://dx.doi.org/10.1097/BOR.0000000000000107] [PMID: 25203116]

[89] Conrad K, Schneider H, Ziemssen T, *et al.* A new line immunoassay for the multiparametric detection of antiganglioside autoantibodies in patients with autoimmune peripheral neuropathies. Ann N Y Acad Sci 2007; 1109(1): 256-64.
[http://dx.doi.org/10.1196/annals.1398.031] [PMID: 17785314]

[90] Sowa M, Großmann K, Scholz J, *et al.* The CytoBead assay – a novel approach of multiparametric autoantibody analysis in the diagnostics of systemic autoimmune diseases. Laboratoriumsmedizin (Berl) 2015; 38(s1): 000010151520150036. https://www.degruyter.com/document/doi/10.1515/labmed-2015-0036/html?lang=en [Internet].
[http://dx.doi.org/10.1515/labmed-2015-0036]

[91] López-Longo FJ, Rodríguez-Mahou M, Escalona-Monge M, González CM, Monteagudo I, Carreño L. Simultaneous identification of various antinuclear antibodies using an automated multiparameter line immunoassay system. Lupus 2003; 12(8): 623-9.
[http://dx.doi.org/10.1191/0961203303lu439oa] [PMID: 12945722]

[92] Fraune J, Gerlach S, Rentzsch K, *et al.* Multiparametric serological testing in autoimmune encephalitis using computer-aided immunofluorescence microscopy (CAIFM). Autoimmun Rev 2016; 15(10): 937-42.
[http://dx.doi.org/10.1016/j.autrev.2016.07.024] [PMID: 27490202]

[93] Tešija Kuna A, Đerek L, Drvar V, Kozmar A, Gugo K. Assessment of Antinuclear Antibodies (ANA): National recommendations on behalf of the Croatian society of medical biochemistry and laboratory medicine. Biochem Med (Zagreb) 2021; 31(2): 210-29.
[http://dx.doi.org/10.11613/BM.2021.020502] [PMID: 33927550]

[94] Liaskos C, Marou E, Simopoulou T, *et al.* Multiparametric autoantibody profiling of patients with systemic sclerosis in Greece. Mediterr J Rheumatol 2018; 29(3): 120-6.
[http://dx.doi.org/10.31138/mjr.29.3.120] [PMID: 32185313]

[95] Fritzler MJ, Fritzler ML. The Emergence of Multiplexed Technologies as Diagnostic Platforms in Systemic Autoimmune Diseases http://www.eurekaselect.comhttps://www.eurekaselect.com/article/2678
[http://dx.doi.org/10.2174/092986706778201639]

[96] Conrad K, Andrade LEC, Chan EKL, *et al.* From autoantibody research to standardized diagnostic assays in the management of human diseases – report of the 12th Dresden Symposium on Autoantibodies. Lupus 2016; 25(8): 787-96. [http://dx.doi.org/10.1177/0961203316644337] [PMID: 27252254]

[97] Maecker HT, Nolan GP, Fathman CG. New technologies for autoimmune disease monitoring. Curr Opin Endocrinol Diabetes Obes 2010; 17(4): 322-8. [http://dx.doi.org/10.1097/MED.0b013e32833ada91] [PMID: 20531181]

[98] Hueber W, Robinson WH. Proteomic biomarkers for autoimmune disease. Proteomics 2006; 6(14): 4100-5. [http://dx.doi.org/10.1002/pmic.200600017] [PMID: 16786488]

[99] Tozzoli R. The diagnostic role of autoantibodies in the prediction of organ-specific autoimmune diseases. Clin Chem Lab Med 2008; 46(5): 577-87. [http://dx.doi.org/10.1515/CCLM.2008.138] [PMID: 18839462]

[100] Bizzaro N, Tozzoli R, Villalta D. Autoimmune diagnostics: the technology, the strategy and the clinical governance. Immunol Res 2015; 61(1-2): 126-34. [http://dx.doi.org/10.1007/s12026-014-8587-z] [PMID: 25398640]

[101] Castro C, Gourley M. Diagnostic testing and interpretation of tests for autoimmunity. J Allergy Clin Immunol 2010; 125(2) (Suppl. 2): S238-47. [http://dx.doi.org/10.1016/j.jaci.2009.09.041] [PMID: 20061009]

[102] Barcellini W, Giannotta JA, Fattizzo B. Autoimmune complications in hematologic neoplasms. Cancers (Basel) 2021; 13(7): 1532. [http://dx.doi.org/10.3390/cancers13071532] [PMID: 33810369]

[103] Breda L, Nozzi M, De Sanctis S, Chiarelli F. Laboratory tests in the diagnosis and follow-up of pediatric rheumatic diseases: an update. Semin Arthritis Rheum 2010; 40(1): 53-72. [http://dx.doi.org/10.1016/j.semarthrit.2008.12.001] [PMID: 19246077]

[104] Tozzoli R, Bizzaro N, Tonutti E, *et al.* Guidelines for the laboratory use of autoantibody tests in the diagnosis and monitoring of autoimmune rheumatic diseases. Am J Clin Pathol 2002; 117(2): 316-24. [http://dx.doi.org/10.1309/Y5VF-C3DM-L8XV-U053] [PMID: 11863229]

[105] Tampoia M, Giavarina D, Di Giorgio C, Bizzaro N. Diagnostic accuracy of Enzyme-Linked Immunosorbent Assays (ELISA) to detect anti-skin autoantibodies in autoimmune blistering skin diseases: A systematic review and meta-analysis. Autoimmun Rev 2012; 12(2): 121-6. [http://dx.doi.org/10.1016/j.autrev.2012.07.006] [PMID: 22781589]

[106] Wajda A, Sivitskaya L, Paradowska-Gorycka A. Application of NGS technology in understanding the pathology of autoimmune diseases. J Clin Med 2021; 10(15): 3334. [http://dx.doi.org/10.3390/jcm10153334] [PMID: 34362117]

[107] Fox RI, Dotan I, Fei HM, Compton T, Hamer M, Saito I. Use of dna amplification methods for clinical diagnosis in autoimmune diseases. J Clin Lab Anal 1989; 3(6): 378-87. [http://dx.doi.org/10.1002/jcla.1860030611] [PMID: 2693667]

[108] Sherer M, Struchen MA, Yablon SA, Wang Y, Nick TG. Comparison of indices of traumatic brain injury severity: Glasgow Coma Scale, length of coma and post-traumatic amnesia. J Neurol Neurosurg Psychiatry 2007; 79(6): 678-85. [http://dx.doi.org/10.1136/jnnp.2006.111187] [PMID: 17928328]

[109] Plebani M, Pittoni M, Celadin M, Bernardi D, Mion MM. Recent advances in diagnostic technologies for autoimmune diseases. Autoimmun Rev 2009; 8(3): 238-43. [http://dx.doi.org/10.1016/j.autrev.2008.07.032] [PMID: 18718878]

[110] Campos Domínguez M, Suárez Fernández R, Lázaro Ochaita P. Diagnostic methods in autoimmune subepidermal bullous diseases. Actas Dermosifiliogr 2006; 97(8): 485-502. [PMID: 17067526]

[111] Tozzoli R. Recent advances in diagnostic technologies and their impact in autoimmune diseases. Autoimmun Rev 2007; 6(6): 334-40.
[http://dx.doi.org/10.1016/j.autrev.2007.01.005] [PMID: 17537377]

[112] Shadmani G, Simkins TJ, Assadsangabi R, *et al.* Autoimmune diseases of the brain, imaging and clinical review. Neuroradiol J 2022; 35(2): 152-69.
[http://dx.doi.org/10.1177/19714009211042879] [PMID: 34490814]

[113] Alvarez Moreno E, Jimenez de la Peña M, Cano Alonso R. Role of new functional MRI techniques in the diagnosis, staging, and followup of gynecological cancer: Comparison with PET-CT. Radiol Res Pract 2012; 2012: 1-11.
[http://dx.doi.org/10.1155/2012/219546] [PMID: 22315683]

[114] Besson FL, Nocturne G, Noël N, Gheysens O, Slart RHJA, Glaudemans AWJM. PET/CT in inflammatory and auto-immune disorders: Focus on several key molecular concepts, FDG, and radiolabeled probe perspectives. Semin Nucl Med 2024; 54(3): 379-93.
[http://dx.doi.org/10.1053/j.semnuclmed.2023.10.005] [PMID: 37973447]

[115] Procaccini E, Chianelli M, Pantano P, Signore A. Imaging of autoimmune diseases. Q J Nucl Med 1999; 43(1): 100-12.
[PMID: 10230286]

[116] Colella G, Cannavale R, Flamminio F, Foschini MP. Fine-needle aspiration cytology of salivary gland lesions: a systematic review. J Oral Maxillofac Surg 2010; 68(9): 2146-53.
[http://dx.doi.org/10.1016/j.joms.2009.09.064] [PMID: 20580145]

[117] Roccarina D, Garcovich M, Ainora ME, *et al.* Diagnosis of bowel diseases: The role of imaging and ultrasonography. World J Gastroenterol 2013; 19(14): 2144-53.
[http://dx.doi.org/10.3748/wjg.v19.i14.2144] [PMID: 23599640]

[118] Primack SL, Müller NL. Radiologic manifestations of the systemic autoimmune diseases. Clin Chest Med 1998; 19(4): 573-586, vii.
[http://dx.doi.org/10.1016/S0272-5231(05)70104-0] [PMID: 9917954]

[119] Saunders TH, Mendes Ribeiro HK, Gleeson FV. New techniques for imaging colorectal cancer: the use of MRI, PET and radioimmunoscintigraphy for primary staging and follow-up. Br Med Bull 2002; 64(1): 81-99.
[http://dx.doi.org/10.1093/bmb/64.1.81] [PMID: 12421727]

[120] Guarneri A, Perrone E, Bosello SL, D'Agostino MA, Leccisotti L. The role of PET/CT in connective tissue disorders: systemic sclerosis, Sjögren's syndrome and systemic lupus erythematosus. Q J Nucl Med Mol Imaging 2022; 66(3): 194-205.
[http://dx.doi.org/10.23736/S1824-4785.22.03463-X] [PMID: 36066111]

[121] Jayaram G, Chew MT. Fine needle aspiration cytology of lymph nodes in HIV-infected individuals. Acta Cytol 2000; 44(6): 960-6.
[http://dx.doi.org/10.1159/000328617] [PMID: 11127753]

[122] Bongiovanni M, Trimboli P, Rossi ED, Fadda G, Nobile A, Giovanella L. Diagnosis of endocrine disease: High-yield thyroid fine-needle aspiration cytology: an update focused on ancillary techniques improving its accuracy. Eur J Endocrinol 2016; 174(2): R53-63.
[http://dx.doi.org/10.1530/EJE-15-0817] [PMID: 26450171]

[123] Mathiot C, Decaudin D, Klijanienko J, *et al.* Fine-needle aspiration cytology combined with flow cytometry immunophenotyping is a rapid and accurate approach for the evaluation of suspicious superficial lymphoid lesions. Diagn Cytopathol 2006; 34(7): 472-8.
[http://dx.doi.org/10.1002/dc.20487] [PMID: 16783780]

[124] Das DK. Fine□needle aspiration cytology: Its origin, development, and present status with special reference to a developing country, India. Diagn Cytopathol 2003; 28(6): 345-51.
[http://dx.doi.org/10.1002/dc.10289] [PMID: 12768643]

[125] Fröstad B, Tani E, Kogner P, Maeda S, Björk O, Skoog L. The clinical use of fine needle aspiration cytology for diagnosis and management of children with neuroblastic tumours. Eur J Cancer 1998; 34(4): 529-36.
[PMID: 9713304]

[126] Lever JV, Trott PA, Webb AJ. Fine needle aspiration cytology. J Clin Pathol 1985; 38(1): 1-11.
[http://dx.doi.org/10.1136/jcp.38.1.1] [PMID: 2578481]

[127] Pinki P, Alok D, Ranjan A, Nanak Chand M. Fine needle aspiration cytology versus fine needle capillary sampling in cytological diagnosis of thyroid lesions. Iran J Pathol 2015; 10(1): 47-53.
[PMID: 26516325]

[128] Barnes PJ. Corticosteroids: The drugs to beat. Eur J Pharmacol 2006; 533(1-3): 2-14.
[http://dx.doi.org/10.1016/j.ejphar.2005.12.052] [PMID: 16436275]

[129] Hench PS, Kendall EC, Slocumb CH, Polley HF. The effect of a hormone of the adrenal cortex (17-hydroxy-11-dehydrocorticosterone; compound E) and of pituitary adrenocorticotropic hormone on rheumatoid arthritis. Mayo Clin Proc 1949; 24(8): 181-97.
[http://dx.doi.org/10.1016/S0025-6196(24)00526-3] [PMID: 18118071]

[130] Liu E, Perl A. Pathogenesis and treatment of autoimmune rheumatic diseases. Curr Opin Rheumatol 2019; 31(3): 307-15.
[http://dx.doi.org/10.1097/BOR.0000000000000594] [PMID: 30920455]

[131] Drachman DB, Brodsky RA. High-dose therapy for autoimmune neurologic diseases. Curr Opin Oncol 2005; 17(2): 83-8.
[http://dx.doi.org/10.1097/01.cco.0000152974.65477.35] [PMID: 15725909]

[132] Alexander T, Greco R, Snowden JA. Hematopoietic stem cell transplantation for autoimmune disease. Annu Rev Med 2021; 72(1): 215-28.
[http://dx.doi.org/10.1146/annurev-med-070119-115617] [PMID: 33106103]

[133] Rouveix B, Blin O. Pharmacological basis of immunotherapy in autoimmune diseases. Clin Neuropharmacol 1993; 16(2): 104-12.
[http://dx.doi.org/10.1097/00002826-199304000-00002] [PMID: 8477406]

[134] Carter PH, Zhao Q. Clinically validated approaches to the treatment of autoimmune diseases. Expert Opin Investig Drugs 2010; 19(2): 195-213.
[http://dx.doi.org/10.1517/13543780903418452] [PMID: 20050823]

[135] Selmi C. Autoimmunity in 2017. Clin Rev Allergy Immunol 2018; 55(3): 239-53.
[http://dx.doi.org/10.1007/s12016-018-8699-7] [PMID: 30051260]

[136] Rosman Z, Shoenfeld Y, Zandman-Goddard G. Biologic therapy for autoimmune diseases: an update. BMC Med 2013; 11(1): 88.
[http://dx.doi.org/10.1186/1741-7015-11-88] [PMID: 23557513]

[137] Selmi C. Autoimmunity in 2018. Clin Rev Allergy Immunol 2019; 56(3): 375-84.
[http://dx.doi.org/10.1007/s12016-019-08745-w] [PMID: 31168760]

[138] Bechman K, Yates M, Galloway JB. The new entries in the therapeutic armamentarium: The small molecule JAK inhibitors. Pharmacol Res 2019; 147: 104392.
[http://dx.doi.org/10.1016/j.phrs.2019.104392] [PMID: 31401212]

[139] Michot JM, Bigenwald C, Champiat S, *et al.* Immune-related adverse events with immune checkpoint blockade: a comprehensive review. Eur J Cancer 2016; 54: 139-48.
[http://dx.doi.org/10.1016/j.ejca.2015.11.016] [PMID: 26765102]

[140] Bellanca CM, Augello E, Cantone AF, *et al.* Insight into risk factors, pharmacogenetics/genomics, and management of adverse drug reactions in elderly: A narrative review. Pharmaceuticals (Basel) 2023; 16(11): 1542.
[http://dx.doi.org/10.3390/ph16111542] [PMID: 38004408]

[141] Neill J, Belan I, Ried K. Effectiveness of non-pharmacological interventions for fatigue in adults with multiple sclerosis, rheumatoid arthritis, or systemic lupus erythematosus: a systematic review. J Adv Nurs 2006; 56(6): 617-35.
[http://dx.doi.org/10.1111/j.1365-2648.2006.04054.x] [PMID: 17118041]

[142] Dean Y, Dépis F, Kosco-Vilbois M. Combination therapies in the context of anti-CD3 antibodies for the treatment of autoimmune diseases. Swiss Med Wkly 2012; 142: w13711.
[http://dx.doi.org/10.4414/smw.2012.13711] [PMID: 23254986]

[143] Neupane YR, Mahtab A, Siddiqui L, *et al.* Biocompatible nanovesicular drug delivery systems with targeting potential for autoimmune diseases. Curr Pharm Des 2020; 26(42): 5488-502.
[http://dx.doi.org/10.2174/1381612826666200523174108] [PMID: 32445443]

[144] Khan H, Sureda A, Belwal T, *et al.* Polyphenols in the treatment of autoimmune diseases. Autoimmun Rev 2019; 18(7): 647-57.
[http://dx.doi.org/10.1016/j.autrev.2019.05.001] [PMID: 31059841]

[145] Kostoglou-Athanassiou I, Athanassiou P. Anti-inflammatory diet in autoimmune diseases. Front Nutr. 2024;11:1497058.
[http://dx.doi.org/10.3389/fnut.2024.1497058]

[146] Long Z, Zeng L, He Q, *et al.* Research progress on the clinical application and mechanism of iguratimod in the treatment of autoimmune diseases and rheumatic diseases. Front Immunol 2023; 14: 1150661.
[http://dx.doi.org/10.3389/fimmu.2023.1150661] [PMID: 37809072]

[147] Chatenoud L. Immune therapies of autoimmune diseases: are we approaching a real cure?. Curr Opin Immunol 2006; 18(6): 710-7.
[http://dx.doi.org/10.1016/j.coi.2006.09.004] [PMID: 17011768]

[148] Doycheva I, Watt KD, Gulamhusein AF. Autoimmune hepatitis: Current and future therapeutic options. Liver Int 2019; 39(6): 1002-13.
[http://dx.doi.org/10.1111/liv.14062] [PMID: 30716203]

[149] Haanen J, Ernstoff MS, Wang Y, *et al.* Autoimmune diseases and immune-checkpoint inhibitors for cancer therapy: review of the literature and personalized risk-based prevention strategy. Ann Oncol 2020; 31(6): 724-44.
[http://dx.doi.org/10.1016/j.annonc.2020.03.285] [PMID: 32194150]

[150] Nosadini M, Mohammad SS, Ramanathan S, Brilot F, Dale RC. Immune therapy in autoimmune encephalitis: a systematic review. Expert Rev Neurother 2015; 15(12): 1391-419.
[http://dx.doi.org/10.1586/14737175.2015.1115720] [PMID: 26559389]

[151] Perez-Alvarez R, Pérez-de-Lis M, Ramos-Casals M. Biologics-induced autoimmune diseases. Curr Opin Rheumatol 2013; 25(1): 56-64.
[http://dx.doi.org/10.1097/BOR.0b013e32835b1366] [PMID: 23114587]

[152] Tiligada E, Ishii M, Riccardi C, *et al.* The expanding role of immunopharmacology: IUPHAR Review 16. Br J Pharmacol 2015; 172(17): 4217-27.
[http://dx.doi.org/10.1111/bph.13219] [PMID: 26173913]

[153] Gleicher N, Weghofer A, Barad DH. Cutting edge assessment of the impact of autoimmunity on female reproductive success. J Autoimmun 2012; 38(2-3): J74-80.
[http://dx.doi.org/10.1016/j.jaut.2011.05.016] [PMID: 21664106]

[154] Bournia VKK, Vlachoyiannopoulos PG, Selmi C, Moutsopoulos HM, Gershwin ME. Recent advances in the treatment of systemic sclerosis. Clin Rev Allergy Immunol 2009; 36(2-3): 176-200.
[http://dx.doi.org/10.1007/s12016-008-8114-x] [PMID: 19132559]

[155] Shu SA, Wang J, Tao MH, Leung PSC. Gene therapy for autoimmune disease. Clin Rev Allergy Immunol 2015; 49(2): 163-76.
[http://dx.doi.org/10.1007/s12016-014-8451-x] [PMID: 25277817]

[156] Evans CH, Whalen JD, Evans CH, Ghivizzani SC, Robbins PD. Gene therapy in autoimmune diseases. Ann Rheum Dis 1998; 57(3): 125-7.
[http://dx.doi.org/10.1136/ard.57.3.125] [PMID: 9640124]

[157] Dunbar CE, High KA, Joung JK, Kohn DB, Ozawa K, Sadelain M. Gene therapy comes of age. Science 2018; 359(6372): eaan4672.
[http://dx.doi.org/10.1126/science.aan4672] [PMID: 29326244]

[158] Ewart D, Peterson EJ, Steer CJ. A new era of genetic engineering for autoimmune and inflammatory diseases. Semin Arthritis Rheum 2019; 49(1): e1-7.
[http://dx.doi.org/10.1016/j.semarthrit.2019.05.004] [PMID: 31146955]

[159] Seroogy CM, Fathman CG. The application of gene therapy in autoimmune diseases. Gene Ther 2000; 7(1): 9-13.
[http://dx.doi.org/10.1038/sj.gt.3301111] [PMID: 10680009]

[160] Furlan R, Butti E, Pluchino S, Martino G. Gene therapy for autoimmune diseases. Curr Opin Mol Ther 2004; 6(5): 525-36.
[PMID: 15537054]

[161] Pan X, Veroniaina H, Su N, *et al.* Applications and developments of gene therapy drug delivery systems for genetic diseases. Asian Journal of Pharmaceutical Sciences 2021; 16(6): 687-703.
[http://dx.doi.org/10.1016/j.ajps.2021.05.003] [PMID: 35027949]

[162] Feldmann M, Maini RN. Anti-TNF therapy, from rationale to standard of care: what lessons has it taught us?. J Immunol 2010; 185(2): 791-4.
[http://dx.doi.org/10.4049/jimmunol.1090051] [PMID: 20601610]

[163] Edwards JCW, Szczepański L, Szechiński J, *et al.* Efficacy of B-cell-targeted therapy with rituximab in patients with rheumatoid arthritis. N Engl J Med 2004; 350(25): 2572-81.
[http://dx.doi.org/10.1056/NEJMoa032534] [PMID: 15201414]

[164] Jones G, Sebba A, Gu J, *et al.* Comparison of tocilizumab monotherapy versus methotrexate monotherapy in patients with moderate to severe rheumatoid arthritis: the ambition study. Ann Rheum Dis 2010; 69(1): 88-96.
[http://dx.doi.org/10.1136/ard.2008.105197] [PMID: 19297346]

[165] Kremer JM, Westhovens R, Leon M, *et al.* Treatment of rheumatoid arthritis by selective inhibition of T-cell activation with fusion protein CTLA4Ig. N Engl J Med 2003; 349(20): 1907-15.
[http://dx.doi.org/10.1056/NEJMoa035075] [PMID: 14614165]

[166] Pushpakom S, Iorio F, Eyers PA, *et al.* Drug repurposing: progress, challenges and recommendations. Nat Rev Drug Discov 2019; 18(1): 41-58.
[http://dx.doi.org/10.1038/nrd.2018.168] [PMID: 30310233]

[167] Kingsmore KM, Grammer AC, Lipsky PE. Drug repurposing to improve treatment of rheumatic autoimmune inflammatory diseases. Nat Rev Rheumatol 2020; 16(1): 32-52.
[http://dx.doi.org/10.1038/s41584-019-0337-0] [PMID: 31831878]

[168] Shoaib M, Kamal MA, Rizvi SMD. Repurposed drugs as potential therapeutic candidates for the management of Alzheimer's disease. Curr Drug Metab 2017; 18(9): 842-52.
[PMID: 28595531]

[169] Fong W, To KKW. Repurposing chloroquine analogs as an adjuvant cancer therapy. Recent Patents Anticancer Drug Discov 2021; 16(2): 204-21.
[http://dx.doi.org/10.2174/1574892815666210106111012] [PMID: 33413069]

[170] Parsons CG. CNS repurposing - Potential new uses for old drugs: Examples of screens for Alzheimer's disease, Parkinson's disease and spasticity. Neuropharmacology 2019; 147: 4-10.
[http://dx.doi.org/10.1016/j.neuropharm.2018.08.027] [PMID: 30165077]

[171] Juárez-López D, Schcolnik-Cabrera A. Drug repurposing: considerations to surpass while re-directing

old compounds for new treatments. Arch Med Res 2021; 52(3): 243-51.
[http://dx.doi.org/10.1016/j.arcmed.2020.10.021] [PMID: 33190955]

[172] Baker NC, Ekins S, Williams AJ, Tropsha A. A bibliometric review of drug repurposing. Drug Discov Today 2018; 23(3): 661-72.
[http://dx.doi.org/10.1016/j.drudis.2018.01.018] [PMID: 29330123]

[173] Ioakeim-Skoufa I, Tobajas-Ramos N, Menditto E, *et al.* Drug repurposing in oncology: A systematic review of randomized controlled clinical trials. Cancers (Basel) 2023; 15(11): 2972.
[http://dx.doi.org/10.3390/cancers15112972] [PMID: 37296934]

[174] Xiang Y, Zhang M, Jiang D, Su Q, Shi J. The role of inflammation in autoimmune disease: a therapeutic target. Front Immunol 2023; 14: 1267091.
[http://dx.doi.org/10.3389/fimmu.2023.1267091] [PMID: 37859999]

[175] Mtewa AG, Amanjot A, Yadesa TM, Ngwira KJ. Drug repurposing for SARS-CoV-2 (COVID-19) treatment. Coronavirus Drug Discov. 2022; pp. 205-26.

[176] Wicht KJ, Mok S, Fidock DA. Molecular mechanisms of drug resistance in *Plasmodium falciparum* malaria. Annu Rev Microbiol 2020; 74(1): 431-54.
[http://dx.doi.org/10.1146/annurev-micro-020518-115546] [PMID: 32905757]

[177] Hess S, Ozoux ML, Gerl M. Biomarker definition and validation during drug development. In: Vogel HG, Maas J, Gebauer A, Eds. Drug discovery and evaluation: Methods in clinical pharmacology. Berlin, Heidelberg: Springer 2011; pp. 223-44.
[http://dx.doi.org/10.1007/978-3-540-89891-7_20]

[178] Krishnamurthy N, Grimshaw AA, Axson SA, Choe SH, Miller JE. Drug repurposing: A systematic review on root causes, barriers and facilitators. BMC Health Serv Res 2022; 22(1): 970.
[http://dx.doi.org/10.1186/s12913-022-08272-z] [PMID: 35906687]

[179] Visvikis-Siest S, Theodoridou D, Kontoe MS, Kumar S, Marschler M. Milestones in personalized medicine: From the ancient time to nowadays—the provocation of COVID-19. Front Genet 2020; 11: 569175.
[http://dx.doi.org/10.3389/fgene.2020.569175] [PMID: 33424917]

[180] Bachiller S, Jiménez-Ferrer I, Paulus A, *et al.* Microglia in neurological diseases: A road map to brain-disease dependent-inflammatory response. Front Cell Neurosci 2018; 12: 488.
[http://dx.doi.org/10.3389/fncel.2018.00488] [PMID: 30618635]

[181] Wei SC, Duffy CR, Allison JP. Fundamental mechanisms of immune checkpoint blockade therapy. Cancer Discov 2018; 8(9): 1069-86.
[http://dx.doi.org/10.1158/2159-8290.CD-18-0367] [PMID: 30115704]

[182] Korman AJ, Garrett-Thomson SC, Lonberg N. The foundations of immune checkpoint blockade and the ipilimumab approval decennial. Nat Rev Drug Discov 2022; 21(7): 509-28.
[http://dx.doi.org/10.1038/s41573-021-00345-8] [PMID: 34937915]

[183] Gianchecchi E, Delfino DV, Fierabracci A. Recent insights on the putative role of autophagy in autoimmune diseases. Autoimmun Rev 2014; 13(3): 231-41.
[http://dx.doi.org/10.1016/j.autrev.2013.10.007] [PMID: 24184881]

[184] Gros F, Muller S. Pharmacological regulators of autophagy and their link with modulators of lupus disease. Br J Pharmacol 2014; 171(19): 4337-59.
[http://dx.doi.org/10.1111/bph.12792] [PMID: 24902607]

[185] Pierdominici M, Vomero M, Barbati C, *et al.* Role of autophagy in immunity and autoimmunity, with a special focus on systemic lupus erythematosus. FASEB J 2012; 26(4): 1400-12.
[http://dx.doi.org/10.1096/fj.11-194175] [PMID: 22247332]

[186] Byun S, Lee E, Lee KW. Therapeutic implications of autophagy inducers in immunological disorders, infection, and cancer. Int J Mol Sci 2017; 18(9): 1959.
[http://dx.doi.org/10.3390/ijms18091959] [PMID: 28895911]

[187] Hunter Z, McCarthy DP, Yap WT, *et al.* A biodegradable nanoparticle platform for the induction of antigen-specific immune tolerance for treatment of autoimmune disease. ACS Nano 2014; 8(3): 2148-60.
[http://dx.doi.org/10.1021/nn405033r] [PMID: 24559284]

[188] Saito E, Kuo R, Kramer KR, *et al.* Design of biodegradable nanoparticles to modulate phenotypes of antigen-presenting cells for antigen-specific treatment of autoimmune disease. Biomaterials 2019; 222: 119432.
[http://dx.doi.org/10.1016/j.biomaterials.2019.119432] [PMID: 31480002]

[189] Getts DR, Shea LD, Miller SD, King NJC. Harnessing nanoparticles for immune modulation. Trends Immunol 2015; 36(7): 419-27.
[http://dx.doi.org/10.1016/j.it.2015.05.007] [PMID: 26088391]

[190] Kishimoto TK, Maldonado RA. Nanoparticles for the induction of antigen-specific immunological tolerance. Front Immunol 2018; 9: 230.
[http://dx.doi.org/10.3389/fimmu.2018.00230] [PMID: 29515571]

[191] Leishman AJ, Sims GP, Sleeman M, Braddock M. Emerging small molecule and biological therapeutic approaches for the treatment of autoimmunity. Expert Opin Investig Drugs 2011; 20(1): 23-39.
[http://dx.doi.org/10.1517/13543784.2011.540569] [PMID: 21118058]

[192] Kalled SL, Ambrose C, Hsu YM. The biochemistry and biology of BAFF, APRIL and their receptors. Curr Dir Autoimmun 2004; 8: 206-42.
[http://dx.doi.org/10.1159/000082105] [PMID: 15564723]

[193] Galgani M, Bruzzaniti S, Matarese G. Immunometabolism and autoimmunity. Curr Opin Immunol 2020; 67: 10-7.
[http://dx.doi.org/10.1016/j.coi.2020.07.002] [PMID: 32784085]

[194] O'Shea JJ, Kontzias A, Yamaoka K, Tanaka Y, Laurence A. Janus kinase inhibitors in autoimmune diseases. Ann Rheum Dis 2013; 72(Suppl 2): ii111-5.
[http://dx.doi.org/10.1136/annrheumdis-2012-202576]

[195] Murakami M, Tomiita M, Nishimoto N. Tocilizumab in the treatment of systemic juvenile idiopathic arthritis. Open Access Rheumatol 2012; 4: 71-9.
[http://dx.doi.org/10.2147/OARRR.S21969] [PMID: 27790014]

[196] Tang Y, Cao Y. Modeling pharmacokinetics and pharmacodynamics of therapeutic antibodies: Progress, challenges, and future directions. Pharmaceutics 2021; 13(3): 422.
[http://dx.doi.org/10.3390/pharmaceutics13030422] [PMID: 33800976]

[197] Said C, Coleiro B, Zarb Adami M, Azzopardi LM, Serracino Inglott A. Cost effectiveness of TNF-α inhibitors in rheumatoid arthritis. Int J Inflamm 2013; 2013: 1-8.
[http://dx.doi.org/10.1155/2013/581409] [PMID: 24324915]

[198] Furie R, Petri M, Zamani O, *et al.* A phase III, randomized, placebo-controlled study of belimumab, a monoclonal antibody that inhibits B lymphocyte stimulator, in patients with systemic lupus erythematosus. Arthritis Rheum 2011; 63(12): 3918-30.
[http://dx.doi.org/10.1002/art.30613] [PMID: 22127708]

[199] Grayling MJ, Bigirumurame T, Cherlin S, Ouma L, Zheng H, Wason JMS. Innovative trial approaches in immune-mediated inflammatory diseases: current use and future potential. BMC Rheumatol 2021; 5(1): 21.
[http://dx.doi.org/10.1186/s41927-021-00192-5] [PMID: 34210348]

[200] Ali T, Bronze , Kaitha , Mahmood , Ftaisi , Stone . Clinical use of anti-TNF therapy and increased risk of infections. Drug Healthc Patient Saf 2013; 5: 79-99.
[http://dx.doi.org/10.2147/DHPS.S28801] [PMID: 23569399]

SUBJECT INDEX

A

B

C

All rights reserved-© 2025 Bentham Science Publishers

D

E

F

G

H

I

L

M

N

O

S

T

U

V

W

X

www.ingramcontent.com/pod-product-compliance
Lightning Source LLC
LaVergne TN
LVHW070950210926
848482LV00002B/162

9798898812362